Naming the Pain and Guiding the Care

The Central Tasks of Diagnosis

Donald D. Denton

University Press of America,® Inc.
Lanham · Boulder · New York · Toronto · Plymouth, UK

Copyright © 2008 by
University Press of America,® Inc.
4501 Forbes Boulevard
Suite 200
Lanham, Maryland 20706
UPA Acquisitions Department (301) 459-3366

Estover Road
Plymouth PL6 7PY
United Kingdom

Library of Congress Control Number: 2008930730
ISBN-13: 978-0-7618-4182-1 (paperback : alk. paper)
ISBN-10: 0-7618-4182-2 (paperback : alk. paper)
eISBN-13: 978-0-7618-4183-8
eISBN-10: 0-7618-4183-0

♾™ The paper used in this publication meets the minimum
requirements of American National Standard for Information
Sciences—Permanence of Paper for Printed Library Materials,
ANSI Z39.48—1984

Dedication

To my grandson Killian James Denton
And
Any further grandchildren who may yet appear
May they play their part in relieving suffering
With
Courage and integrity

Table of Contents

Foreword

The field of psychiatric diagnosis, like many others within the mental health disciplines, has known peaks and valleys in terms of conceptual and theoretical foundations, quality of accumulated knowledge, and practical applicability. Its trajectory over centuries has earned praise and recognition for positive accomplishments, as well as criticisms and objections to ambiguities and contradictions. This is not only because the very etimology of diagnosis covers a wide variety of areas, but also because its purpose, structure, and use have been the subject of increasingly complex research and scientific advances, themselves open to debate and controversy (1, 2). Traditionally, the scope and impact of diagnosis focused on the systematic delineation of clinical symptoms and syndromes, and on some implications of causality. Furthermore, the historical role of diagnosis implied generic indications and guidelines for treatment, as well as the estimation of prognosis or outcomes whenever possible (3).

The 21st. century, almost one decade old already, savors the progress brought about by consistent clinical and heuristic work. Contemporary psychiatric diagnosis is the foundation of large and deep epidemiological surveys (and epidemiology is, indeed, the basic science of clinical practice), the basis for the elucidation of risk and protective factors, the reflection of the dynamic roles of families and communities in mental health and mental illness and, most importantly, the repository of initiatives in policy-making and delivery of services. Last, but by no means least, diagnosis in the mental health field now recognizes culture and cultural variables as essential components in the assessment of real clinical entities occurring in really suffering human beings (4-6). Thus, present-day psychiatric diagnosis encompasses a multitude of areas, and forces the mental health practitioners to view their work from a broad, comprehensive, and consistent perspective.

In the United States, and indeed across the world, the highest expression of the "state of the art" in psychiatric diagnosis is the current Fourth Edition-Text Revised of the American Psychiatric Association's Diagnostic and Statistical Manual (DSM-IV TR) (7). The creature of expert groups' consensus with innumerable printings over the years, translated into all languages on Earth, in short, another symbol of the multicephalous hegemony that this country exerts -- not always wisely, we must say --, DSM-IV-TR is now on the spot. The initial steps toward the development of DSM-V are taking place: the APA has already appointed the Task Force as well as different Work Groups, international conferences have taken place (coordinated by

APA, with the participation of the World Health Organization, National Institute of Mental Health, and World Psychiatric Association), new field research and contributions of representatives of the public health and academic communities are being planned. The new Manual is expected to see the light around the year 2011 (8, 9). Needless to say, the stakes are high, expectations are intense, and people involved in the work towards the DSM-V are looking forward to very exciting four or five years.

Everybody agrees that for a diagnosis to be effective and useful, it has to be thorough and comprehensive. Historically, the field of psychiatry has been a productive, at times chaotically so, setting of efforts to break down the barriers of an old-fashioned Cartesian dualism (10, 11). At this stage, suffice it to say that the old debate between categorical and dimensional approaches will regain center stage (12). The contributions from basic neurosciences will be an important ingredient of forthcoming diagnostic conceptualizations (13), as will the obvious needs and demands of public mental health (14).

This latter development will take place because issues such as poverty, inequality, social injustice, stigmatization, diversity, prejudice, and repression reside (whether we like it or not) at the core of what we call mental illness. And practically all of the above concepts are part and parcel of culture, understood as a set of meanings, behavioral norms, and values or reference points utilized by members of a particular society as they construct their unique view of the world, and ascertain their identity (15). The concept of culture enriches the notion of a multidimensional definition of health, beyond the now old-fashioned biopsychosocial umbrella (16, 17). Why? Because culture goes beyond material or nonmaterial elements (language, traditions, values, social relationships, financial philosophy, or the ascertainment of technology). It implies context, meaning, and integration, not only for the internal consistency of a diagnosis but also for the external presentation of its multiple variations. And culture is a vital and decisive notion because it also entails religious beliefs, spiritual needs, moral thoughts and structures (18, 19).

It is in this crucial area that *Naming the Pain and Guiding the Care* by Donald D. Denton, not only builds on his first volume, *Religious Diagnoses in a Secular Society*, but advances the field both conceptually and pragmatically, a rare and notable accomplishment indeed. In the manner of an initial reflection about the book, one has to say that the spiritual and religious experiences of a human being, touch the most sensitive cord of the science vs. humanism dichotomy. And thereof a number of questions emerge. Shall such experiences be considered an element – or product-- of the cognitive apparatus and functions of the individual? (20, 21) Or are they mostly phenomena of the highest order, resulting from the thirst for transcendency and search for meaning in everyone's life? (22) Shall spiritual and religious aspects of the individuals suffering be evidence-based or, more than that, value-based so that the true humanistic entity of psychiatry and mental health be vindicated? (23) How do the spiritual and religious aspects of human life apply to the so-called "special populations" reflected in ethnic diversity, age differences, gender interactions, and the like? And finally, to what extent do spiritual and religious matters play a role in what we call clinical symptomatology, a varied body of manifestations, both physical and psychological, that must be systematized not only in the name of "diagnostic accuracy," but also because our job is to deal with the "whole" human being asking for help? (24)

Twenty-two chapters (each one of them well designed, well written, exciting texts) give shape to the book. With the premise that "spiritual pain is the most personal of human suffering," the structure of diagnosis as a cultural product is described from three "world views": the ontological, the teleological, and the integrative. The first "tends to see disease as being built into the nature of reality, in categories such as the 'wrath of God'." The second attempts to accomplish the most difficult task of "accurately identifying the etiology of the disease"-in the author's view, something that is at the core of DSM. It advocates the use of instruments of evaluation and treatment, technology and psychometrics in a way that may be as yet unreachable as it is ambitious. The integrative world view, as the name implies, "attempts to take into account the importance of issues related to being and quality of life (ontology), as well as health factors that are objectively verifiable and responsive to a course of care that can be replicated across cultures (teleology)." In the author's assessment, the evidence-based clinical practice is an example of efforts at integration. Needless to say, effectiveness of management is emphasized, and ending the polemics between science and humanism, while practicing a truly person-centered treatment, are duly recognized needs. Ultimately, the provision of "humane care" becomes the main goal of a good diagnosis.

Not surprisingly, the book proposes a "clinical interview with spiritual implications," and provides itemized points of exploration. Those bulleted lines in several pages of Part One, particularly chapters 3 and 4, are welcomed gems of clinical pragmatism, usefulness, and wisdom. One of the most original contributions of this volume is the proposal of "systems of faith" that approach the diagnosis examining "the inherent tensions between various clinical and non-clinical models." Parts II, III, and IV present all these perspectives quite cogently. The first, ethical guilt or the feeling of blame is a component that, from a clinical point of view, cuts across different entities. The second perspective addresses idolatry or the feeling of betrayal. It has to do with "naming the Gods in diagnosis," an effort to set the stage for "the soul of pastoral counseling." The description of "secular gods of cultural religion," the gods of ambiguity shaping up clinical features (primarily of personality disorders), the fusion of a particular world religion with a culture or nation, are scary pathogenic routes. Thus, "helping individuals name such terror for what it is, becomes a part of the healing task." Nothing could be more truthful.

Dread or the feeling of defilement, puts both the patient and the diagnostician/therapist straight into the "care versus cure" dilemma. The language of defilement evokes self awareness at its most tragic scope. Defilement may symbolize stain and stigma, a sense of abandonment, but also entails the promise of cleansing, "transforming the soul" into the unique personal experience of happiness or inner serenity that comes as liberation, yet not without a "saving sacrifice."

Denton moves from metaphor to clinical discussions with ease and elegance. His three axes of a "theological model" (that, some would rightly assert, goes beyond theology), are rounded up by illustrative case vignettes. They enrich the theoretical concepts, present real-life situations, and respond to the needs of clinical practitioners as much as anything else in the book. Part Five addresses "special cases" such as children, substance abuse, stress disorders, and bereavement. Each subsection keeps a straight eye on faith needs, spiritual concerns, experiential debacles, and existential hopes.

The therapeutic value of a spiritually-oriented diagnostic work is undeniable (25, 26). Caregivers get frustrated at the limitations of neurology and physiology, but also at their own inability to achieve the total erasure of suffering. In such context, the instillation of hope is certainly one of the most extraordinary contributions to the effectiveness of any kind of psychotherapy (27), its spiritual and profoundly human origins and repercussions being difficult to ignore. Thus, the achievement of forgiveness, reconciliation, and restoration is both, a precious goal of a good diagnostic work, and an essential and rather critical ingredient of psychotherapy or counseling. The assessment and management of a "crisis of religious belief, triggered by a life crisis or chaos in life created by an overly pious practice of a religion's central tenets," could lead to lofty goals such as the search for meaning, provision of creative values, foster self-esteem, or stimulate growth of inner freedom and autonomy.

The book ends with a suggestion and a challenge. The first is the conceptualization and inclusion, in any forthcoming diagnostic manual, of either an Axis VI, or an original spiritual/theological multiaxial diagnosis with Axis I as guilt, Axis II as idolatry, and Axis III as dread. The challenge comes through a question: Will there be any intentional integration of the spiritual or religious diagnoses within the official lexicon of diagnosis? I have to agree with the notion that nosology of the DSM-IV-TR "hardly does justice to the anguish of all concerned." In agreement with APA's pronouncements about the recognition of cultural variables, and specifically religious and spiritual aspects of human suffering into the diagnostic task, the author hopes for an end of the "clinical bifurcation" noted in the last two or three decades regarding the religious dimensions of human distress and human equanimity, deplores the lack of bibliographic support (that *Naming the Pain and Guiding the Care* undoubtedly provides), and supports going beyond an essentializing, disease-centered approach driven almost exclusively by biomedical technologies.

Nevertheless, the book also urges the pastoral counselors and professionals involved in spiritual and religious care, to abandon their own isolation, fight extremisms, and go beyond diagnosis in an authentic search for integration and integrity. Providing "diagnostic criteria" for individuals with "unhealthy or faulty awareness of providence, grace, and/or dependence" becomes a crucial task. The need for primary research is rightly proclaimed, and the summary chapter of this volume offers a book, Caldwell (31) elucidates faith as obedience, guilt as transgression, ostracism, disgrace and death. One wonders about the pathogenic power of such formidable entities – faith, as a potentially rigid, supra-rational dictum, guilt as the perhaps unplanned result of the dominance of inexhaustible "immoral impulses." It is therefore clear that diagnosis, its role and implications, go far beyond clinical considerations, if we accept the moral dimensions of behavior.

One final point. Let's reiterate another unequivocal reality: globalization is a fact, a concept, and a practice (32, 33). Therefore, together with its recognition, keeping a vigilant, critical eye on the term's genuine meaning of balance and equity must be everybody's task. Religious and spiritual needs respond to the communal, globalizing needs of humankind. Yes, fundamentalism should be rejected, but this rejection should not be used as an excuse for violation of the rights of many other groups or communities throughout the world. I read this book – beyond its nuclear purpose-- as a proclamation of real integrative humanism, trying to put an end to artificial divisions and separations, emphasizing values that are inherent to our human condition, rejecting intolerance, protecting privacy, and caring for the public good (34). La Rochefoucauld, the 17th century French thinker, praised the coexistence of human beings in a social conglomerate because it restricts "immoderate appetites," and fosters the learning of reciprocity, a social ideal that overcomes selfishness and irresponsibility. This balanced recognition in social life, is as important as an objective diagnosis is for our patients. Naming the pain and guiding the care are examples of how psychiatry and mental health transcend medicine, and the bureaucratic scope of the professions. One of our fundamental missions in this noble effort is to see the human through spiritual lenses, and to see the spiritual through human lenses. *Selah!*

Renato D. Alarcón, MD, MPH
Rochester, Minnesota
August 2007

Preface

This work builds on my first work in the field of diagnosis. That book took ten years to formulate and produce. Interest in enlarging the multi-axial system described in *Religious Diagnosis in a Secular Society: A Staff for the Journey*, surfaced almost at once. Having just completed that volume, I wanted a significant amount of time to pass before producing a second volume. I hoped the multi-axial system would bring some conversation between the clinical and 'non-clinical' diagnosis.

This direct collaboration has yet to happen. Instead, the non-clinical side of the discipline of humane care has continued to produce more models of diagnosis. One reason to write a second volume is to therefore include a more thorough review of these various systems and to re-state my call for collaboration between these spiritually oriented writers if not between them and their secular colleagues.

I also knew that the task of clinical and religious diagnosis would continue to advance. Neurobiology, pharmacology and social psychology have provided helping professionals with more nuance as we seek to understand the factors and forces that create and relieve human suffering. A second reason to write is to incorporate these advances in the field of diagnosis.

A third reason for a second volume has been the march of events in this intervening decade. Events have created challenges in trying to understand, and therefore name, the disorders, distress or factors that prompt people to fly airplanes into buildings, murder their fellow students sitting attentively in their classrooms, and prolong a loved-one's biological processes in the face of overwhelming evidence they are deceased. It remains my belief that the clinical diagnosis structure of the DSM-IV-TR is too narrow when applied to such situations.

Finally I wanted to re-name my work to make it more accessible. The title of the first volume seemed cumbersome and reinforced the notion that religious practice and sentiment is mainly a thin veneer over a more basic secular culture. The title of this volume more clearly describes the nature of the work at hand. The title of this volume also makes plain that humanity remains a spiritual creature whose need for affiliation with the Divine remains undeterred by the forces of secularization. Diagnosis is incomplete if it fails to take this need into consideration, as the mental health research of the past decade now shows with irrefutable clarity.

My wife, Dr. Nedra Voorhies, has been a primary mover in the production of this second volume. Her intellectual stimulus, her uses of the first volume in her own work as an educator, her editorial suggestions and personal encouragement have been invaluable.

Donald D. Denton
Richmond, Virginia
October, 2007

Acknowledgments

There are a number of individuals and institutions that have contributed to my effectiveness as a clinician and success as a writer. I want to identify them here, hoping the reader will credit them only for whatever strengths and graces they find in this volume. The errors in print and the 'growing edges' in my life remain mine alone.

Dr. Renato D. Alarcón, MD, MPH, Medical Director of the Mood Disorders Unit of the Psychiatry and Psychology Treatment Center at the Mayo Clinic graciously wrote an integrative and perceptive Foreword.

The Brett-Reed Memorial Foundation provided financial support for pre-publication activities and its members have been encouraging of my writing.

Dr. Donald Michenbaum for his thoughtful pre-publication review of the entire manuscript.

Dr. Everett Worthington, Professor of Psychology at Virginia Commonwealth University, for being a good friend, professional colleague and fellow-traveler in the field of integrating psychology, religion, and spirituality. His pre-publication review was very helpful.

Dr. Orlo Strunk, managing editor of The Journal of Pastoral Care and Counseling, has continued to encourage my professional writing and provided pre-publication review of this book.

John Hinkle, Ph. D., has mentored my understanding and use of psychological testing and clergy assessment.

Esteban Montilla, D. Min., utilized my earlier book and provided pre-publication review of this book.

My brother, Michael J. Denton, M.S., CADAC, LMFT is a Clarian Health Program Manager of Alcohol and Drug Services. He is an inspiration to me as well as a ready source of professional consultation. His pre-publication review was immeasurably helpful.

A number of professional colleagues at Virginia Institute of Pastoral Care, Chris Bowers, M. Div., Sandra Hamilton, D. Min., and Marjorie Smith, D. Min., read specific chapters and made helpful suggestions.

D. W. Donovan, Manager of Operations Bon Secours Richmond Pastoral Care, provided consultation on end-of-life concerns

The Working Group on Pastoral Diagnosis of the American Association of Pastoral Counselors contains a number of dedicated colleagues who have offered me their critique and encouragement over twenty years. They and the group remain a ready venue for exploring this entire area.

Clients and members of congregations who have trusted me to walk with them in their search for both cure and care continue to inspire me. Although their names and circumstances have been altered in this volume to protect their identities, they names and faces remain in my heart.

Basic Types of Pastoral Care and Counseling, Howard Clinebell, 1966, Abingdon Press. Used by permission.
Stages of Faith: The Psychology of Human Development and the Quest for Meaning James W. Fowler Harper&Row, 1981. Used by permission
The Symbolism of Evil, Volume Seventeen of the Religious Perspective Series, by Paul Ricoeur. Beacon Press, 1967. Used by permission
Religious Ethics and Pastoral Care, Don S. Browning. Augsburg Press, 1983. Used by permission.

Introduction: The Status of Diagnosis

In my prior volume on diagnosis I identified two themes in diagnosis that would need attention: the continued professionalization of religious care and the continued spiritualization of secular care. The challenge for religious providers of relational care would be to find a unified language of diagnosis with which they could communicate among themselves and also speak effectively with the wider community of human care. The challenge in the secular clinical community was somewhat similar, growing out of the culture's emerging desire for care that includes sensitivity to spiritual values: finding a nosology for diagnosis that would honor the dilemmas of the human heart we recognize as 'spiritual' without denigrating them or simply retranslating them into psychological categories.(1)

These two challenges remain. In the decade since the publication of *Religious Diagnosis in a Secular Society* the religious clinical community has continued to design and publish diagnostic schema. While at least one effort looks hopeful of usefulness beyond that author's immediate circle, generally the religious clinical community has remained unsuccessful in developing and utilizing a unified way of speaking professionally of human spiritual pain. Within the secular clinical community there has been a similar want of progress. There has been a proliferation of quasi-spiritual 'therapies' offered by mental health clinicians who seek to incorporate their own religious sentiments into their clinical practice. These approaches are more or less helpful. But a more primary pattern still exists within the secular clinical community: it remains much less conversant with the diagnostic resources of the religious clinical community than the reverse. We are still faced with two parallel diagnostic universes. (2)

The Diagnostic Rhombus

These two challenges form two sides of the diagnostic rhombus within which professionals attempt to relieve human suffering through the primary tasks of diagnosis. I have formulated those two tasks as *naming the pain* and *guiding the care.* Recognizing that people of good will must accomplish these two tasks regardless of their clinical approach, this volume seeks to approach this portion of the diagnostic rhombus through these two lenses and continue the professional conversation Two other cultural discussions inform the other sides of the diagnostic rhombus. The professional debate over whether one is conducting *assessment* or *diagnosis* along with who is providing this service and the wider cultural debate around the definition of and distinction between *spirituality* and *religion* all impinge upon the two tasks of diagnosis. The intensity and even fury with which some of these discussions are conducted seems to be unhelpful to the more primary task of providing relief to another human's suffering. This volume will also attempt to bring more light rather than more heat to this conversation.

The tasks of diagnosis are aided by the continuing march of medical technology. Through the use of various brain imaging technology and continued sophistication in genetic research clinicians in all the helping disciplines now have available to them – and thus can make available to their patients or clients – new ways of perceiving and new levels of understanding the etiology and complexity of their patient's condition. The way in which this information is understood and then employed to relieve human suffering, along with the way in which this utilized data is communicated to the human seeking help is influenced directly by the first task of diagnosis (*naming the pain*) and will influence the second task of diagnosis (*guiding the care*). This volume will address the influence of this technology and make suggestions on ways to utilize this rapidly growing clinical technology.

Almost as soon as the current *Diagnostic and Statistical Manual –IV* was published, the American Psychiatric Association laid plans for the publication of a fifth edition. The six white papers developed in preparation for DSM-V's publication will be utilized in the following pages. In my earlier work I noted that for diagnosis to be complete 'there needs to be an assessment of the positive values of a person's life.'(3) This is the practice of spiritual direction in a nutshell. Thus while there is a white paper for DSM-V that addresses cross-cultural issues, it remains to be seen how much the next manual will provide indicators of healthy functioning or genuine spiritual wholeness since one fundamental goal of DSM-V appears to be 'the development of an etiologically-based, scientifically sound classification system.'(4) In a similar vein while the white paper on cross-cultural issues does recognize that 'for any psychiatric diagnosis to be truly comprehensive and culturally valid, it has to take account of a multitude of variables, from race and ethnicity to the more encompassing notions of language, education, religion, habits, values and gender and sexual orientation.'(5) It appears to leave out age and weight as factors that influence the psychological and spiritual components of one's overall care. As the reader might expect from a pastoral counselor, the reader will find I give the developments in this cultural area of diagnosis special attention.

The Voyage of Diagnosis

The naming of human pain remains a journey rather than a destination. Thus disorders, the religious clinical community has also continued to look for ways to more adequately name pain and guide the care of persons. Since the publication of my initial volume in this area several other writers have put forward diagnostic schemata in either journal articles or in book form. The works of Paul Pruyser and Wayne Oates retain their usefulness in part because of their descriptive capacities and in part because seminaries continue to use their works rather than what is most current in the professional literature. I will offer critiques of these schemata in a separate chapter.

The question of how to adequately diagnose the spiritual or religious concerns of children arose almost immediately after the publication of *Religious Diagnosis in a Secular Society*. Since that volume's publication there has certainly been events that created spiritual distress for even young children beyond the traditional spiritual anguish caused by parental divorce, family dysfunction and the child's own coping with disease. Children have questions related to the meaning of life and the destiny of those around them that arise from such events. Providing adequate care for children includes assisting them in naming their own pain around such events; offering tools to their parents and other adults with the responsibility for the guidance of children is likewise responsible professional practice. This volume makes some initial effort to assist in this effort.

The terrorist attack of September 11, 2001, our overall national response to terrorism and what is cast as 'unprecedented' natural disasters have created a new context in which humane care must be provided. Mass deaths and the inevitable deaths that result from active military activity are only the most obvious alterations in the context of human care. The increased role of National Guard and Reserve forces in combat as well as the utilization of the active duty military units in post-disaster relief efforts within the confines of the continental United States has increased the stress on military families and is expanding the expectations on mental health providers. The consequent spike in anxiety and stress disorders appears to be rising in part from both objective events and a rupture of civilian expectations that their lives will be totally secure that result from natural disasters. This two-pronged rupture in the expectation of security requires care providers to address the role such expectations play in exacerbating stress beyond mere symptom relief. Caregivers have a public role to play in bringing realism to a community's expectations of security and a civic duty to assist in maintaining public calm rather than adding to the anxiety that naturally results from public disasters. The pain of bereavement goes well beyond assisting individuals and communities in naming their immediate losses to include what is likely to include a generational shift in family identity and national self-understanding.

While the demand for illegal drugs is undergoing a slight decrease at present, the increase use and overuse of prescription medication by youth remains troubling. While helpful, the use of spectroscopic imagery as an educative adjunct to providing care for impaired individuals does not address the more basic lack of meaning or provide the behavioral lifestyle skills that lead to – and

While the demand for illegal drugs is undergoing a slight decrease at present, the increase use and overuse of prescription medication by youth remains troubling. While helpful, the use of spectroscopic imagery as an educative adjunct to providing care for impaired individuals does not address the more basic lack of meaning or provide the behavioral lifestyle skills that lead to – and result from – prolonged misuse of narcotics and drugs. Naming the pain and guiding the care of individuals impaired by substance abuse remains a chronic feature of the landscape, including continued debate over what constitutes 'addiction' and 'dependence.'

These last three areas of children, stress disorders and substance abuse will be addressed in separate chapters. While naming the pain in such settings is relatively straightforward, providing care in these instances is made more complex by the presence of outside factors that effect both the course of care as well as the framework of meaning in which the care is provided. Providing care for others while living in a community devastated by a natural disaster and assisting families coping with a child's severe organic or developmental disorder requires the clinician to work collaboratively with an increasingly complex web of institutions over a lengthy period of time. Providing care for individuals impaired through substance abuse along with addressing the ravages such abuse wreaks upon their families is a task going well beyond the sacred 50-minute hour of psychotherapy. The burden of care falls primarily on individuals within the extended family and community institutions such as churches, schools and community service boards. These chapters will be written with an eye toward equipping these care providers with a language to name the pain and guide the care of their loved ones.

Concluding Considerations

The text that follows is organized along the following lines. Five parts divide the topic of diagnosis into matters of structure, guilt, idolatry, dread and special considerations. These topics exist whether one uses the current psychiatric diagnostic system or some schema of spiritual assessment. Each part has four chapters that examine the topic in detail, concluding with illustrative vignettes. These vignettes will be enriched at each part with additional information. The vignettes have been altered to insure confidentiality. A final part will revisit the tensions between secular and spiritual diagnostic schemas.

I have continued my practice of using single sex pronouns to describe both human pain and the delivery of humane care. Anguish is personal not androgynous.

Understanding spiritual concerns within a secular care setting and recognizing clinical syndromes in a religious context remains a thorny thicket. In my experience these two communities of humane care still do not read one another's journals or draw on whatever research each community develops. Third-party payers continue to be the elephant in the consulting room and hospital settings whose presence shapes the description and delivery of care. How human pain is named and relieved in the public square is guided much more by who is paying for the treatment rather than the judgment of the clinician. While it is doubtful these two areas of tension will be resolved quickly, the practicing clinician must take seriously the mandate to deal responsibly with human spirituality while also working effectively within our existing system of mental health care. As a consequence, it remains my experience that the mystery of Spirit ultimately finds a way through this thicket to infuse the care we provide one another to move toward health. Dr. Martin Luther King, Jr. once said, "The arc of the moral universe is long but it bends towards justice;" in my experience it also bends towards wholeness. *Selah!*

Part I-The Structure of Diagnosis

Chapter 1

The Purpose of Diagnosis

"Mary's leg has carried her for nearly seventy years," commented the surgeon. "Now it is killing her. In order to save her we have to remove this leg." His voice was calm but touched with compassion. He had known Mary for over a decade, caring for her as her diabetes took its toll on her body. She was in severe life-threatening pain. Competent compassionate care dictated amputation.

We have little trouble identifying an individual's physical disease. We have a well-defined compendium of physical maladies that seems to grow by the day with ever-increasing precision. The same is increasingly true for the anguish that tears at the human mind and heart. Thanks to the patient work of thoughtful professionals and the advances in psychological care we now understand much more about the sources of human suffering.

These efforts build upon millennia of experience in naming human pain and guiding the care of our fellows. As the introduction to the DSM-IV makes quite clear this history is both 'extensive' and nevertheless quite varied in its focus. The only criteria which has remained constant is the recognition for the need for such a 'classification system.' (1) Whether we called them a physician, priest, shaman, *curandero,* or monk, we have always gathered near the warmth and wisdom of another human being for healing. Our ancestors saw these individuals as a representative of the gods and we came with the expectation that such a representative of the gods would both understand our pain and be an agent of relief from our suffering. Regardless of the public myth about how the healer restored our health, we know that their practice was based upon a system of diagnosis that guided treatment

Our understanding of disease and health has advanced. The technology currently available for the healing of our bodies is breathtaking. Yet the deeper burdens of the human condition remain fundamentally unchanged. These burdens may result from illness and lead us into physical disease. Our burdens may also result from the human condition, what Shakespeare called 'the slings and arrows of outrageous fortune.' The source of our distress does not matter.

We expect the healer to both understand and do something about our suffering. This is true whether our pain is from a tumor on the brain or from the ache of loneliness, whether the sadness comes from grief or from a malfunctioning thyroid, whether the confusion in our cognition arises from mercury in a childhood serum or from the trauma of incest. Methods for understanding the nature of these ailments as well as directing our care of others can be very complex or very simple. All seem to have some efficacy for some persons.

The efficacy of religious care, quite apart from formal therapy by a religiously oriented clinician, is increasingly recognized by secular agencies. The DSM-IV became the first secular diagnostic system to recognize <u>Religious or Spiritual Problem</u> as a specific diagnosis. There is hope the newer DSM-V will build upon this sensitivity. The various 12-Step recovery programs that address a variety of human problems, while maintaining a religiously neutral stance, nevertheless encourage a *de facto* spiritual consciousness through the imagery of the Higher Power. Thus it is common for even the average parish pastor to have within a congregation at least one person who has had experience with the therapeutic use of spiritual imagery through such a lay-directed group. It is also common for secular therapists to be treating people who are being assisted by one of these 12-Step programs. Hopefully by now all clinicians will have had exposure to such rubrics for care as a part of their formal training.

For all providers of human care the question is not so much "will I encounter human anguish and ecstasy?" but rather "how will I understand and respond to the sweep of human experience?" In broad form, this is the question of diagnosis and care. An adequate diagnosis is "transformational knowledge...heavily influenced by wisdom emerging from praxis and is affected by the technical mandate to 'do something' to urgently alleviate...suffering." (2) Adequate diagnosis assists us in evoking the terror and appreciating the beauty inherent in our life. Diagnosis can shape our response to tragedy and to triumph.

Naming the Pain

Pain is the universe telling us something is weak if not broken. If faced directly with the proper resources pain and its concomitant weakness can be driven from body and confusion banished from the mind. Although taking longer to achieve, anguish in the soul can be soothed with peace and injustice within society can also be restored. Pain is not something most of seek out or invite. Naming the etiology, intensity, extent, and implications of pain all play a part in the thorough naming of pain and completing this primary task. This necessity is contained in the requirement that treatment plans be based upon a thorough *biopsychosocial* (and spiritual) assessment. Naming the pain is the primary task of diagnosis. Professional boundaries of craft and club are drawn around who has the 'authority' or 'privilege' to name pain officially. But all of us know when we hurt and we revere those who have the capacity to not just confirm our pain but to also to eliminate our pain

The interplay between these four quadrants of human distress in the task of diagnosis was recognized within the DSM-IV. Effective providers of humane care utilize wise judgment in whatever setting they encounter a human in distress. "A compelling literature documents that there is much 'physical' in 'mental' disorders and much 'mental' in 'physical' disorders," the manual notes. The manual continues, "Although this manual provides a classification of mental disorders, it must be admitted that no definition adequately specifies precise boundaries for the concept of 'mental disorder.' (3) This volume shares this viewpoint The author recalls a seminar on diagnosis in which Allan Francis, the chairperson of the DSM-IV task force predicted those assembled would, 'this very week,' encounter a new patient or client whose 'mental disorder' was most likely caused by either the misuse of some legitimately prescribed medication or some physical ailment that we were not recognizing because we were focused on diagnosing a 'mental' state of distress.

Biological or physiological pain causes us the most anxiety and calls for the most prompt response because of its signal that our distress might end our life. Physicians name such pain quite thoroughly and the care of such pain consumes much of our individual and community resources. Our sophistication in naming pain now extends to the sub-genetic level thanks to MRI's, spectrographic tomography and the use of remote-controlled fiber optic technology. As a result overall life expectancy in highly developed countries has risen to dramatically.

Psychological pain of both a co-morbid condition with biological disease as well as a signal of relational, emotional, or developmental distress in its own right now receives similar precision. Such brokenness is named by a host of mental health professionals utilizing the DSM-IV / ICD-9. A plethora of surveys and assessment instruments back up the skilled eye and ear of a practicing clinician in addition to the increasingly exacting nomenclature of these two diagnostic compendiums. In the end what often decides the 'naming' of psychological pain is not the precise fit with diagnostic rubrics but the wise employment of a clinician's life experience. This lack of precision frustrates the suffering person, their loved ones and the professional. The difficulties inherent in making such an exact determination, along with the still-devastating social consequences of being tagged with the label of poor mental health, makes professionals frequently reluctant to fully name an individual's true psychological condition.

Societal pain is named or at least witnessed by mental health professionals as well as politicians, attorneys, teachers, law enforcement and emergency responders. These disciplines utilize a variety of tools that assist them in this task. Because distress in a societal setting carries the risk of affecting an individual's liberty there is the need for exceptional caution when trying to identify the source of pain within an individual. It is tempting to engage in speculation as to the source of an individual's distress and there are frequently powerful but misguided incentives to label the troubling behavior of an individual as crazy, sick, sinful or seditious. Within an increasingly pluralistic society these incentives must be balanced within the wider interplay between anindividual's culture of national origin and the culture in which they now seek to live. Nevertheless, the connection between psychological distress and social policy finds explicit expression in the vision statement of the *President's New Freedom Commission on Mental Health:*

> We envision a future when everyone with a mental illness will recover, a future when mental illnesses can be prevented or cured, a future when mental illnesses are detected early, and a future when everyone with a mental illness at any stage of life has access to effective treatment and supports – essentials for living, working, learning, and participating fully in the community. (4)

Spiritual pain is the most personal of human suffering. Although it may be named officially by religious leaders and eloquently portrayed in public by artists of all types, its presence is pervasive throughout all venues of human distress. The persistence of spiritual pain too frequently remains in spite of whatever drug, touch or rite a caregiver or community might offer. The key element in naming the spiritual component of human agony lies in the recognition of being somehow separated from God. The 'naming' can result from violating a divine edict or religious standard. The more pervasive diagnosis is frequently the individual's belief they have run afoul of some divine imperative that is resulting in distress in some other aspect of their life as well as the interior experience of guilt, shame, terror or dread. This belief is seen most poignantly in the ancient epigram 'whom the gods destroy they first make mad' or in the Biblical story of Adam and Eve. (5)

A thorough diagnosis occurs only when one fully identifies the scope of human pain in each of these areas. Such thoroughness is not necessary for care to begin or for profound suffering to be alleviated. But as human agony subsides in the dominant quadrant, awareness of pain's existence in the other areas becomes a more important focus of scrutiny. This is especially true as one makes the transition from simply providing enough care to relieve the dominant symptoms to providing sufficient care for there to be either complete healing or at least a substantial improvement in the quality of life. This type of diagnosis occurs when those charged with the responsibility of healing collaborate; fortunately our healing does not ultimately depend upon such collaboration, but only upon our receiving the appropriate care.

Guiding the Care

"I wanted to let you know that I have completed my second decade of being cancer free," she said in a voicemail. "My doctor will not say I am 'cured' and I still must go in every five years for a check up. But I am grateful to God for my health."

Dr. William B. Oglesby was the first person I heard who distinguished between 'care' and 'cure.' As indicated above, diagnosis implies that one will *do something* to relieve suffering as a consequence of naming the pain. At the very least there is the expectation that the agent of healing will not make the situation worse. Some maladies, diseases and disorders can be cured. I will never again suffer from chicken pox, having had it during childhood. Many more conditions and syndromes must be endured or managed. Multiple sclerosis, chronic depression, the aftermath of divorce and the existential condition of addressing the status of having survived Pol Pot's killing fields are all conditions that one must cope with throughout the remainder of life. While there may be extensive knowledge about such conditions, what can be done to relieve the suffering attendant to many human diseases varies with the distress, the resources of the individual and culture as well as the skill of the caregiver. The title of one volume illustrates how the effort towards a cure in any of these quadrants is more of a quest than a destination (6) although our contemporary expectation is that 'recovery will be the common, recognized outcome of mental health services.'(7)

Within the biological realm we have an extensive health care system that devotes uncountable resources to the outright cure of disease and relief of the human suffering that attends disease. This system sets the gold standard for precision in diagnosis, success in cure and compassion in care. When physical pain begins to grab our attention our initial expectation is of the cessation of pain through the outright cure of the underlying disease. Disappointment frequently attends the announcement that there is no known cure for our disease.

Our attitudes and efforts toward care and cure in the psychological are neither less ancient nor any less varied. The move to separate psychological treatment from both medicine and religion has its roots in the Enlightenment philosophers who 'believed science would provide a breakthrough in the quest for a cure to mental illness.'(8) Indeed the initial criteria for admission to America's first public hospital was restricted to those deemed either 'curable or dangerous' and long-term residents were 'not welcome. '(9) The rise of public hospitals during this period of history represents a step forward in the care of psychological distress. As crude as those methods of both diagnosis and cure seem to us today, they were guided by a mixture of compassion and fear that remains in our contemporary response to mental illness. It is not hyperbole to note the sense of stigma that impedes the provision of mental health care.(10) Just as today, these early treatment efforts were guided by the diagnostic understanding of the source of human pain.(11) Our emphasis on scientific research and verifiable outcomes for both diagnosis and delivery of care remain the driving forces in our approach to a system of care that emphasizes increasing humanity's 'ability to successfully cope with life's challenges, on facilitating recovery, and on building resilience, not just on managing symptoms.' (12)

If the second overall effort at diagnosis fluctuates between strategies for cure and efforts to provide care, the working out of these strategies in the societal arena appear to swing between tactics of control and tactics of autonomy. The former efforts at their worst are driven by fear and prejudice while the latter, at their worst, result from either societal anarchy or the surrender of legitimate familial responsibility. The early recognition that alcoholics were 'a nuisance to the community' but were thus more appropriately the responsibility of the care of local churches has now swung in the direction of greater control that can result in incarceration plus psycho-educational efforts. This care is now backed up by the force of the law when an individual's use of alcohol produces intoxication while operating a motor vehicle.(13) Substance use disorders and the necessity of providing effective care remain a concern of contemporary mental health care.(14) More broadly these societal efforts at care are influenced by both changing understanding of the source of human pain as well as fluctuations in the basic social contract within a nation or community.

The societal aspects of care and cure, as well as their link to the first task of diagnosis (naming the pain) is seen the overall goal of a transformed mental health delivery system:

> When a serious mental illness or serious emotional disturbance
> is first diagnosed, the health care provider – in full partnership
> with consumers and families – will develop an individualized
> plan of care for managing the illness. This partnership of personal-
> ized care means basically choosing *who, what and how* appro-
> priate care will be provided. (15)

This study mandates that 'new, relevant research findings must be systematically conveyed to front-line providers so that they can be applied to practice quickly.'(16) Implementing such a vision, along with the technological support and improved access to care to underserved areas encouraged in Goal 6, underscores the way in which societal factors either enhance or impede the delivery of competent and timely care. Unfortunately, 'the lag between discovering effective forms of treatment and incorporating them into routine patient care is unnecessarily long, lasting about 15 to 20 years.'(17)

The role of religious faith and spiritual sentiment in both the care and cure of distress is well known to the average person while being formally absent from most academic and social policy discussions of care delivery. Yet in spite of the millennia of care begun and provided by religious communities, the inspiration to hope and the behavioral strictures promoting health that are the hallmarks of healthy religious faith, this document mirrors our contemporary discomfort thinking about spiritual care in the public square. It avoids any explicit mention of this wellspring of hope. Although the New Commission on Mental Health's report speaks of 'hope playing an integral role in an individual's recovery,' as well as defining resilience as 'the personal and community qualities that enable us to rebound from adversity, trauma, tragedy, threats or other stresses,' the report is silent about one of the chief sources that develop such hope and resilience: religious faith and the communities that preserve and promote such spiritual awareness. (18)

I noted this absence in my first work on religious diagnosis as well as the abiding hunger in humanity for 'care that combines the unspeakable dimensions of the self along with the very recognizable maladies of body and mind.'(19) This absence is all the more noteworthy eight years later due to the increasing visibility of spirituality in the popular culture and the demand for such care in people as they seek relief from their caregivers, regardless of the venue. It is long past the time when we can afford to maintain the tension and mutual deafness between the hospital and the church, the physician and the pastor as to who is the 'dispenser of hope and care.'(20)

Conclusion

The couple, long divorced, sat in my office on opposite couches. Their mutual concern is the conduct of a son. Approaching middle school, his anger erupts at home in nearly uncontrollable bursts. I am the third counselor brought in to attempt a 'cure' for this youngster's 'anger management problem.' A colleague in another practice had produced a well-written summary of diagnosis and treatment goals. It was professionally accurate; nevertheless it was ineffective. In a burst of candor the father says to the mother, "if we could just get our act together in spite of our divorce, his anger would subside. He reacts to our tensions."

The boy's mother nods even as her tension mounts. She had provided me with a multi-page description of their conflicts prior to this session. She would later state she is 'afraid to be alone' with the boy's father because of their shared history of combat. So I know there is little chance of truly 'curing' their conflict; thus their son's care must focus on helping him manage his way through this thicket of family life and the increasing demands of public education for docile students. A stimulant is already being used to manage the child's apparent attention deficiencies. Behavioral rewards to reinforce positive conduct will accompany parallel behavioral consequences to reduce if not erase negative conduct. Activities in the community and church will hopefully expose him to positive values and a variety of males for the times when his father is absent.

But how can the father's sense of injustice at 'having to pay everything and drive six hours just to be with my children' be assuaged? How will the mother's fear of the man who once promised to cherish her be reduced? What can a therapist realistically achieve in such a setting with such a child whose one-hour every-other-week appointment is sandwiched in between a grieving professional and an overly anxious young adult? These are the realities of outpatient care, whether the clinician is a secular or religious counselor. Naming this young man's pain and equipping him with the tools to manage his distress as well as whatever genuine neurological impairments exist will be a challenge. To truly cure this youngster's hurt that lies behind his angry dyscontrol makes those who labor in this vineyard periodically long for either a magic wand or hope somehow to provide two parents with words that will assuage this child's feelingof abandonment and fear to an extent that he will refocus his considerable energy on a more productive path.

Ultimately it will be a combination of competent technique, wise compassion and warm companionship employed toward this entire family system that may bring some relief to this hurting child. We may trust that father and mother may find enough maturity to put aside their continuing conflict to act in concert with their son. Naming their shared pain, guiding their care and hoping for cure will no doubt remain a lifelong journey for the professionals who will periodically address this child's circumstance or the circumstances of his yet-to-be-born children. The approach used to name his pain and their efficacy will also depend upon the system of diagnosis utilized by the professionals he has yet to meet. It is to a review of these various diagnostic systems that we now turn our attention. *Selah!*

Chapter 2

The Types of Diagnostic Systems

The pencil-scribbled note was left on my desk. "Came by to see you," it began. "Just got out of jail. Trying to do better. You R the best. Helped me. Living in Wilson hotel for now." I didn't need to look at the signature because I knew who it was. She had a knack for showing up unannounced, sometimes having ridden a bike or walked. It has been years since she has driven a car. During the past twenty years she has held a variety of entry-level jobs. All have ended due to tardiness, conflict with co-workers or supervisors, or being drunk while working.

Frequently she will spend several days without sleeping, alternating her incredible energy between writing a novel, hunting for agates to polish, running 'to get rid of my middle,' or looking for a new job. Other times she will sleep for twenty-four hours straight. When this storm of energy rises and falls over her it is impossible for her to keep focused on getting to work. Or she will find someone for a casual sexual encounter. Or she will call my office and swear at the secretary who's polite 'I'll put you into his voice mail' is more frustration than she can bear at the moment.

To the contemporary clinician, Jill meets the criteria for Bipolar Disorder II along with Alcohol Dependence (Chronic) as the most immediate foci of treatment. This overlays what is likely a Borderline Personality Disorder. She is surprisingly physically healthy but her chronic problems with the legal system almost preclude her finding any meaningful work.

But individuals with Jill's profile just didn't appear once the Western professional culture began producing the first Diagnostic and Statistical Manual. How would she have been viewed and helped during Colonial America? Or in France during the 12th Century? Or by an African holy woman? One of the true legacies of our post-modern era is the recognition that the value system we bring to a situation determines to some extent who and what we perceive as well as how we respond.

This chapter explores the variety of diagnostic systems. My purpose is two-fold. The first is simply to enlarge and hopefully enrich our understanding of how varied this task of diagnosis has been over the millennia. My second purpose has the aim of providing caregivers with additional resources through which to view – and respond – to the suffering humanity who comes to them for assistance. For while we may have to use the latest Diagnostic and Statistical Manual for official work, some of the more ancient diagnostic systems have insights into the etiology of our human condition and the course of our distress that are more helpful in providing care than our current Western model of treatment. Whether we prescribe a magic pill to control an individual's dyscontrol or if the 'magic pill' is the iron bars of a sanitarium that isolates someone like Jill from the bulk of the community depends much more on what the clinician brings to the conversation by the well in the heat of the day than what the person brings to the clinician. (1)

The Structure of Diagnosis

The task of diagnosis is derived from the basic worldview of the community or individual who is the instrument of healing. How the individual understands the source of the human suffering and distress determines to a great degree how pain will be named and what they will recognize as effective care, whether the agony is their own or that of a fellow citizen. In general there appears to be three general worldviews that determine the structure of diagnostic systems. The wider community gauges the effectiveness of these structures if it meets or exceeds the culture's expectation for understanding the dilemmas of the individual and relieving the suffering of the individual.

The Ontological Worldview

A worldview that focuses on the meaning of life and enriching the being of citizens tend to produce diagnostic systems that are *ontological* in structure. A diagnostic system derived from within an ontological structure tends to place the emphasis on adequately understanding the individual's overall life, the role which disease plays in their life and the way in which a person develops long-term resiliency in responding to the disease. The spiritual or religious component of ontological diagnostic structures tend to see disease as being built into the nature of reality in categories such as the 'wrath of God' and health being the consequence of God's mercy or grace.

Approaching the human situation from an ontological viewpoint has produced some fine diagnostic models that are rich in evocative power and sensitive to the nuances of human development across the lifespan. Gregory the Great, using an Aristotelian understanding of life, viewed diagnosis as discerning the person's distortion of some Golden Mean and viewed care as assisting the individual in returning to the mean between two extremes. Psychologist Paul Pruyser devised a developmental model influenced by Eric Erickson's understanding of human development. Thus health or anguish was perceived as the way in which an individual responded to the challenges of maturity posed by questions such as 'Is life trustworthy?' and 'Is life purposive?' and 'Is life valuable?' An ethical model of diagnosis, developed by Donald Browning, views pain as a failure in the person's ethics or value system. Browning assesses pain along lines ranging from a recognition of specific ethical lapses to the wider issues of examining a person's fundamental values. Merle Jordan and many other theologians utilize an anecdotal model that seeks to utilize either a sophisticated theology or philosophy or religious story to explain the person's dilemma. The implication in such a model is that the road to health is found in responding as faithfully to life as the icon of faith responded to a similar challenge.

Western psychology has been heavily influenced by ontologically based theories of diagnosis and care. Although founding members of modern psychology such as Sigmund Freud, Carl Jung and Mortimer Adler were medically trained, they were also deeply influenced by western classical literature. Thus while they used medically oriented categories for disorders such as hysteria and depression, their fundamental categories of diagnosis and approaches to care tend to focus on issues of meaning and being. Freud's explanation of human pain as deriving from the struggle between our super ego, ego and id or Jung's discernment that humanity approaches life through the personality types of introversion or extroversion are primarily ontological schemas of understanding the human condition. More current founders of psychological care such as diverse in theoretical orientation as Bruno Bettleheim, Karen Horney, Irving Yalom, Carl Rogers, Virginia Satir and Rollo May maintain a foundational emphasis on improving the being of individuals and families through understanding familial antecedents or personality structures.

This worldview, along with these founders of personality theories and the diagnostic models influenced by them have either produced or recommend utilizing a number of assessment instruments. Psychological assessment instruments, relational assessment approaches and spiritual inventories that seek to assess an individual's personality or overall approach to life may be said to have an ontological theoretical underpinning. I draw this conclusion because these particular instruments tend to focus on the nature or being of the individual rather than focus on their specific conduct or the impact their conduct is actually having on others. Instruments such as the Myers-Briggs Type Indicator, the 16 PF, Edwards Personality Preference and the Adjective Check List are some examples of pencil-and-paper assessment instruments. Richard Gardner's *Mutual Storytelling Technique* with children, the Draw-A-Person, Kinetic Family Drawing, Thematic Apperception Test and perhaps even the Rorschach Test are examples of ontological ways of making an effort to name the pain and also suggest intervention strategies for proceeding in a clinical setting. Theologically oriented inventories of spiritual gifts or tools that make an effort to ferret out an individual's religious orientation are also likely to be based upon an effort to learn the quality or direction of someone's being or character and are thus ontological in worldview. Effective care and much good can be provided to individuals and families from these instruments and this overall diagnostic structure, regardless of the specific diagnostic approach.

The Teleological Worldview

A worldview that we would recognize as 'scientific' (even if is ancient) tends to produce diagnostic models that are *teleological* in nature. The emphasis in this worldview is on accurately identifying the etiology of the disease, specifying the course of treatment and in some fashion building case studies, research libraries and encyclopedias for care. Thus the practice of bleeding, which we now see as absolutely barbaric, arose from a diagnostic viewpoint that perceived human troubles as caused by an excess of a specific quality within the blood and that relief would come from reducing a measurable amount of the afflicted blood from the person. The religious or spiritual component of teleological structures will focus on human flaws in action or inaction ('what I have done and left undone' in the words of historic confession) and prescribe specific sacrifices or rites through which pain may be alleviated and health restored. Denigrating these religious practices as 'magical thinking' or 'primitive,' especially when they share the same basic teleological worldview as some of the early medicinal practices are ironic; such arrogance overlooks the more basic human effort to relieve human suffering that stands behind the practice.

Although the medical community provides us with the most extensive example of this overall approach to diagnosis and treatment, psychology, societal structures and religious communities have also developed sophisticated diagnostic models that prescribe specific courses of treatment for disease. The use of drugs to alleviate pain or promote well-being are clear examples of a teleological understanding of diagnosis where the goal is restoration of health and cure rather than just care and coping with disease. The effectiveness of medicine is based upon producing verifiable results although there is some recognition within this worldview that human compliance with the mandated treatment plays an important role in producing health. It should be noted that such compliance may have much more to do with an individual's personality and being than with their capacity to passively submit to an invasive procedure.

The *Diagnostic and Statistical Manual* in all of its editions provides us with the clearest example of the teleological worldview's approach to the diagnosis and treatment of mental illness. The manuals provide specific criteria by which one can rule in or rule out not just specific categories of human distress but also distinguish between sub-categories of major conditions. The multi-axial system, first introduced in the third edition, also offers lenses through which a care provider can gauge the intensity or severity of an individual's distress as well as delineating broad classes of disorders within which this distress may be lodged.

Thus an *Adjustment Disorder* is recognized as something that is a normative response to the events of life while a *Personality Disorder* is identified as both more severe in terms of effect on an individual's quality of life as well as having its source more in the character structure of the individual, i.e. it is a state an individual *brings to* life rather than something solely that life brings to the individual. The manual's recognition that medical conditions and treatment can in and of themselves exacerbate if not produce mental and spiritual distress underscores the teleological worldview's effort to be as comprehensive as the ontological worldview.

As with the ontological worldview, so the teleological worldview has also produced powerful instruments that attempt to discern the presence of mental anguish and quantify the intensity of mental distress. Two widely used instruments the *Minnesota Multiphasic Personality Inventory* (MMPI) and the *Millon Clinical Multi-axial Inventory* (MCMI) are the paradigms for this worldview's approach to diagnosis. The linkage between the latter's developer and the current multi-axial approach to diagnosis, Theodore Millon, underscores how precisely this worldview makes the effort to both categorize the existence of human pain as well as prescribe specific clinical interventions. Some instruments, such as the *Beck Depression Inventory* or the *Strong Vocational Inventory* are highly accurate at detecting the presence of a single mental state or discerning a career path where an individual will find the most congruence between their interests and their work. The resources of time and talent, money and effort that go into the design, development, marketing and revision of psychological instruments underscores how deeply rooted is our desire to precisely name human distress as well as an indicator that we are as fearful that we will unwittingly come into contact with the stain of mental illness as we are fearful of some physical contagion.

The teleological worldview is now the dominant approach to the tasks of both diagnosis and treatment. As just one example, *NeuroPsychiatry Reviews* touts is mission as offering psychiatrists 'the latest news in biological psychiatry.' Regular features include a Clinical Trial Digest that reviews 'findings from recently published randomized controlled trials' and a Literature Monitor that summarizes research studies published in other professional journals. Whether treating combat-related PTSD, pediatric bipolar disorder or seeking to validate prescribing pet ownership for better mental health, a clinician will find helpful information in the plethora of reviews or newsletters that condense the turgid prose of the more technical research-based professional journals. (2)

The teleological worldview can also be found within the world of religious or spiritual care. The clearest example of this comes from the practice of pre-vocational screening rather than the delivery of parish pastoral care. Religious communities of all persuasions have always had standards by which they assessed both the character and conduct of their candidates for ordination. Initially these standards were more ontological or practical in nature.(3) People might just show up and proclaim their readiness to be of service; but history is replete with examples of what happens when religious communities fail to exercise due diligence in screening candidates. However since the advent of empirically based psychological testing some religious communities have added this testing to their assessment or discernment process. While one might argue this is not diagnosis *per se,* at this point my purpose is to simply acknowledge that religious values need not exclude a teleological worldview. Today many mainline denominations and local religious community utilize objective tests such as those noted above to both screen for psychopathology as well as evaluate an individual's overall fitness for the task of ministry. A more thorough discussion of this evaluative process will be offered in a later chapter. The fact that in spite of such screening people of poor character and questionable conduct nevertheless wind up in positions of trust underscores the limits of even the best psychological testing and the most savvy clinician. This is unfortunately true whether the position of trust is in the religious world or within the worlds of law enforcement and intelligence service.

Whether assessing for vocational readiness, academic ability, developmental maturity, or basic intelligence, objective psychological testing has a role to play in the provision of care even if one is not attempting to name a specific disorder or current pain. Thus chapters in a current textbook on psychological testing begins with chapters on principles of testing before proceeding to chapters on the application of specific tests and then on to concerns related to test bias and the overall ethics of psychological testing. (4) As this or any other introduction to psychological testing makes clear, the chief concerns of a psychological test focus on issues of reliability and validity regardless of whether one is utilizing an pure objective instrument such as the Wechsler Intelligence Scales and the California Psychological Inventory or a more subjective instrument such as the Rorschach Inkblot or Thematic Apperception Tests.

While these latter two instruments have a strong ontological component in that they seek to assess an individual's being, one textbook provides a teleological critique of these instruments. This critique illustrates the teleological worldview's approach and its dominance in today's clinical environment. "The Rorschach has been called everything from a psychological X-ray and perhaps the most powerful psychometric instrument ever envisioned to an instrument that bears a charming resemblance to a party game and should be banned in clinical and forensic settings." (5) The underlying concern is to provide both the clinician and the client a measurement of their abilities and distress. In a teleological worldview the *adequacy* of such instruments and their *usefulness* in being helpful are based upon their statistical *accuracy* in naming the individual's anguish, resiliency or demonstrated success in a chosen vocational field. "Scientific inadequacy" thus becomes this worldview's damning assessment of ontologically based instruments despite their ability to be helpful in the accomplishing the two central tasks of diagnosis: naming the pain and guiding the care. Throughout the history of humane care each worldview has had periods of ascendancy and decline, periods during which the just-replaced worldview is either denigrated or at least its proponents viewed as primitive by the newly ascending worldview.

The Integrative Worldview

At various periods there has been some effort to develop a third worldview that is more comprehensive than an exclusive focus on ontology or teleology provides. Such a worldview might rightly be called *integrative* in that it attempts to take into account the importance of issues related to being and quality of life (ontology) as well as health factors that are objectively verifiable and responsive to a course of care that can be replicated across cultures (teleology). In my assessment the current interest in *evidence based clinical practice* is one such effort at integration.

At first blush, the teleological core of evidence based clinical is obvious, as the name more than suggests. However, at least one resource notes 'the importance of the patient's individual experience and narrative…so that it has become clear that many clinical questions and uncertainties in mental health are best answered using clinical epidemiology and informatics.' This source continues, 'the goal of evidence-based practice is to *integrate* the best currently available evidence into clinical decision-making' (emphasis added). (6)

The best way to grasp the integrative effort of this approach is to review an example of how an evidence-based worldview of diagnosis and treatment approaches a specific disorder. Since depression in some form is the number one mental health concern most clinicians treat, a quick review of this worldview's methodology will be enlightening:

> We found no reliable direct evidence that one type of treatment (drug or non-drug) is superior to another in improving symptoms of depression. However, we found strong evidence that some treatments are effective, whereas the effectiveness of others remains uncertain. Of the interventions examined, prescription anti-depressant drugs and electroconvulsive therapy are the only treatments for which there is good evidence of effectiveness in severe and psychotic depressive disorders. (7)

What follows in this source is a twenty-three-page review of the entire range of diagnosis and treatments of depression. The language speaks repeatedly of 'care pathways' rather than cure as well as noting that in some types of depression ontologically oriented approaches to care (bibliotherapy and non-directive therapy) are as effective as teleologically oriented approaches to care (cognitive behavioral therapy and combining anti-depressant medication and psychological treatment). (8) Significantly this worldview notes the etiology of depression is 'uncertain' but 'includes childhood events and current psychosocial adversity,' an assessment not unlike what is offered for generalized anxiety disorder. (9) The measured approach of evidence-based treatment in its review of both diagnosis sources and avenues of care suggest an integrative worldview rather than a more restrictive teleological or ontological worldview.

There are also integrative efforts toward diagnosis and care within the domain of religious counsel and pastoral research. In an excellent article entitled *Pastoral Research: Past, Present and Future* John J. Gleason outlines the antecedent tension between 'scientists who would like to explain all the mysteries by empirical inquiry' (teleological worldview) 'over against the faithful, who fervently believe in spiritual forces immeasurable by any meter' (ontological worldview). (10) He briefly describes the seminal work of John L. Florell who delineated a variety of approaches to pastoral research and then cites Florell's integrative conclusion:

> A working definition of pastoral research is the disciplined study of religious experience by pastoral practioners toward increased effectiveness in ministry within the larger context of religious research (work conducted by persons representing many disciplines: theology, medicine, nursing, psychology, psychiatry, sociology and so on. (11)

It is Florell's and Gleason's inclusion of those 'many disciplines' in their view of what constitutes pastoral research that makes their viewpoint integrative rather than either teleological or ontological. Gleason continues to note the motivation for such research appears to be coming from 'religious researchers from many disciplines' but 'not clinical clergy pastoral researchers.' (12) While this is not good news for the narrow discipline of pastoral care research, it documents this present desire among providers of humane care from all disciplines to integrate religious or spiritual insights in naming the pain and guiding the care that are effective in reliving human suffering. Gleason rightly notes the seminal work of David B. Larson as the source of this shift in consciousness. Larson's untimely death was a blow to this integrative effort but not before he was able to state unequivocally and presciently this assessment of where this research would lead:

> A growing number of studies demonstrate that spiritual commitments associated with clinical benefit for both mental and physical health status. Results are so consistently positive and so contrary to prevailing academic ideas that we believe that the mental and physical health professions may be on the verge of a transformation in perspective in the next few years. (12)

I noted both a similar interest by 'secular' care providers and a similar paucity of research by 'religious' counselors in my prior volume on religious diagnosis. It is an interest that now appears to be at full flood stage – and religious researchers appear to have completely abandoned the field of quantitative research that would enhance the integrative dialogue. It appears that the bulk of writing by clinical clergy continues to address the same two questions I noted in my earlier work: 1) what unique insight and care does your profession provide to those who suffer and 2) can you speak to the other health care professions about this uniqueness in a way that enhances patient care? (13)

Clinical-Secular or Religious-Spiritual Diagnosis?

Within the religious world, the edge upon this query extends at least as far back as Augustine's polemic, "What has Jerusalem to do with Athens?" The execution of Socrates for the crime of corrupting the youth by getting them to question the stories of the gods speaks of a similar hostility beyond the Christian worldview. This tension is as current as a contemporary hospital administrator and senior hospital chaplain arguing over the efficacy of a pastoral care department, especially when the chaplain's assessment of the patient's 'spiritual need' sounds very much like it was written by Sigmund Freud or Carl Rogers rather than Moses or Mohammed. This dichotomy is ancient, exists today in both venues, is maintained by purists on both 'sides' and shows no immediate sign of ending.

These two approaches to the tasks of diagnosis exist within the teleological, ontological and integrative worldviews. While it is relatively easy to discern their presence within the first two worldviews, too often attempts at integrating these approaches ends with someone pronouncing this is a false dichotomy with little further attempt to truly integrate these approaches into the effort of naming human pain and providing compassionate care to human suffering. "I'm an eclectic clinician," thus becomes a stopgap code word for individual efforts at finding a way between the two dominant worldviews without doing the hard intellectual work genuine integration requires. As I noted in an earlier work, this genuine division highlights a 'division between those who view care from a teleological viewpoint (where *facts* are pre-eminent…and those who view care from an ontological viewpoint (where *values* are pre-eminent.'). (14) Nevertheless, a discussion of the definitions, strengths and limitations within these two approaches is a necessary prelude to any genuine effort at integration. Efficacious care requires that practicing clinicians of all persuasions be conversant with these concerns regardless of their primary orientation to the tasks of diagnosis. There is nothing inherently wrong with approaching diagnosis from either primary worldview; the fault comes only when the efficacy of one approach is judged by the epistemology of the other approach.

The secular side of this tension maintains the glaring absence of providing basic information to trainees on how to diagnosis or assesses religious or spiritual concerns. Textbooks on psychological testing, assessment and report writing simply do not mention the topic. At all. This does not stop clinicians who lack theological training or formal connection with a religious community from writing about what they deem to be 'spiritual values.' It probably doesn't stop practioners from checking off the box designating a religious orientation in their counseling on the insurance credentialing application if it offers them the option. But this topic is almost entirely absent from peer-reviewed clinical journals; within more popular clinical magazines what is passed off as 'spiritual' is most likely to be simply giving the client advice. Nothing is wrong with giving a client or patient wise counsel, especially if it is helpful! But dispensing it without training can be as risky as the minister who assumes one course in pastoral care qualifies her to identify paranoia.

The religious side of this tension is no less at fault in maintaining this divide. Seminary classes in pastoral care typically focus on identifying the parishioner's 'point of need' and instructing them in how to do reflective listening. These are helpful skills as far as they go. But the average religious professional does not receive the depth or breadth of training necessary to equip them to adequately diagnose or respond to the parade of human pain that frequently comes through their door. Mercifully they are urged to refer to clinical specialists or pastoral counselors and many do so, especially after their first year in parish ministry. Surveys of people seeking mental health assistance continue to identify either ministers or religiously oriented clinicians as their either the initial source to which they turn to for aid or their preferred source for succor.

Do pastoral researchers or clinically trained chaplains have anything to offer to this discussion? The answer is a qualified 'yes.' There have been numerous efforts to identify the term 'spirituality' in its present uses. The most helpful review comes to the conclusion 'that the quest for the true essential meaning of spirituality is a fool's errand.'(15) In addition to the numerous survey instruments and assessment tools developed by chaplains to diagnose spiritual concerns, two pastoral clinicians have offered models built around the concept of DSM-IV-TR axis. (16)

Writing in *The Journal of Pastoral Care and Counseling*, Dr. Lucy Bregman makes this point about the use of the term 'spirituality' at the conclusion of her essay:

> Spirituality ...is used for the *personal* side of religion, by those who pit it
> Against 'institutional' or 'public' or 'organized religion *a la* Shelia Larson.
> And it has taken over the 'existential core human dimension' once the
> identified domain of humanistic psychologies. It works so well precisely
> because these different and separable meanings and uses flow into one
> another and carry with them connotations and implications as they travel
> from one of these niches to another. Spirituality does multiple jobs, and
> keeping its meanings vague and shifting helps to continue this handy
> situation. (16)

I agree with Dr. Bregman's assessment of how this term functions in the present clinical environment. Most providers of humane care benefit from this vagueness, whether in 'secular' or 'religious' counseling settings. But only the citizens of *Wonderland* get to make words mean 'whatever I say they mean.' Professional care providers should rightly demonstrate a higher and more consistent standard. Thus I find these definitions useful in both the clinical-secular and in the religious-spiritual setting. *Spirituality* is the practice of the presence of God. *Theology* is the thinking about that practice. *Religion* is the ritualizing of that practice. *Faith* is the belief in that practice. These definitions can help all care providers speak clearly about the ineffable dimensions of our common humanity in a way that helps us attend to the pain of those who come for aid without our clients and patients having to go through the looking glass to find out what ails them or what will assuage their distress.

As many writers and researchers note, 'people desire to make meaning in their lives through their connectedness with the transcendent or other persons.' In a yet-to-be-published research paper two Canadian writers have developed a Holistic Spirituality Scale that shows some promise for use in theistic, non-theistic and atheistic settings. (17) Linkage of this term to the traditional triad of cardinal moral virtues of faith, hope and love may position clinicians and researchers of all worldviews in a way that allows for conversation across some common ground. The authors provide definitions of these virtues that are helpful.

- Faith is theistic spirituality, God, gods and faith in a Transcendent Other
- Hope is existential spirituality and meaning, fulfillment, purpose of life
- Love is community spirituality and connection, relationship and love of self, others and the world.

These authors position spirituality within a continuum that allows for personal faith as well as 'a socially-influenced perception of either some divine being, or some sense of ultimate truth or reality.' Moreover these definitions allow for clinicians to assess both the nominative function of these virtues (what is held as the *content* of faith, hope and love) as well as the active function of these virtues (what is *done* as an expression of faith, hope and love). As with the above insight these linkages move the term spirituality away from solipsism and toward a community definition. (18) The usefulness of the Canadians' scale remains to be seen. Unless employed by clinical-secular researchers, my fear is their scale will become one more idiosyncratic instrument whose use is limited to a single hospital, seminary pastoral care curriculum or scattered religious congregations whose clergy have an affinity for research.

It remains an open question whether or not it will be possible for an integrative worldview to develop a diagnostic schema for religious and spiritual concerns that is at once truly helpful to the diagnostic needs of both patient and clinicians of all persuasions and also practically accepted among the more narrow worlds of the clinical-secular and the religious-spiritual clinicians. In the development of the new DSM-V there appears to be little communication from the clinical-secular side of the divide with the religious-spiritual clinicians. Moreover, in a most recent review of this discussion within a premier journal of the religious-spiritual clinicians it appears this arena still has elements steadfastly opposed to any type of specificity in diagnosis (19) in spite of the efforts of several other clinicians to bridge this divide. (20)

Conclusion

Nonetheless, like my just-cited colleague Wesley Brun, I too remain hopeful that such an integrative system of diagnosis will eventually come forth. My optimism springs from three sources: people in distress continue to demand it of clinicians who are charged with the responsibility of relieving their pain, the literature on the health / cost benefits to individuals and institutions of an active religious-spiritual orientation push health care plans to refer to religiously sensitive counselors and the continued insights from neuropsychiatry on the interplay of brain function with the more ineffable areas of the values people hold and the choices they make based upon those values. It is because I am optimistic about the interplay of these three factors to ultimately produce an integrated model of diagnosis that I have written this second volume on the topic.

The interplay of these three factors is already leading to some integration in professional education and clinical practice of care providers on both sides of this divide. Primary care physicians and other medical caregivers continue to both write about this area of assessment as well as refer to clinically oriented religious counselors. Licensed professional clinicians must now receive enough training in religious or spiritual concerns to be able to correctly answer questions on state licensure exams that address this area. A number of seminaries and universities now offer dual degree programs in social work and ministry, with the primary tension now focused on whether the individual is a minister with social work training or a social worker with ministerial training. The day is rapidly disappearing when these two disciplines viewed one another with antipathy.

The next two chapters will continue to address structural concerns around the two central questions of diagnosis. In my view the chatter between 'is it diagnosis or assessment?' is more than semantics debate but less than an ultimate division within the practice of those charged with the obligation to relieve human suffering and guide human decision-making with something approaching wisdom. Likewise it will serve all sides in the discussion to review the non-clinical models of diagnosis that nevertheless are effective in achieving the primary tasks of diagnosis: naming the pain and providing care for the person in need. Once these two tasks are addressed, the remainder of the volume will explore what I continue to view as three seminal areas of diagnosis as well as offer the reader an approach to several special areas of clinical concern: children, substance abuse, stress disorders and mass bereavement. *Selah!*

Chapter 3

Is It Diagnosis or Assessment?

The hearing room within the juvenile and domestic court was filled with a larger than typical number of professionals, family members and various co-workers. As was all-too-typical in such settings, each former spouse was now attempting to demonstrate the other parent was less qualified to be the primary custodian of their children. A bevy of psychologists, physicians and guardian ad litems each made their way to the witness box, were duly sworn in and cross-examined by the other side's counsel. In each case the conclusion of professionals was the same: while both parent showed signs of distress, neither of them fit the diagnostic criteria for a mental disorder.

The judge was getting exasperated. "The concern here is not whether either parent is crazy," she said. "The concern is this: is either parent either fundamentally incompetent or at least a greater risk to the safety of the children?" None of the professionals would budge.

Until each attorney placed their own client on the witness stand. Under the prodding of their spouse's attorney, one parent quickly became hostile, sarcastic and at one point stood up in the witness box. She grew aggressive enough that the bailiff went over to stand next to her. The opposing attorney then recalled one of the psychologists. "Based on what you have just seen, is Ms. Smith likely to be overly aggressive with her children?" He asked.

"Based on what I have just witnesses, I would have to amend my recommendation to the court," she replied. "Ms. Smith is more likely than Mr. Smith to be overly aggressive with the children and appears to need education in anger management," she continued. While not afflicted with a diagnosable mental disorder, the mother failed to demonstrate a primary attribute of effective parenting: self-control under duress. The court ordered the mother to attend anger management and parenting courses as well as having her visitation monitored by another adult. The father retained physical custody and the parents were to consult with one another regarding decisions related to the children's health and education. The final disposition of custody was deferred for six months.

Neither assessment nor diagnosis is a purely academic consideration. Thus how we define these two tasks and whom we empower to conduct the tasks have direct implications for many lives beyond the individual whose situation is under consideration. While we might like a sterile field within which to make such determinations, according to our most ancient of stories we lost that option millennia ago.(1) We now have the obligation of discerning not just good from evil and illness from health in all their many manifestations but also recommending to our fellow travelers what pathway is likely to increase their life and enhance their wisdom. Assessment procedures fall into four broad categories, of which diagnosis plays only a part: personality testing, ability testing, informal assessment and the clinical interview.(2) A review of ability testing is beyond the scope of this volume. The concerns in the remaining three areas as they relate to the two tasks of diagnosis will be discussed in this chapter.

Objective Assessment With Subjective Concerns

Most graduate programs in professional counseling and all state licensing programs require some familiarity with objective psychological testing. Although psychologists retain the legal responsibility for the technical scoring and interpreting of many of these instruments, the rise of both computer-scoring and the Internet make these instruments accessible to all professional counselors. The most widely used instruments are quite helpful in identifying the presence of Axis I and Axis II disorders, an individual's degree of resiliency, and an individual's vocational interest. Some objective tests are also useful in couples counseling in that they either help couples identify areas of the relationship where there is conflict (parenting, finances, sexual expression) or where there is a basic difference in personality style that is likely to lead to conflict (introversion, extroversion, tough-mindedness).

Here are several of the most widely used objective assessment instruments and their general use:

- Minnesota Multiphasic Personality Inventory (MMPI-2) identifies psychopathology and Axis I disorders.
- Millon Clinical Multiaxial Inventory (MCMI-III) identifies personality disorders on Axis II and their symptoms.
- Beck Depression Inventory (BDI-II) identifies the presence and severity of depression.
- Myers-Briggs Type Indicator (MBTI) personality types based on Carl Jung's theory of personality (non-clinical population).
- 16PF sixteen personality factors that influence individual personality, couple relational satisfaction and vocational fit.
- PREPARE / ENRICH provides four inventories for couples that focus on twenty areas relevant to relational strength.

- Strong Interest Inventory identifies six general occupational themes based on the work of Holland's personality theory.

For the practicing clinician the primary tasks with objective instruments concern the selection and interpretation of the appropriate instrument. Beyond being familiar with the specific instruments, the decision of which instrument to select as well as interpreting the results of such an instrument will be done in the clinical setting. Thus the clinician's capacity to gain the client's trust is essential to the entire process.

This is particularly true when the information developed by an objective instrument identifies a serious personality disorder, significant vocational miss-match or poor marital satisfaction. Denial is one feature of the most serious Axis II disorders (narcissism, paranoia, sociopath) that renders test interpretation to such clients a delicate matter. In highly conflicted couples it is equally difficult to utilize results of an objective instrument in a way that will be helpful. Even though a divorce may be the most helpful outcome, the results of an objective instrument in such a troubled relationship are likely to become ammunition for the negotiation of opposing attorneys.

There are a host of professional issues with which one must be familiar if they intend to use or benefit from psychological testing in their practice of counseling. All texts on psychological testing and clinical training programs now include forthright discussion of matters related to the theoretical design of testing, their adequacy and matters related to the tension between actuarial vs. clinical prediction. Underneath these concerns lie fundamental ethical considerations related to human rights, the matter of labeling an individual and the potential for dehumanization that occurs whenever powerful psychiatric diagnosis are utilized.

These subjective implications have profound impact on the basic tasks of diagnosis. On the one hand a licensed clinician is obligated to provide clients with an adequate understanding of their distress and a treatment plan that will actually alleviate their suffering. On the other hand a licensed clinician is also obligated to protect a client's privacy from undue invasion and not overly pathologize their condition so that all hope of care is removed. Readers should regularly review these concerns, especially if they use objective testing in their counseling practice. An annual reading of the Ethical Principles of Psychologists and Code of Conduct of the APA or your professional association is also a helpful reminder that 'the clinician retains responsibility for the appropriateness of the analysis' of all psychological testing and the adequacy of any diagnosis. (3)

Informal Assessment With Serious Implications

Let me say at the outset that the term 'informal' intends to show only that this part of an assessment procedure does not use formal psychological testing. In no way should the reader conclude that 'informal' means 'inaccurate' or 'casual' or 'unofficial.' Indeed since one of the 'informal' methods of assessment (the clinical interview) is used to confirm or disconfirm two of the 'formal' methods of assessment (personality and ability testing), the competent professional must be familiar with all four areas of assessment and at least be able to utilize their results in a manner consistent with the standards of care promulgated by the particular discipline.

"Are you an investigator?" asks the younger sister of a middle school boy as we leave for the ritual walk I take at the beginning of every counseling session with boys. As we walk and talk together about his school, his friends, the squirrels and single hawk that inhabit the land around office park, I am conducting observational assessment. While I am not Sherlock Holmes, I do notice if he is dressed properly, how he walks, what he volunteers in conversation, and who he avoids mentioning. How he responds when parents or family members enter the room is also diagnostic information.

Observational assessments carry the same significance for adults in much the same way, once new clinicians get past the 'don't be judgmental' attitude they seem to have acquired in public education and their initial professional formation. Noting the presence or absence of jewelry, tattoos, type and quality of clothing are as significant as the individual's capacity to express or contain emotion and the content of their thoughts. I will say more about the significance of observation in the following section.

"Just how intense is the migraine today?" I asked. The young man replied, "today it isn't that bad. Probably a 7 on a 10-point scale." According to his self-report, the pain had never reached a 9 or 10. It is significant that his verbal report of his pain is in contrast with the number of the rating and illustrates the presence of denial.

The use of self-reported rating scales is another important informal assessment tool. In terms of naming the pain, self-reported rating scales provide the clinician with information about the client's interior awareness of their situation. In terms of guiding the care, such scales help the client or patient step outside of their situation for a brief moment, assess their own resources and participate in their care. Whether measuring the intensity of anger, physical pain or any other subjective state they can be quickly used to provide what one writer describes as 'homegrown' information that is quite useful to the overall assessment process.(4)

The Internet provides clinicians with all sorts of informal but nevertheless very effective self-reported rating scales. This is especially true in the areas of marital or couples therapy and alcohol abuse. Marriage Builders and the Gottman Institute are but two of a plethora of sites with tools that help get couples started in the direction of naming their pain in a non-threatening but effective manner. The same is true for websites such as Alcoholics Anonymous and even the Substance Abuse and Mental Health Services Administration (SAMHSA). These informal inventories help people participate in their assessment as well as get them started in the direction of health.

"I want you to read these e-mails I printed off," she said quietly. "All these years I thought I was crazy." She plucked two pages out of a large folder that detailed her husband's affair with a co-worker. Obviously devastating, these records and personal items and documents helped her gain some resolution on distressing thoughts and spousal behavior that otherwise made her 'feel crazy.' Talk about 'naming the pain!' For any clinician such moments are profoundly sacred times of being with someone in an anteroom outside of Hell.

"It hurts to have betrayal confirmed," I said. "But it must also be something of a relief. What are you going to do?" Whether reviewing such damning documents of a marriage's demise, listening to a client review their journal entries from the week or having a child bring their favorite toy to an initial session these are frequently highly personal moments of conversation between a therapist and a client. Responding appropriately to them builds the trust so essential if any healing is to occur; exploring their meaning aids both the clinician and the client in naming the depth of the pain they bring as well as providing some clues to the way forward.

One final 'informal rating scale' deserves special mention: The Adjective Check List. While this instrument has apparently fallen out of favor with hard-core psychometric clinicians, I believe it or any compilation of self-reported adjectives to be an invaluable assessment tool. These lists have some 300 adjectives equally balanced between complimentary (assertive), neutral (thoughtful) and uncomplimentary (greedy). For over twenty years I have reviewed roughly 100 such lists each year of candidates for the professional ministry.

A general pattern has emerged that assists in overall vocational assessment, made powerful due to this fact: the candidate is describing themselves in their own words. Not only does it become clear what constitutes acceptable character traits for professional clergy that includes an ability to be somewhat self-disclosing with uncomplimentary adjectives but also the reaction of some candidates to asking them during the clinical interview, "so tell me, how will your trait of 'stubbornness' affect your ministry?" For many candidates such an inquiry into their uncomplimentary or complimentary adjectives provides a moment of significant self-reflection. For a few it is not just embarrassing but also provides them with the opportunity to complain to the judicatory how insulted they felt that they would be 'accused' of being 'stubborn' or 'cynical' or 'greedy.' This response is diagnostic about the candidate and, if the judicatory takes the side of the candidate's wounded narcissism, is also diagnostic about the judicatory.

Informal assessment plays an important role – and sometimes a pivotal role – in naming someone's pain as well as providing insight into their capacity for personal change and professional effectiveness. Clinicians who have philosophic problems with informal assessment instruments or observations because such assessment seems judgmental or subjective should ask themselves this question: would I want a lawyer defending me who described themselves as 'insecure' or would I trust the care of my child to someone whose body odor was nauseating? If the answer to questions such as these is 'No,' then why avoid drawing conclusions on such observations that will likely help relieve human suffering?

Clinical Interview With Spiritual Implications

As the reader will have noted by now I utilize 'clinical' and 'spiritual' diagnosis or assessment as integrative rather than exclusive categories. Indeed one of the primary purposes of this volume is to redress the continued demonstration in most professional texts that one side of the caregiver world is almost completely unfamiliar if not outright suspicious of the tools and methods of the other side of the entire enterprise of assessment and humane treatment. In one text detailing how to arrive at an assessment report based on a clinical interview, here is author's only reference to religion or spiritual concerns: "I got a job as an outpatient therapist at a mental health center. I was compulsive about conducting thorough clinical interviews, and religious about dictating my case notes, my intake summaries and my quarterly summaries." (5) (emphasis added)

The overall categories of any assessment, whether formal or informally conducted, contain similar categories. In a formal mental health setting the clinician gathers information from a wide variety of intake documents such as self-reporting demographic information, objective testing, taking a thorough history and conducting a mental status examination. While people do not fill out a ton of paperwork or answer explicit questions during a home visit by a minister or social worker, a professional should nevertheless be able to acquire some information in the following areas:

- Demographic information
- Presenting concern or need
- Family background
- Significant medical or counseling history
- Substance use and abuse
- Educational and vocational history
- Other pertinent information
- Mental status

Based on the initial interview or visit the use of some assessment instrument may be indicated. Long before the insurance companies stopped routinely paying for psychological testing, I was asking myself this question: "Do I need a psychological test to tell me this client is depressed / anxious / a major substance abuser / introverted / confused?" Answering 'No' to this does not automatically rule out the use of testing for a seasoned clinician. Rather, it helps me frame how the use of a test or inventory will be presented to the client.

"You've already told me you are having nightmares, you scan the environment for threats and you jump at loud noises," I will say. "Your sleep is disturbed. Your mood fluctuates between irritability and sadness and your husband complains you have slept with a knife under your pillow ever since the assault three years ago. We do not need a test to confirm the presence of post-traumatic stress and depression. But a test will help us gauge your resilience." Naturally psychological testing is indicated if the client seems resistant to any suggestion of relational or personal flaw, if a formal report needs to be written or if the setting is forensic in nature. Clergy rarely if ever have to provide such documentation but other counselors have to provide both the client and a host of third parties with such reports more than any of us care to admit.

Yet since the DSM-IV-TR mandates awareness of religious or spiritual concerns in the provision of care, how does one go about gaining such information and making responsible judgments about the information provided? Gathering basic religious information can be accomplished on a standard demographic face sheet. Yet what is the clinical and diagnostic significance of answering such a line 'Episcopalian' or 'Baptist' or 'Buddhist?'

To me it is an open question whether or not a clinician can gain enough knowledge of religious life beyond their own spiritual practice to adequately have sufficient information so that they can assess the role in which a person's spiritual life plays a role in diagnosis. Taking an adequate spiritual or religious history with a professional eye that is equivalent to taking their sexual history, substance abuse history, educational or vocational history requires more than just going to a two-day workshop on spiritual assessment. Given the DSM-IV-TR mandate and the continued desire of individuals to have a counselor who shares their religious or spiritual values it is insufficient to assume this information fits somehow under the heading of 'other pertinent information.' All too often some of the most powerful resources in an individual's life, their capacity to access the spiritual virtues of faith, hope and love as well as the ability to utilize their religious practices to name their pain and direct their care either gets left to chance or remains under-utilized due to our bifurcation of 'clinical' care and 'spiritual' care.

Responsible diagnosis and care involves making sufficient inquiry of an individual or couple's religious life and spiritual practices so that one can determine the answer to two questions:

- What role does religion or spiritual practice play in their life?
- What assets and liabilities does this area offer to their name their present pain and assist them in their long-term care?

Only as a clinician answers these questions responsibly can they then assess the resiliency of their client. Only as a clinician learns the breadth and depth of these areas can they reasonably know whether or not to refer the person to a pastoral specialist.

So what helps this inquiry take place? Beyond having a line on the client's demographic information sheet about 'religious preference / membership,' here are some open-ended questions one might ask:

- How often do you attend your church / synagogue / mosque?
- Has their been any recent change in your religious life?
- Do you pray or regularly read devotional literature?
- Who is your favorite religious hero or leader?
- Do you have a favorite passage from the Koran / Torah / Bible; if so, what is it?
- What resources does your faith or spiritual practice offer you as you face this present dilemma?

Remember that in asking these questions your task is to gather information that will assist you in helping the person. Your task is not to critique their beliefs. Nor should you avoid engaging them in exploring their beliefs if those beliefs either directly bear upon the reason they are seeking your aid or have within them resources that will assist in reliving their suffering. Whether or not the client is comfortable answering this line of inquiry as well as the content of their responses to such open ended questions provides us with significant information about the client's mental status, affective stability, capacity for relationships and overall level of maturity.

Using a five-point scale the workbook accompanying the PREPARE / ENRICH testing offers these suggestions for discussion as a couples exercise that can be utilized in a clinical session:

- My partner and I agree on how we practice our spiritual beliefs
- Religion has different meanings for each of us.
- My partner and I agree on the level of religious involvement in our marriage.
- Regular attendance at a place of worship is important to me.
- Our spiritual beliefs help us feel closer as a couple. (6)

Spiritual compatibility is a key factor in marital satisfaction. This is underscored by the fact that 89% of 5,153 self-reported happy couples in a study responded positively to the statement 'I am satisfied with how we express our spiritual values and beliefs' and only 36% of 5,127 self-reported unhappy couples in the study responded positively to this statement. (7) A clinician conducting mari`al therapy who does not inquire about this area of marital satisfaction is failing in their responsibility to conduct a thorough assessment of the couple.

Conclusion

Whether our primary approach to diagnosis is teleological, ontological or a genuine effort at integration, clinicians have a fundamental obligation to provide effective care to those who seek relief of their suffering. This obligation applies to all clinicians whether their office is in a hospital, community service board, in a mental health center, a freestanding private practice or religious community. I continue to believe that secular clinicians have as much obligation to receive training in religious or spiritual diagnostic categories prior to utilizing them as religious clinicians have to receive training in clinical diagnostic categories and psychological testing prior to providing professional care.

Thus while I wholeheartedly agree with a recent article that concludes, 'to exclude God from a consultation is a form of malpractice. Spirituality is wonder, joy and shouldn't be left in the clinical closet,' it is both noteworthy and tragic that the author of this article does not cite one religious, theological, or pastoral clinician in making his well-researched point regarding the healing efficacy of religious practices as a part of overall patient care.(8) This author's professional myopia is reinforced by his observation noting this statement comes 'from other limited-care sub-specialists who expediently claim that it is in the patient's best interest to always be referred to themselves.' (9) To decry that such 'assertions are usually not accompanied by outcomes-based research' and then not cite readily available research in journals of pastoral clinicians illustrates the depth of the problem. This is especially troubling since this particular author makes the point of having taught 'more than 6,000 health care providers on incorporating spirituality or religion into their clinical practice.' (10)

As this just-cited author notes, 'the first editorial published in the British Medical Journal wrote about the faith that heals.' The editorial then adds 'nothing in life is more wonderful than faith...faith pours out an unfailing stream of energy while abating neither jot nor tittle of its potency." (11) The use and efficacy of those age-old tools was known long before evidence-based practice began. Those tools include resources to assess the overall health and maturity of people as well as diagnose specific maladies of body, mind and soul. It is to a review of some of these age-old resources that we turn in the next chapter. *Selah!*

Chapter 4

Non-Clinical Diagnostic Systems

The counseling center where I began my internship had the practice of the clinical staff reviewing all intake interviews in a Thursday morning group. A consulting psychiatrist joined the pastoral counseling staff and staff psychologist. Diagnosis, the initial treatment plan and the treating clinician were decided by consensus. After one particularly complex and rather grisly presentation, the consulting psychiatrist said, "The correct diagnosis is NAWP."

"NAWP? What on earth is that," asked one of the senior staff.

"Not A Well Person," he replied. "This individual is not well at all and unlikely to get better any time soon." An apt diagnosis as well as an assessment of the likely course of treatment! Such a diagnosis isn't in any manual and certainly wouldn't receive reimbursement from any insurance company. But it captured more of the clinical situation and prognosis than any fully formed case presentation.

In addition to this rather humorous off-the-cuff assessment, it is necessary to be reminded that people have been conducting the two tasks of diagnosis long before the DSM-IV-TR and ICD-9 arrived on the scene. This is especially true in the area of spiritual or religious life. While it may be linguistically correct that whenever the word 'diagnosis' is used we have begun using a medical model to understand in individual's distress, such reductionism seldom serves the best needs of the person. Particularly when the setting for care is the local religious community or one is simply encountering individuals in a social context.

This is especially true in the continued tension around screening for spiritual concerns that are likely to bear directly on their care and recovery. Thus neither consultation with the individual's religious leader nor referral to a chaplain are as routinely made as referrals to medical specialists. As one source notes, "because many clinicians do not routinely inquire about spirituality and do not appreciate the frequent patient relevance, such referrals often are not made."

The source continues, "The lack of appropriate clinical spiritual referrals can constitute a form of negligence." (1)

While the work of such medical educators such as Harold G. Koenig and Walter L. Larimore provide physicians with training in the area of spirituality, such training is necessarily reductionistic. The religions of the world are much more complex than can be covered in a single course during the press of medical school or a two-day seminar. Thus the resources they bring to the diagnostic enterprise as well as the difficulties religious beliefs create in people just about mandate the need to consult with those who Larimore calls 'pastoral professionals' if there is to be genuine understanding of someone's spiritual needs.

Thus the goal of this chapter is to acquaint the reader with some of the non-clinical diagnostic systems that are likely to be used by pastoral professionals. This chapter also has the goal of reminding pastoral professionals that those who come to them for help do so out of a desire to hear their distress placed in a spiritual context and have their care motivated by the dynamics of faith. While a local religious leader may be thoroughly trained in clinical diagnosis, they had still better be able to speak the language of spiritual assessment to their people if they expect to be effective.

Some of these systems are quite ancient while others are more contemporary. While this review is only suggestive the diagnostic models in this chapter are nevertheless highly effective in the non-clinical realm and they provide a value-added layer of understanding within the clinical environment. Thus it is especially important for all professionals charged with the responsibility of providing humane care to understand the efficacy of non-clinical models from within the major religious tradition or spiritual practice as thoroughly as they recognize the power of the current clinical model of diagnosis.

Moral Models of Diagnosis

The connection between moral fault and disease is ancient. The connection is also real and carries with it an ability to both explain the source of our distress and guide us into a better life. Thus a group of religious leaders ask Jesus of Nazareth a diagnostic question, "Rabbi, who sinned, this man or his parents, that he was born blind?" (2) In another encounter Jesus links forgiveness of sin with healing of disease. (3)

As much as our contemporary post-modern sensibility wants to readily announce our distress 'isn't anybody's fault,' often the facts of the matter are very different. Certainly the emotional and spiritual response to human pain typically begins with a feeling of being blamed. I will review this dynamic in Part II but for now I want to briefly highlight several moral models of diagnosis that may be operating within both the person suffering and the person delivering the care.

The Ten Commandments and Seven Deadly Sins

The Ten Commandments signal the fundamental moral nature of the universe. (4) Insofar as we allow ourselves to be guided by them in our personal lives and public vocation they are an integrative worldview. The first three commands instruct us about the nature of the Deity and its relationship to our being (ontology), including what takes place when we violate the primary moral order of the universe.

The fourth through tenth commandments shift their focus onto our relationship with one another. There are profound relational consequences for overwork, disrespect to parents, murder, adultery, theft, lying and coveting (teleology). There are also significant relational consequences for obedience. (5) As much as our contemporary sensibility may be uncomfortable with the language of compliance and rebellion in the diagnostic enterprise, a significant amount of human pain rises from violating one of these principles and an equal amount of improved care results when we bring our lifestyle back into alignment with these moral boundaries.

Pride, avarice, lust, anger, gluttony, sloth and envy are likewise responsible for significant human suffering. These Seven Deadly Sins are named thus as a tribute to their life-ending power. They are entertaining in the theater; they are devastating in our souls and around our dinner table. Using them as diagnostic categories can add a layer of illumination to the struggles of an individual as they wrestle with drug addiction, as their spouse attempts to live with their personality disorder, or as their co-workers make efforts to solve complex problems with them.

Studying these seven character flaws and writing about them in a personal journal can lead to a major reorientation of an individual's life. This is as valid and effective a care plan for personal transformation as completing the fourth step of Alcoholics Anonymous or facing the results of an MCMI-III. Although these 'deadly sins' are again ontological in nature insofar as they speak of our being, their existential consequences are teleological and historical. Their presence speaks volumes about our alienation from the 'Self' so dear to object relations as well as the havoc we wreak upon others across the generations so well examined by strategic and systemic family therapies.

Moral Decision-Making

An educator who teaches at a community college had given his first on-line test but allowed the students to take the test at their home. Suspecting the classes of cheating, he gave the second one in the school's computer lab. "The questions on each test were entirely random in order," he said. "The consequences demonstrate that most of the students had 'unauthorized assistance.' But it is what I expected. The students are at Kohlberg's third stage of moral development. They will get away with whatever they can and do what is right only to avoid being punished."

The teacher was conducting a diagnosis of his class. Of course among the some ninety students there were individuals whose moral code prompted them to study effectively. Their higher grades demonstrated the benefits of maturity. The teacher is doing what instructors have always done: provided character formation to the students through his bearing as well as offered them information about the specific subject matter. Parents, pastors, political leaders, physicians, psychologists and nurses enhance their guidance of others if they take the time to assess an individual's stage of moral development before they attempt to guide them.

In his work *Religious Ethics and Pastoral Care* Don Browning outlines five levels of practical moral thinking. (6) Browning is quite explicit that this schema can be used to assess or diagnose an individual's pain as well as guide their care. (7) Although a contemporary provider of care may be uncomfortable with moral categories and ethical thinking, I believe it is as negligent to avoid a discussion of moral categories with a client if such categories are helpful to them as it is negligent to avoid a discussion of their sexual orientation, drug use or lack of proper diet. Browning argues that 'our traditions of care, both within and outside the church, need to be reconstituted under the guidance of a critical practical moral theology or religious ethic.' (8)

Thus a provider of humane care can enhance both the naming of their patient's pain and guidance in the direction of their care by evaluating the situation within Browning's moral framework. While a full presentation of his system is beyond the scope of this work, consider the following question: how would care of any particular client or patient be enhanced by reviewing their situation through these five questions?

- What kind of world or universe constitutes the ultimate context of the client's action?
- What is the client obligated to do?
- Which of all the client's human tendencies and needs are they obligated to do?
- What is the immediate context of their action and the various factors that condition it?
- What specific roles, rules and processes of communication should they follow in order to accomplish their moral ends? (9)

Browning cites the work of Lawrence Kohlberg as influential in his search for a practical way to recover the moral dimension to the provision of care. He then makes the following point about the use of any diagnostic system, regardless of its worldview or the setting in which the diagnosis is delivered: "no ethical, sociological, reformist or praxis point of caring discipline whether religious or secular should ever forget the people within them." (10) One thing is certain about these moral models: they notify us of our primary connection with both our neighbor as well as signal that the Deity is a partner in every action or thought. There is no such thing as a 'victimless crime;' the Person of God is the Ultimate and Eternal Victim of our rebellion.

Anecdotal Models of Diagnosis

An economist who works on anti-trust issues and the economics of the beer industry teaches at the nearby University of Virginia. He also writes murder mysteries whose hero (Henry Spearman) 'is very much like the real-world Milton Friedman.' In discussing his creative writing with an interviewer he commented, "Over and again, as Bill and I worked on our three books, we would ask ourselves what might Milton Friedman say in this situation." (11)

This is the essence of effective training, parenting, teaching, mentoring and creative writing. We hope that at crucial points in an individual's life they will ask themselves, "what would Mom do?" They recall in their heart the guidance of a favorite teacher, sometimes even recalling the tone of voice and posture. This is also the heart of the anecdotal method of diagnosis.

One of my earliest supervisors had a cross-stitched plaque in his office. He had positioned it so that only he could see it. The plaque read, "Sometimes you have to shoot your own dog. Don't farm it out. That will only make it worse." At crucial decision points in my own clinical work I recall those words and share the entire story with the client. The story has the effect of allowing the client to acknowledge their situation (name their pain) as well as recognize the seriousness of the action that they must take if they are to become whole (guiding the care).

Whether the anecdotes come from within the community that supports the care provider or simply rises out of the shared wisdom of the human community, the dynamics are the same. The clinician identifies a story or anecdote that approximates the situation of the client, then shares the anecdote with the client for the purpose of transforming the client's situation. Thus the central feature of this method is its hortatory nature. The assent of the client through personal insight and a change in direction confirms the accuracy of the diagnosis.

Biblical Counseling

One can grasp the hortatory and anecdotal nature of Biblical Counseling through reading an essay by one of this movement's chief proponents, Wendell E.

Miller. In an essay entitled *Providing an Alternative that is Not an Alternative* he makes the following appeal:

> Biblical counseling might be though of as an alternative to secular counseling. However, it is so important that Christians obtain biblical counseling and not secular counseling, that for Christians who need help with their problems, biblical counseling should not be thought of as an alternative but an imperative. (12)

Thus the focus of biblical counseling 'is God-centered' and those who provide biblical counseling are directed thusly: 'The reason for man's existence, and the goals to be achieved in counseling, are centered in God and His revealed word. In addition, both knowledge with regard to Man's nature and counseling principles are God-given through Scripture." (13) While secular counseling is derived from 'man's philosophies' and 'utilizes man's principles,' this approach to counseling 'utilizes principles that are God-given in the Scriptures.' (14)

Although both tasks of diagnosis (naming the pain and guiding the care) are to be found in Scripture, since this method views Scripture as the source of God's revelation, this approach to diagnosis is ontological. Thus this approach 'is dedicated to helping people solve the problems of their lives through the teaching of biblical principles.' This is a thorough-going approach to assisting people develop strong marriages, react to provocation from others and otherwise assist Christian people with the task of 'progressive sanctification.'

This approach to counseling has an accrediting association, a newsletter, training centers and annual conferences. Clinicians and pastors will encounter individuals who hold this worldview. They expect to hear this language from the pastor or therapist to whom their pastor refers them. In a society that prides itself on being pluralistic and tolerant regarding beliefs, this method of addressing human suffering must be treated respectfully albeit with caution: sincerity of belief does not necessarily lead to the belief being true. Nevertheless the clinician who blindly dismisses this approach as 'fundamentalist' or worse is as negligent as the clinician who uncritically embraces any approach or seeks to alter a counselee's belief without their consent.

Mutual Story-telling Technique

The use of stories and anecdotes is as ancient an approach to naming pain and guiding care as the discovery of fire. Because this technique is so ancient and affects the individual's self-fabric across the lifespan as well as its use by clinicians of all persuasions, it is most accurately recognized as reflecting an integrative worldview of diagnosis and treatment. Whether in the privacy of a consulting room, by a hospital bedside or in the more public domain of corporate worship, school classroom or political rally the timely use of the appropriate story can either relieve suffering and promote health or energize entire nations to wreak havoc on their neighbors.

Richard Gardner developed the use of stories as an explicit therapeutic technique in the 1971. (15) That this approach is still used to both assess a child's distress as well as guide the care of a child is a tribute to its efficacy. (16) It begins with a straightforward request for the child to tell a story. The therapist 'listens for themes and conflicts in the child's story and then retells the story, using the child's characters but incorporating adaptations that resolve the conflict in a healthy way.' (17) The story becomes the instrument of the child literally 'naming their pain' through the characters and plot of the story. The therapist's retelling of the story is the provision of care. The author of this paper notes, "the effective use of narrative psychotherapy, directed toward helping children and adolescents construct positive life stories, requires clinicians to sensitively align narrative approaches with each child's developmental abilities and interests.' (18)

It is Gardner's use of specific stories for discreet developmental challenges or relational distress that makes this an explicit diagnostic approach. The approach is virtually unchanged since Gardner's first formulation and illustrates the integrative worldview behind the approach:

- The therapist attempts to determine which figure or figures in the child's story represent the child himself.
- The therapist attempts to determine which figure or figures in the story stand for significant people in his environment.
- The therapist 'gets a general feel' for the atmosphere of the story.
- The therapist identifies the most pertinent psychodynamic interpretation that will be helpful for the child at this particular time.
- The therapist re-tells the story in a way that provides the child with new avenues not considered in the child's scheme of things. (19)

Gardner provided therapists with a full demonstration of this technique throughout the course of therapy as well as suggesting its usefulness to a host of 'common clinical problems.' These problems included traditional psychodynamic formulations such as oedipal problems and super-ego deficiencies as well as the situational concerns of anger inhibition, death of a parent and traumatic surgery. The epigram stating 'the pen is mightier than the sword' speaks only one-half the truth.. The pen or spoken word is also mightier than the scalpel. As explored in another article, "story-telling techniques after abreaction of (traumatic) memories allow several important restorative functions to take place:"

- The therapist bears witness to the patient's experience, ending the
  the isolation and secrecy in which the trauma has existed,
  and rendering the recast experience a social one.
- A narrative subtext is created, making the memory available for future
  accessing and conversations.
- New identity formation is facilitated out of the story being told in a
  transformative vein, allowing the shift from a victim identity to one of
  being a survivor. (20)

Therapeutic techniques as diverse as Critical Incident Stress Management and
traditional psychoanalytic psychotherapy recognize the healing power of one
human being telling the dimensions of their pain in an empathic relationship.
Even therapists whose training precludes them from 'giving advice' will
nevertheless listen carefully to the nuances within a client's story – and time
their brief interventions carefully – to essential provide interpretations that are
essentially a pithy recasting of the patient's story.

The power of the story's capacity for both naming the pain and being curative
is frequently enhanced when done in a group setting. This is the genius behind
self-help groups of all stripes. Indeed one might say that developing the third ear
is only half the task of becoming an effective healer. One must also acquire a
variety of voices so as to adequately speak the curative story at the proper
moment if one would use this technique in its most powerful incarnation.

Developmental Models of Diagnosis

The recognition that humanity is a developmental creature fueled the riddle of
the Sphinx. "What creature walks on four legs, then two and finally three?" she
asked those who traveled across her path. Philosophers reflect upon these
transitions and artists portray the transformations humanity undergoes
throughout the lifespan. Thus developmental models of diagnosis and
assessment by definition grow out of an ontological worldview. Jesus of
Nazareth told parables that nudged us to recognize how differently people
respond to the same information and how an individual's character can be
discerned by the way in which they treat others. (21)

The work of Piaget on the stages of human development renewed the modern
recognition of humanity's developmental stages. Two writers, Eric Erickson and
Lawrence Kohlberg, have played significant roles in the way therapists of all
worldviews understand human needs and the resources they have for meeting
their needs. Added to this is the long-standing recognition within legal theory
that youth under a certain age are to be held to a less-stringent moral standard
than fully matured adults. Our contemporary concern over whether or not a

person is sane enough to understand the charges against them and assist in their own defense is an enhancement of this developmental recognition.

Even within the clinical field of diagnosis and psychological testing there is a different set of standards for maturity. Indeed within all the contemporary diagnostic manuals there have been separate categories for disorders unique to childhood and adolescence. There is also the recognition that roots of some adult disorders can be perceived in childhood as the person develops. Thus it should come as no surprise that within the field of non-clinical diagnosis there are developmental approaches to diagnosis; far too many to review in this volume. What follows is a brief review of two such methods.

The Minister as Diagnostician

Dr Paul Pruyser provided my introduction to the task of diagnosis within pastoral counseling. Speaking at a regional retreat, he spoke directly to a gathering of some forty clinically trained clergy. I recall him saying something to this effect, "Don't give away your own professional identity or the power you have to visit in the home simply because you perceive psychologists as being more sophisticated or competent." It was a thesis he elaborated in his slender volume that is still in use today throughout the world of pastoral caregivers: "That pastors, like all other professional workers, possess a body of theoretical and practical knowledge that is uniquely their own, evolved over years of practice by themselves and their forebears." (22)

He then adds this caveat that current pastoral clinicians seem to have forgotten and secular clinicians never seem to be quite be able to embrace, "adding clinical insights and skills to their pastoral work does not – should not – shake the authenticity of their pastoral outlook and performance." (23) That his volume is still in use is a tribute to his scholarship and perspicuity. That these two professional communities still do not speak a common diagnostic language honoring the pastoral or developmental insights of Pruyser is a witness to our personal stubbornness and professional protectionism.

Pruyser promulgated five guidelines by which he hoped pastors would assess those who came to them for assistance. His insight was that these areas exist across the lifespan, throughout various cultures, and could potentially be used by a variety of religious sentiments. For those unfamiliar with he work, here are the guidelines:

- Awareness of the Holy – what is sacred?
- Awareness of Providence – what is the divine intent?
- Awareness of Faith – what is believed and what difference does it make?
- Awareness of Grace – does the universe ever smile?

- Awareness of Repentance – what is the capacity for change?
- Awareness of Communion – with whom is there connection?
- Awareness of Vocation – what is life's guiding purpose?

In one short chapter spanning nineteen pages Pruyser lays out a perfectly useful schema for understanding an individual's spiritual concerns. These categories are effective for both the developmental spiritual challenges one faces as we mature as well as a tool for discerning the unique distress in a discreet situation for an individual, a community or even a nation. The lack of awareness of Pruyser's model and of the efficacy of involving hospital chaplains and pastoral professionals in the provision of care by the medical profession (let alone utilization of a model such as Pruyser's) remains a chronic black hole in medical education and practice. (24) Including these nineteen pages in a physician's medical education could do much to begin overcoming this prejudice by introducing them to the late twentieth century's understanding of competent pastoral assessment rather than the late nineteenth century's pathological viewpoint about religion. (25)

List of Virtues

While the work of Erickson and Kohlberg assist clinicians in recognizing the developmental nature of assessment, both ancient and contemporary communities value a core set of cardinal virtues. These virtues are faith, hope and love. They speak ontologically to an individual's maturity across the lifespan as goals for maturity. They also provide meaningful albeit soft measures of an individual's conduct, especially when they are enhanced by other character traits such as honesty, trustworthiness, peace, patience, kindness, gentleness, compassion and self-control.

Such virtues become significant adjuncts to clinical diagnosis, especially in attempting to recognize the presence of personality disorders or arrive at an assessment of vocational fit. It is frequently the demonstrable absence or lack of development in one or more of these character traits that help elaborate the reason for an individual's chronic and pervasive failure to cope effectively throughout their life. Such failures in adequately exhibiting these virtues come as the consequence of failures either in primary attachments, socialization or a toxic mixture of inadequacy in these two areas.

At its best a list of such virtues can be used in a self-reflective manner under the guidance of a sponsor in a recovery program, counselor, minister or spiritual director. Reflection on these virtues demonstrates the quality of courage and has been the grist for personal diaries as well as conversational wisdom by parents and between friends throughout millennia. In a more public arena these virtues form the matrix that measures a person's fitness for and advancement within a variety of jobs and elected offices. Advancement in youth service organizations such as the Boy and Girl Scouts frequently depend as much on the young person exhibiting these virtues as in demonstrating some specific skill or gaining knowledge of a subject.

Writing in the Middle Ages, Gregory the Great developed a system of diagnosis that is essentially a list of virtues. Utilizing the ethical theory of Aristotle, Gregory guided his priests to measure the presence of these virtues by assessing the balance between two extremes. (26) Given our current culture's distaste for making formal assessments of individual virtuosity, it is unlikely that we will see a resurgence of interest in such a diagnostic approach. Nevertheless a clinician or spiritual guide may wish to keep such a list of virtues nearby when reflecting on the scope of human pain that people bring to them for relief.

Qualitative Models of Diagnosis

As should now be apparent there are numerous resources available to clinicians of all persuasions that will enhance the task of diagnosis. The resources in this section take the current clinical standards elaborated in the DSM-IV-TR as a given. Nevertheless these three models of qualitative diagnosis seek to provide either a more relationally satisfying way of recognizing specific disorders in a non-clinical setting or of guiding caregivers to conduct interviews that will tease out the religious and relational details essential for an adequate diagnosis.

My own multi-axial system of diagnosis is also a qualitative model of diagnosis. First elaborated in a prior volume upon which this present volume is built, the remainder of this volume will be an updating of my model. Thus to say much about it at this point would be premature.

Behind the Mask of Sanity – Wayne Oates

The bulk of our life is not lived in a mental health clinic or hospital. We work, play, serve the community, worship and raise our children in settings devoid of the demand for diagnostic understanding and clinical precision. This does not mean we do not encounter individuals and systems that are toxic. It only means we find ourselves embroiled in tangled relationships with individuals whose personal flaws we find out about too late – after we've entrusted our daughter to them on a softball team, moved our family across the country to work for them, or become married to them. Our instinct as well as the calamity they begin to wreak in our life tells us something is profoundly amiss in their psyche. But we have trouble naming that pain and then knowing how to respond to the hurt and havoc that comes from being in relationship with them.

In a helpful book entitled *Behind the Masks: Personality Disorders in Religious Behavior* Wayne Oates attempts to integrate the world of clinical psychiatry and ordinary parish experience. This volume is helpful beyond even the narrow focus of the parish. He enhances our recognition and understanding of the clinical DSM system by noting as pastors and people we are often called to respond to or live with deeply troubled persons who nevertheless serve on church committees, sing in church choirs, teach adults and shepherd children in the congregations we join and serve. He observes that 'no amount of helping them seems to have any lasting effect. As we look around and see how these persons relate to other people, we see that we are not alone. They relate to others even as they do to us.' (27)

Oates indicates that as we read the Bible 'we find vivid portraits of persons who lived like this.' Using the work of Theodore Millon and the DSM-III-R he aids us in seeing our families and co-workers if not ourselves. This is a valuable use of both clinical and religious literature. The ability of a clinician to accurately depict the features, behavior and dilemmas of an individual is an important step in recognizing an individual's pain and guiding their care. (28) This work is focused on personality disorders rather than the broad range of distress indicated by mood and developmental disorders.

Oates reminds us that while personality disorders result from a fundamental failure in attachment, human beings nevertheless seek out ways of becoming whole. As a consequence, this hopeful human quest for health is precisely what places such individuals in our lives. Personality disorders are thus signaled, according to Oates, by conflicting experiences of closeness and distance with the person. It is almost as though they are saying, 'I love you; please leave!' or 'I need a job; please fire me!' As such awareness dawns in our relating to individuals, we have come a ways toward naming the individual's pain.

Near the conclusion of this volume, Oates makes as perceptive and eloquent an assessment of the long-term quandary around the issue of 'cure vs. care' as any author one might care to consult:

> With the exception of the borderline, the paranoid and the schizotypal, these disorders are ways of life the person has learned to reenact in adult life. They do not seem to involve specific abnormalities in the central nervous system or other organ systems of the body. Psychiatrists do not ordinarily consider these disorders in living as requiring the use of psychotropic medications They have little opportunity to do psychotherapy aground in the troubled waters of home, school, marriage, workplace and church. with such persons because these persons seldom see the necessity for insight, understanding, or instruction. Unteachability runs through these persons (29)

What then about guiding the care of such persons? As I have worked with Oates' system and personality disorders over the years I have come to a basic conclusion. We 'help' persons with personality disorders by reflecting back to them the very paradoxical nature of reality they are attempting to resolve. Our refusal to solve their dilemma puts the responsibility squarely where it belongs (on the individual) and positions the caregiver precisely where we need to be (alongside but without shouldering their dilemma). As uncomfortable as this approach is to a mental health system that focuses on 'cure' rather than 'care,' our religious traditions and life itself tell us repeatedly that the suffering and struggle with our character flaws is a primary way that God is disclosed to us and that genuine maturity occurs.

Beyond the Genogram – David Hodge

Although a study cited earlier highlighted the hesitancy of medical students in Virginia 'that consideration of religion in academic medicine is not appropriate, even when involving such issues as end-of-life care and prayer with terminal patients,' (30) medicine is not the only discipline that suffers from this myopia. An article in the Journal of Marital and Family Therapy makes the same point: 'most marriage and family therapists …appear to have received little training on the topic.' While marriage and family therapists now appear to have a high interest in recognizing the importance of religious information in the treatment of families, the articles surveyed in this study 'included some reference to religion and, in most cases, the references were peripheral to the article's primary theme.' (31)

   This author reminds us all that 'JCAHO generally recommends that a brief,, initial spiritual assessment be conducted *with all clients*' (emphasis added). The author continues that the first goal of such an assessment is to 'emphasize the functional nature of spirituality in clients' lives-how spirituality acts as a personal and environmental strength.' He further states, 'the second goal of the initial assessment is to determine whether an additional, more comprehensive spiritual assessment is required.' He then provides us with two guidelines for making the determination for conducting a more comprehensive assessment:

- When the norms of the client's faith tradition relate to service provision / client care, as might occur with Pentecostalism and mental illness.
- When spirituality plays a central role, functioning as an organizing principle in the client's life. (32)

The author then offers a review of five complimentary approaches that therapists may wish to consider. One is a verbally based spiritual history approach. The other four are 'diagrammatic or graphic approaches (spiritual life-maps, spiritual genograms, spiritual ecomaps and spiritual ecograms).' These are not new approaches but are the adaptation of traditional family therapy diagrammatic tools to acquire and utilize religious or spiritual information. This information bears directly on the effective care of families for 'the concrete depiction of spiritual strengths an foster the adoption of new salutary narratives as clients see an array of assets physically depicted in front of them.' He continues, 'the approach often gives therapists ample content that can be used to help clients rewrite their narratives.' (33)

Citing another study, this author suggests that the hesitancy to use such qualitative resources results from a lack of training. (34) Perhaps this is the case. It is as likely to be the result of an academic training model that continues to view religion as a barrier rather than a benefit since it appears to take roughly twenty years for relevant research to actually make it into the halls of training programs. This hesitancy may also be the result of something else: the lack of involvement by mental health professionals in the religious life of their community. When it comes to the area of spiritual assessment it is difficult to adequately gauge something about which you have no first-hand experience.

Believe the Evidence – Robert T. Lawrence

So if a physician or clinician does not intuit whether or how to conduct a qualitative spiritual assessment, are there practice recommendations for a 'natural set of principles for consistent clinical decision-making regarding spiritual or alternative adjuncts to medical therapy?' (35) This author notes that while physicians and others are encouraged to utilize qualitative or spiritually oriented assessments, the practice of such assessments 'can be ethically complex.'

Presenting a paradigm of guidelines that focuses on principles of evidence, belief, quality care and time, Lawrence proposes using these principles as a matrix for assessing whether, when and how to gain spiritual or qualitative information as well as how to intervene. Like other authors cited in this chapter, Lawrence reports 'guidelines for acting on a patient's spiritual history were not found in a Medline search of the medical literature, including articles and letters from peer-reviewed publications of the last 15 years that refer to or assess the clinical relevance of spirituality, prayer, clergy, religion or faith.' So how does a clinician utilize these four principles?

Lawrence urges clinicians to first 'evaluate the evidence that supports a therapeutic advantage to such action.' Thus one is to ask two questions: 1) does sufficient evidence exist to recommend the action, and 2) what is the quality of the evidence? After gathering the evidence, he follows with this caution, 'evidence alone does not establish an ethical imperative to address a patient's spiritual or faith-based practice. The physician's belief, medical and patient values, and available time must also be taken into account.'

Next comes the principle of belief. Recognizing that 'belief in a given therapy, by both the patient and the physician, is a major part of successful doctor-patient interactions.' Noting that 'a spiritual adjunct to therapy is maximally beneficial when congruence exists between the patient's belief, the caregiver's belief and the relevance of that shared belief to therapy.' He wisely notes that even in situations of incongruence, 'using this model may lead to serendipitous therapeutic options as a caregiver and patient work together to find common ground for relevant recommendations.'

Obviously a 'patient's spiritual beliefs are most appropriately incorporated into therapy when and if doing so improves the quality of care received by the patient.' The emphasis here is on the clinician assessing the *patient's* definition of quality of care rather than a more narrow definition that the clinician may have for quality of care. This means clinicians must pay attention to the patient's values. He makes a strong case for treading lightly in making such accommodations to a patient's beliefs for quality of care. Compulsory care or deficient care can be avoided by the use of consultation with hospital chaplains or an ethical consultant.

Finally there is the principle of time. While the lack of time appears to be a major barrier to family physicians utilizing religious or spiritual assessments, this is likely to reflect more the clinician's hesitancy than the actual lack of time. He cites research that documents 'brief physician advice can lead to changes in a patient's health behaviors.' This principle of time states, ' assessing spiritual issues with patients who wish to do so is most appropriate when these issues can be entertained and any actions completed within the time constraints of clinical practice.' He then continues, "Lack of time should not be used routinely as an excuse to withhold care."

I find the tone and direction of this article to be quite helpful and hopeful. This is a practical matrix that can be used to evaluate the decision to gather qualitative spiritual information for use in the delivery of clinical care. The article also maintains a hopeful tone in suggesting not just collaboration between the treating clinician and the community's religious professionals but also concludes with the following caveat: "conscience trumps all other principles. Caregivers should not compromise their own values. Nor should a patient be put into a potentially compromising position concerning his or her spiritual beliefs."

Conclusion

The primary strength in non-clinical diagnosis efforts is their evocative power. They are rich in empathy-rooted imagery that creates connection with the individual's painful suffering. This same imagery is high in nuance so that treatment can be quite personalized. Treatment can thus build on the individual's own wisdom and make use of the relationship that inevitably develops between any caregiver and the person in need. Despite research that documents the necessity of this relationship as a pre-requisite for healing, our medical and clinical training programs still do not emphasize this crucial ingredient in the provision of care.

This evocative detail is also the primary weakness in non-clinical systems. Many of these systems make data acquisition, retrieval, and transmission difficult. These systems require a training experience that emphasizes professional acquisition of wisdom in addition to the use of psychological techniques. The inability of non-clinical systems to guarantee that a specific well-told story will provide the same degree of measurable relief each time runs counter to our culture's need for verifiable results.

In the post-modern age there is an absence of genuine exposure to – and belief in-the ancient classics of culture and religion as sources of personal meaning. Consequently clinicians do not value them as instruments of either explanation or care. Clinicians appear to be more comfortable seeing the 'spiritual' value of art, music, relaxation techniques, support groups, gardening and journal writing. But these practices, as helpful as they are in the provision of care, exist within the penumbra around well-established systems of faith that can be crucial to the recovery of an individual or the restoration of balance within the life of a family. One thing should be clear by now: the lack of utilizing non-clinical qualitative or religious resources in the two tasks of diagnosis does not result from a lack of resources or research. In the chapters that follow I will be elucidating an approach to diagnosis that takes seriously the inherent tensions between these various clinical and non-clinical models. As clinicians understand an individual's ethical matrix, religious beliefs and existential circumstances we may become more confident in our utilization of these qualitative resources. We might even begin to embrace them for our own care and self-understanding! *Selah!*

Part II – Ethical Guilt: the Feeling of Blame

Chapter 5: Realistic and Subjective Guilt

Three times a week I meet with men and women whose combination of alcohol or another mind-altering substance with driving a car has resulted in either the suspension or revocation of their driving privileges. In addition to immediately spending a night in jail, paying a heavy fine and having a breath interlock device installed in whatever automobile they wind up driving for the next year, they must attend an Alcohol Safety Action Program (ASAP) Program. These are on-going psycho-educational groups, with people entering and graduating at different times. As each new member joins a group, everyone has an opportunity to revisit the facts of their conviction.

Revisiting the night of their arrest has two significant components. The objective fact of their Blood Alcohol Content (BAC) that can range anywhere from .08 percent to as high as .32 percent of alcohol in their bloodstream is sometimes a source of amazement. But as the class progresses and, in the language of Alcoholics Anonymous they are 'restored to sanity,' the second component becomes active: the subjective reality of profound guilt as they explore not just their responsibility for whatever damage their impaired driving may have caused but as they begin to recognize the fuller impact that substance abuse has had throughout their lives.

By the end of the sixteen week of mandated classes, most individuals have at least come to terms with some of their realistic guilt, for they are able to mark off completing this program as one step in redressing the objective grievance society has against them. Addressing the more subjective reality of guilt and the long-term consequences of making different choices as they live into a new future is a more permanent challenge. They fear those around them will continue to punish them for their past mistakes long after regaining their driver's license and remaining responsible with their alcohol use.

Try as we might to tell ourselves we have done nothing wrong, the feeling of being punished persists whenever loss afflicts us or calamity strikes those we love. Coupled with the feeling of being punished is the inner scrambling to search for the blemish, sin or mistake that we can redress to avoid the continuing consequences of punishment. Such a frenzied scramble robs life of joy and creativity long after whatever objective consequences have passed. If the losses

53

occur at crucial developmental junctions, one's life can assume a quality of guarded anxiety or depression that cripples for decades.

Worthy and Unworthy Ends

Guilt is not equivalent with fault, especially moral fault. (1) Yet our practice as caring persons places us at the sword points of guilt and fault. The sting of guilt is one's inner presumption of fault, typically communicated through the dynamic of conscience. Again, while the full treatment of the ethical theory of conscience is beyond our present work, the caregiver may be assisted in the tasks of diagnosis and treatment by becoming familiar with the work of a single ethical theorist. Nicolai Hartmann argues persuasively, "Values are not only independent of the things that are valuable, but are actually their prerequisite." (2)

This has immediate implications for the concrete tasks of diagnosis and treatment. First, the person's feeling of guilt is linked to a value which is ethically real and is antecedent to whatever behavior or attitude the person struggles with in counseling. Second, the ethical struggle itself is "a journey along the edge of an abyss." (3) The person who seeks ethical direction in counseling may not be avoiding feelings and relationships. They may be telling the caregiver about a very genuine fight within their soul. Our modern age wishes to believe that human beings name values. But the wrecked hearts in our offices and sanctuaries remind us that what we value names us and maims us. This is not new ethical ground for the religiously sensitive caregiver. Within one's religious tradition there is a recognizable moral code and attendant feelings of guilt whenever one violates the objective moral code. While the caregiver may wish to maintain a morally neutral attitude in the presence of a client's guilt, this may be an affective fiction on the part of the therapist, whether the therapist works from a secular or religious framework. Hartmann reminds us that "not all valuable things are of equal value. The standard of moral goodness indicates exactly the boundary between worthy and unworthy intentions." (4)

The application of this principle to the task of diagnosis is this: we seek to discern the *client's* "boundary between worthy and unworthy intentions.' At a later phase of care we may be invited to assist the other person as they evaluate the place of this boundary. We may even be invited to assist in the birth of a new boundary. However, the *initial* diagnostic task is to discover simply if, and how, the person's own value boundaries contribute to their current dilemma.

The connection between guilt and fault is made complex by the multiple sources that inform any of us about this boundary between worthy and unworthy intentions. Thus we may be in a setting with another person who has done nothing illegal or overtly immoral and yet who carries within a great feeling of pursuing unworthy ends. We must recognize in our diagnosis the legitimacy of realistic guilt that results from the violation of transcendent values. The basic outline of philosophic debate on transcendent values has not substantially changed since Kant's *Groundwork of the Metaphysic of Morals*. *If* we can know transcendent values, *how* we know them and *what we must do* in their presence is the gritty substance of ethical debate. Ethics still attempts to discern and promulgate the laws of free moral action. (5)

One addition to this complex discussion is the ethical theory of James Gustafson. He notes persuasively our life is in a world where values "are grounded in an objective reality of which human life is a part." What is so significant for our purposes here is Gustafson's recognition that our "experience of the ultimate power . . .bearing down upon, sustaining and creating possibilities for action induces or evokes piety." This response of piety "requires that attention be given to deeply *affective* aspects of moral agents." (6) Thus the presence of strong affect becomes the signal of deeply held worthy ends.

The provider of care should not attempt to compile a definitive authorized list of transcendent values. Yet religious and secular communities typically do have such an authorized list. Modern liberal theology notwithstanding, there seems to be fairly common agreement among the various traditions about the values enshrined on such lists. Not many communities center themselves around values such as theft of property, taking another's life, speaking falsely or breaking promises. The diagnostic and treatment issues may be pointed around such ethical questions as "what do I do when two such values conflict?" as well as the primary ethical question of "what is the right and the good?" The employer who must fire a single mother for incompetence, knowing that her children will innocently suffer feels such pain. So too does the nurse whose oath binds her to care daily for the comatose patient whose family members never visit. For the care provider whose central source of these transcendent values is grounded within the Judaeo-Christian tradition, one source of worthy ends is the Ten Commandments. These are typically subdivided into commands that define one's relationship with the Holy and one's relationship with the neighbor (who is also holy). These values were aptly summarized by Jesus of Nazareth (7) and dynamically summarized by Immanuel Kant, "act only on that maxim through which you can at the same time will that it should become a universal law." (8)

A person of the other major religions, Buddhism, Muslim and Hindu share in this inner experience of being "borne down upon" by similarly compelling transcendent values. (9) Such values may be encountered in the arena of family life, culture, religious dogma or the privacy of the heart. But rest assured, they shall make themselves known to each of us. It can be helpful to both diagnosis and treatment for the caregiver to become conversant with these other traditions.

It is unhelpful and dishonest for the clinician to either mix all such values into an eclectic ethical soup or to deny *a priori* a transcendent legitimacy of any value. Indeed such a carefully crafted posture of ethical "neutrality" in a pastoral setting may impede the formation of the very therapeutic alliance that we know to promote healing empathy. The person with religious sentiment may be dismayed at a caregiver's perceived distance from the values of her tradition while the secular person may be confused by a religious caregiver whose moral affect is masked.

Those whose ethical pain compels them to seek care do so within a moral framework. An important part of both diagnosis and care is to allow the individual an opportunity to articulate their moral framework, re-evaluate their framework if necessary, and continue their life's direction. Such an enterprise will involve all aspects of the person's life, including personal cognition, emotions and piety. This process will also envelope their wider family and societal relationships. Such a re-evaluation will necessarily move beyond the consideration of ethics and guilt, but these can be places to begin the inquiry.

Being Punished

Our language is full of metaphors that we 'do not measure up,' we "haven't made the cut," and that we have "missed the mark." Sometimes the mark we miss is tangible, like the "Stop" sign we run or the sales percentage we do not meet. Sometimes the measure we fall short of is an inherited standard about "the way our family ought to be" or "a Christian always begins the day with prayer." This is, indeed, our "first conceptualization of sin" which is "radically different from that of defilement" which is outlined "on the symbolic level." This particular way of symbolizing sin and fault "suggests the idea of a relation broken off." (10) Regardless of the standard's realism or origin, when we fail to meet the standard we feel guilty. We flinch. We brace ourselves for the punishment that our training has taught us to anticipate. Sometimes the anticipation is legitimate and the punishment that ultimately comes our way is real. At other times one is plagued by an anticipated punishment that never truly arrives except in the form of our own sleeplessness and worry. In any event the standard has become at least a minor god in the pantheon of human consciousness, for the person is adjusting both their self-perception and possibly their conduct to escape the punishment they fear comes with violating the standard. We will leave aside an examination of the inherent idolatry of this conclusion for Part III.

One early religious story details the blessing and the curse at the core of human life. (11) Our first experiences with life tell us there are forbidden objects that produce direct and immediate consequences if we touch, spill or trespass upon them. (12) We fall away from the origin of our life. Our falling away produces in us the anticipation of punishment coupled with the feeling of guilt and shame. (13) This anticipation of punishment is more than a theoretical nicety. One needs look no further than our sweaty palms whenever a police car follows us in traffic. Whether the moral law is written primarily upon our heart or remains externally focused, one does not help another's suffering by dismissing the anticipation of punishment as childish or irrational. The child we once were, and the creature of the universe we remain retains a fundamental awareness of vulnerability related to the things we may not touch or we shall surely die.

Although there may be connections between one's background and current painful behavior, it is dishonest to equate empathy with justice. Adequate diagnosis must be ethically real. The emotional fact that a man suffered taunts from his mother and finally struck back at another woman's verbal taunts must not obscure the physical reality of his woman's broken jaw. Part of this man's healing journey involved finally putting a realistic name on his mother's taunts. An equally important part involved his facing real legal guilt. Sometimes punishment is more than a feeling. There are situations when legal punishment is a legitimate component of the healing journey.

The estrangement of pastoral care from ethical thinking is well documented. (14) A clinician's lack of moral clarity or attempt to appear ethically neutral is particularly problematic in the task of diagnosis. Part of the pain that brings persons into counseling may be the long-standing failure to adequately name the wrongs done to them when they were vulnerable. A caregiver's reluctance to enter this ethical discussion creates two problems. Foremost it prevents the person from fully naming their pain. Second, it is re-traumatizing. Once again the individual in distress must put aside their own distress in order to take care of someone else rather than attend to their own need and obtain genuine healing. Only this second time it is the therapist's ethical softness that the wounded person must soothe.

Caregivers have been hesitant to engage in ethical conversation due to awareness that we are not judges, lawyers or juries. An undue emphasis on ethics can reduce the healing journey to an attempt to shape revenge or avoid relieving the relational pain resulting from current or past events. Thus it is tempting in the substance abuse groups to allow individuals to ramble on about how their troubles result from the bartender, the police, their poor attorney or any other person besides themselves. But effective care must begin with the accurate naming of their pain: "I should not have gotten behind the wheel of my car with a BAC of over .08." Don Browning's work in the field of ethics and pastoral care outlines this pitfall very well. (15)

Ethical realism in diagnosis means a willingness to assess the client's behavior, attitudes and life history within a recognizable and consistent framework of values. That a caregiver may immediately hear the internal post-modern supervisor query, "But *which* framework of values?" does not exempt us from this significant task. Unfortunately the religious caregiver often feels they must lay aside their very rich tradition of values in the interest of some ethereal standard of moral neutrality. (16)

The person in pain before us will not be helped by moral neutrality. If anything, many persons bring the acute moral pain of discovering that actions based on a supposed morally neutral world suddenly cause very real guilt and the attendant feeling of being punished. Post-abortion counseling is only one area where this dynamic is surfaced. Certainly the legal proceedings which may ultimately be initiated by a variety of hurting persons, or which may have begun to be brought against them, rise from very real assumptions about the moral nature of the human community.

A complete treatment of ethical theory is well beyond the scope of this volume. However, the caregiver can be aided in the task of diagnosis by acknowledging a single category of ethical reasoning: *prima facie guilt* that results from the failure to execute one's *prima facie* duty. (17) Coming from the ethical theory of W. D. Ross and others, this concept bids us realize that certain behaviors and attitudes are, *on their face,* either morally binding or are, *on their face,* unethical and needing redress. Examples of a *prima facie* moral duty would be the duty to do something because of my own previous actions. Such a duty might include an act of reparation or an expression of gratitude that would rest upon previous actions. Examples of a *prima facie* moral wrong, according to Ross, might include a violation of the *duty of non-malfeasance,"* which would include child abuse in its many forms, taking a human life, or violating another's trust." (18) In short, the astute reader may recognize this list as the Ten Commandments.

Ethical realism also involves recognizing that the mere fact of some personal difficulty does not explain away the emotional anticipation of punishment or necessarily exempt one from real consequences of illegal action. Thus a parishioner who paid off one credit card by charging the debt to another credit card not only finally caved in with paralyzing fear but also had to contend with the very genuine demands of creditors. No amount of psychotherapeutic talk about weak ego boundaries or an addictive personality disorder would either satisfy her creditors' rightful claims or ultimately soothe her inner moral pain.

Recognizing the Fear of Punishment

The most obvious indication of a person's fear of punishment is the sentence that begins "I should have..." and continues with a statement outlining the standard that has been missed. Whether the person could have reasonably met the standard or fulfilled the *prima facie* duty is a matter to be considered as care unfolds. Initially it is important to hear the person's genuine moral anguish as well as their emotional pain. Emotional pain does not exist in some rarefied portion of the brain apart from a framework of values. "I should have covered the swimming pool," "I should have unplugged the coffee pot," I should have read the fine print," and "I should have listened to her," are all statements that express the pith of pain and the limits of abilities. Assisting the individual in identifying this framework of values is as important in their care as providing sufficient safety in which they can express their emotional pain.

Most frequently the sadness or regret at violating an internal moral standard will deepen into remorse or anxiety. These, in turn, fester into an inner posture of hyper-vigilance and accompany the fear of punishment. These affects typically wind up with a clinical category of diagnosis of a *Condition Not Attributable to a Mental Disorder*, one of the specific Adjustment Disorders or the behavioral components of the more serious affective disorders such as Dysthymia, Bipolar Disorder and Anxiety Disorder. The personality disorders and the various addictions inevitably have ethically realistic components to the life-long pain associated with such grievous developmental psychic wounds. While such ethical realism cannot be the terminus of care, neither can these ethical dimensions be overlooked. If one's addiction has roots in a parent's allowing him to drink at age five or because her parents still used marijuana recreationally well into her adolescence, a part of the urgent mandate of care does involve an adequate naming of these *prima facie* failures in parental nurture. These failures were ethically shattering to a vulnerable moral agent, i.e. a small child. It can be diagnostically helpful to note any conjunction between a person's punishment-directed affects and their recounting of major parental figures and settings. One can inquire about genuine events, with an eye toward relieving guilt, without necessarily casting oneself as a Grand Inquisitor.

Fear of punishment can also paralyze an otherwise competent person's ability to make a timely and effective decision. A recent loss, such as being fired from work, can make one hesitant to venture forth on a job search. Here the caregiver will need to gauge with the person the extent to which their discomfort is understandable tenderness vs. a revisiting of previous times when failure brought with it an experience of punishment. Such past experiences may find a voice in expressions such as "I just don't want to be hurt again," "I need some space," or "the last time I was in charge, somebody got killed."

A diligent caregiver cannot initially assume that an individual's reluctance to come to closure with a situation is simply a matter of personal style. In my experience healing begins only through helping an individual distinguish between realistic guilt (for which one is responsible and which one can redress) and subjective guilt (for which one is blamed and which one can seldom redress). No amount of psychobabble that 'it isn't your fault' seems capable of truly soothing the wounded conscience. Even heroes have a limit to the punishment they can withstand. Crushing and repeated rejection can turn a once proudly competent person into someone haunted by an unseen but powerful punisher.

Fear of punishment can also lead someone to be overly decisive. In some particularly brutal households children and spouses can find themselves confronted by an enraged person whose hostility ceases only when an answer, *any* answer, has been provided to their interrogator. Since our American culture tends to value decisiveness, this fearful footprint's damage is more difficult to discern. Inviting out the memory which fuels the fear of punishment may take months of careful listening. Once again a part of the healing journey can be the mature reappraisal of the ethical setting in which the person made those first rapid decisions, as well as the lifesaving decision to 'give the bastard *some* answer that will stop the punishment.'

"Sinners in the Hands of an Angry God"

This is the basic description of the fear that we clinicians must touch if we are to deal spiritually with the feelings of punishment. Even the most theologically sophisticated individuals come to a point in life where they feel positively stalked by a Malevolent Force who has come for them. The Greek goddess of righteous anger, Nemesis, personifies this primal fear. It is a fear that seemingly drives narcissists the hardest. Well it might, for it was Nemesis who executed the binding punishment upon the original Narcissus for rejecting true love. (19)

One need not know the content of such primal fear in another in order to hear and respect the fear. But one must be alert so as to respond to it when it is voiced. The core of such fear is not merely an emotion of vulnerability but, more commonly, such a feeling rests upon some violation of a promise that the person has made to herself. If the caregiver can even tease out the shadow of this broken promise, one has come a great way toward soothing the fear of punishment that cripples many people.

The author remembers getting a telephone call from another Vietnam veteran. There had been an electrical fire in his home. His wonderful, life-filled daughter had been found cringing under her crib. She would live, but death would have been a mercy.

"I need someone to walk through the ashes with me," he said.

I went and we walked.

We walked in silence for several moments. They seemed to take us both back to another land and another time.

Finally he spoke. "This is the payback." It was all that he said.

We embraced.

"Then it looks to me like the debt has been paid in full," I said through our tears. "May God's mercy come to you and to your daughter!"

We need not look solely to the mythological traditions for this primal fear of punishment. It goes back to our own earliest heritage as Biblical people. Prior to this literary datum, our limbic memory of glowing eyes waiting in the darkness outside of our dwelling remains a terrible reminder of the predatory danger waiting for us when we violate the basic rhythms in the universe. Thus regardless of our views on the literary sources for many of Scriptural writings we must acknowledge the ethical reality of punishment meted out by a Just God as a potential factor *within the client's consciousness.* In our rush to deter the human action of revenge or our own implicit worldview that perceives the Deity as always warm and loving, may prompt us to overlook the moral force in the verse "vengeance is mine, says the Lord." (20) There are times when it is basically more healing to acknowledge the legitimate dynamics of justice exacted upon a person than to seek always to explain away their fear of being punished. In cognitive-behavioral terms this is simply allowing the individual or couple or teenager to recognize that conduct has consequences.

There are a host of behaviors that carry very real but unfortunate consequences. There are attitudes which, when they become the basis of one's behavior, exert a damaging impact upon the lives of individuals and communities. As much as we might like reality to be different, it appears that there is something built into the nature of things such that a time of justice ultimately arrives. The Apostle Paul calls this "the Wrath of God." (21) It is our basic recognition of this dynamic that drives us behaviorally and ethically, whether our recognition is informed by a religious or moral tradition or the simple brutality of hard life experience. (22) Assisting the person or couple in naming the reality of this particular pain and assisting them in outlining their culpability in creating this pain, are necessary prerequisites for helping them find any dynamics of genuine mercy.

Conclusion

It is the author's clinical experience that some persons who seek care do so out of a desire to have their own re-emerging moral bearings confirmed. I hear this desire for moral clarity expressed most often in the youthful repetition of the phrase, 'does this make sense?' That this catchphrase has come to infect much of the interpersonal conversation of their parents may be more a signal of the age's lack of moral and spiritual insight than a mere conversational way of maintaining connection. The clinical enterprise will be helped if the caregiver responds to such repetitive requests for reassurance by saying, 'I wonder what it means that you keep asking me if your words make sense. Could we explore this a bit?'

When a counselor or chaplain uses their considerable empathic skills to create a setting of safety in which the person may explore their fear of punishment and lack of moral clarity, then a part of the healing journey can truly be undertaken: the acknowledgment of legitimate guilt and the release from the fear of unmerited punishment. But if we do not assist the individual in this moral and spiritual quest for clarity then we have only put a band aid upon a wound they intuitively know goes to the core of their soul. *Selah!*

Chapter 6: Punishment and Seeking Redress

"I went to court on Friday," she said slumping into the couch. "The judge said I was guilty of simple assault and I was placed on two years probation. If I'm a good girl and don't say anything nasty to the jerk for two years, my record will be expunged."

"So where does this leave you?" I asked.

"Right now I'm still very angry. I know I didn't do what he said I did. But he told the judge *every*thing that happened that day, and *yes*, I was pretty upset. We both were. I had called him several times that day and I probably sounded pretty outraged. But I didn't throw the cup of coffee at him. It slipped from my hand and it burned his thighs," she said. She then concluded, "I still think I'm right."

Support from a caregiver, especially during the initial anguish of one's effort at gaining relief from punishment can help lift the weight of guilt. Our empathic stance communicates to the person "I am here with you. Your pain and confusion does not frighten or offend me." Such empathy is crucial if the other person is to ever reassess their moral values. Only from a stance beside another can we begin to see their world, understand the forces that bore down upon them so heavily that no other choice seemed possible, and help them find their own voice instead of the mute suffering of guilt or the humiliation of 'now having my own probation officer.' (1) We must not, however, allow our empathy for the client to cloud our own moral values any more than we would allow the client to misperceive our empathy as a wink-and-nod toward continued illegal or immoral conduct.

Guilt is soothed most completely when an individual joins a new community of moral formation and discourse. Whether they join a non-abusive family through marriage, a caring cadre of companion sufferers such as Narcotics Anonymous, or a vital and receptive religious congregation, such a transition feels like nothing short of a rebirth. It is within such a community that one is not only 'born down upon' by a new set of transcendent values but, more significantly, they find new values and companions who lift them up. Membership in such a community provides an alternative to punishment and can open within the soul the recognition of the necessity to redress a moral wrong. Sometimes people arrive at the doorway to such a community by court order. While the court may assign them to attend classes or orders them to stay away from certain people or places as a part of rehabilitation, the individual at first experiences this order as punishing and restrictive. This is due to the simple fact that they lack the moral insight and emotional maturity to understand their conduct is harmful to others. Historically caregivers both within the religious community and secular clinic have resisted contact with the courts. Some professional providers of pastoral care and legal counsel asks clients to sign a document which states, in part, "I understand that the counselor is not required to testify in a court proceeding, and I further agree that I shall not request my counselor to testify." While clergy and pastoral counselors can claim the tradition of holy writ (2) and the sacrament of confession and absolution, recent exposures of professional abuses and laws mandating reporting of child abuse bring the threat of exposure and its consequent punishment into the counseling relationship. Certainly such pressures can complicate the entire process of redressing any realistic grievance.

Thus contemporary caregivers face a multifaceted dilemma. First, some clients come to counseling with awareness that they desire some type of redress. They look to the therapist as someone who can confirm a layer of damage by another that may help them shape the level of redress that will lead to a measure of healing. This delves right to the heart of our personal and institutional life as providers of humane care. Second, feminist research on counseling in matters related to sexual molestation and rape suggest the therapeutic value of victims actively pursuing those who perpetrated the injury through either the civil or criminal court. This goes to the core of a therapist's institutional stance of not wanting to serve as an officer of the court. Third, although we make much in theory about the sanctity of the confessional, it is quite another matter to have someone who, after some conversation in our office says, 'I must tell you now about the body I buried fifteen years ago . . . or 'we have been distributing cocaine for years. I want to stop, but if I leave the organization, I'm sure I'll be killed. Can you help me?'

Such confessions make good novels. For some care providers, these words are more than a writer's fiction. When these words are spoken in your office, one quickly realizes that there can be more to counseling than the affective relief of suffering. We may not have heretofore construed our role as one that offers more than such relief. Until such words are spoken! Regardless of how we initially define our role, once such words *are* spoken in our presence, the matters of diagnosis and treatment take on an additional degree of seriousness. The matters of 'how do we name this pain?' and 'how might this pain be relieved?' now involve the caregiver and seeker in a journey which includes the broken soul of society. We may be compelled to enter the arena in which this brokenness awaits like a roaring lion to consume all who enter.

Naturally the matters of redress also relate to a person's responding in a new way toward those they have wounded. Healing can bring one to a new level of awareness of their own capacity to change their life's direction. A part of the healing journey may include acts of restitution or words of apology to those one has wronged. This step brings an added layer of subjective relief from the feeling of punishment and whatever degree of realistic guilt that still afflicts the mind. An act of redress also moves one back toward reconciliation if not restoration of a relationship. Thus redressing a grievance shifts the identities and balance of power within the immediate social network of the person who comes for care.

The author remembers dozens of veterans from several wars for who a significant part of their healing involved a return to the land of battle. While combat is frightening to the soul, sometimes the battle within a family or an institution can be more corrosive to the soul because it is unexpected and lasts much longer than a firefight. Thus while not all combatants need to return to the original site of brutality and wounding, redressing the wounding one has done as an expression of gratitude or receiving the amends of another can bring the deepest solace one can witness. Identifying the necessity of these movements and guiding individuals or families through this legal, moral and spiritual thicket is part of the work of naming their pain and guiding their care.

When One Has Been Wronged and Waits for Redress

"The abuse started when I was two, I think. Certainly by the time I was three, my older cousins had already had fights over who got 'first dibs' on me," Paul continued quietly. "I can sort of understand their actions, because they're what we called 'half-wits.' But who can give back to me the trust that my uncles and my aunt took away from me? I am terrified of getting close to men and not too fond of women, although they're a bit easier."

Paul took a deep breath. Then came a cry from his depths, "they stole my childhood and God *damn* them! They ought to *pay!*"

We would journey together through these painful swamps of his torn childhood. No matter how far he roamed into the depths, he returned to this theme: somehow there should be justice, if not for him then justice upon those who had inflicted such continuing horror upon his soul. He felt torn between the desire for these wrongs to be made right and his religious training that apparently compelled him to forgive the ones who were unaware of the depth of damage their humiliation had wrought upon him.

Persons seek to redress their wounds out of a desire to move beyond their roles as victims. Seldom is their motive entirely pure. Seldom does one obtain a complete cure for the damages endured in life. Even though justice and healing may be incomplete, which of us would choose the running sores of continued victimization over the tangible relief that might be gained through redress? Indeed some argue that the transcendence of suffering includes active behavior which helps reshape the person's situation. (3)

As indicated earlier, for many persons it is redress enough to simply acknowledge that they were wronged. For others, there can be a widening circle of persons to whom they acknowledge their woundedness and current degree of healing. From the privacy of a therapeutic relationship to public disclosure to transformation toward a new vocation, many find satisfying avenues to reshape the gashes in soul, psyche and soma.

Thus Paul came for support during his last year in medical school. He struggled with these obvious wounds from childhood that tore at his very soul. As he returned to the anguish of the wounds, he wondered aloud "what must I do now, with the children who remain near to these people?" Not an idle question for either this soon-to-be pediatrician or the now-grown adult who could just as easily be driving a truck. The ethical and behavioral dimensions of redress would remain the same: what is his current responsibility toward those who might yet be victimized? This too is part of the urgent mandate that brings wounded people to the place of healing.

It does help to examine real alternatives, come to some practical decisions about future action and then implement the plan while in a supportive or therapeutic relationship. This had two benefits for Paul. First, it legitimated his concerns in a way that affective symptom relief would not. His feelings were tied to historical events and the current actions of real people. He did not wake up one fine morning deciding to be depressed and full of rage. Second, as care progressed he became able to negotiate his way through the complex web of decisions related to these continuing social and family relationships. He no longer needed to accept uncritically the victimizing demands of his family or the terrorizing rage of his still-wounded memory.

But there are times when the only way of redressing a wound is the court system. We may be requested to provide care for any number of persons who have been wronged by a person or an institution. Whether the request comes from the person wronged or through an attorney, the underlying matters of care remain essentially the same: how can we assist this person in naming his pain within this new arena and how does this context of pain guide our care?

For Rosalie, a tender second grader, the fondling by a grandfather previously convicted on charges of child molestation brought feelings of sadness, poor grades and rebellious conduct at home. She and her mother first sought redress through counseling and a family intervention. This intervention was guided by a local private therapist. It was agreed during this session that "Pa-Paw" would pay for Rosalie's counseling. He also agreed to re-enter group counseling. After a brief investigation, the department and Rosalie's mother sought redress through the courts. At a formal hearing, the charges of molestation was certified and Pa-Paw's probation was revoked. He was remanded to counseling and to pay up to $1,000 for Rosalie's counseling.

Did action through the court help Rosalie and Pa-Paw? The resolution seemed to relieve Rosalie's depression. She seemed to regain her playfulness. She commented that although "it was scary" seeing the judge, it was no more scary than being fondled by her grandfather. Primarily she felt believed by someone powerful. Adults she did not previously know (judge, therapist, social worker) took her seriously and trusted her word. This posture took her out of the role of victim and restored her to the role of citizen. She learned that she could take initiative and respond to a serious problem. Obtaining redress through the court system provided a significant if not complete response to the developmental wounds produced by her molestation.

The provider of religious counseling as well as the secular clinician may have theoretical difficulties with such a case. If so, referral is the ethical course of action. We have no right to attempt to talk someone else out of their legal right of redress simply because we believe that healing may lie in another direction. There is one additional matter that the provider of care must face: when is the perpetrator finally held responsible for their wounding behavior? Is it always someone *else's* failure of attitude, incomplete parenting, underpaying job, etc. to which we redirect our attention? Such social questions impinge on the initial decision whether or not to offer care to one who may become involved in legal action.

When One Has Been the Agent of Wrong and Makes Amends

But what of Rosalie's Pa-Paw? How might he redress the pain inflicted by his own hand? Clearly it was his inability or unwillingness to do so, or to face his guilt, that resulted in an extreme measure being taken. Unless the provider of care, whether pastoral or secular, works within a prison setting, few clinicians will have significant or sustained contact with persons who have been brought to this level of redressing their wrongs.

More typically, the clinician will encounter people who come to some level of self-awareness that they have caused another person significant, life-altering pain. At such a point the person may cry out "what must I do? . . .what *can* I do?" Such moments are poignant to be sure. This is also a moment in which a caregiver can adopt a posture of walking with the person through concrete options for behavioral change.

The levels of redress when one has been an agent of pain parallel the avenues of healing for the victim. For some, the most that can be hoped is that they obtain some private level of soothing for their own hearts and minds. Supportive and insight-oriented therapy as well as the traditional rites of the faith community such as confession and penance can help. For others, there are avenues of genuine contact with those who have felt the impact of their prior behavior. Such contact can be guided during a therapeutic process or through one of the Anonymous programs. The Eighth and Ninth Steps of Alcoholics Anonymous can be effective guides in such a journey: "Made a list of all persons we had harmed, and became willing to make amends to them all; Made direct amends to such people wherever possible, except where to do so would injure them or others." To begin to *wonder* about such steps is healing. To *walk* with another who decides to take the steps is indeed a holy quest for client and clinician. (4)

Assessing the avenues for redress open to one who has been the perpetrator, the clinician may once again choose to walk with the person through cognitive moral inquiry. To help the person articulate the promise that was broken, the boundary that was crossed, the perceptions that were so skewed they led to unfortunate actions can be healing. Clinicians using either cognitive or affectively oriented therapeutic techniques achieve beneficial results.

As the landmark work of James Fowler illustrates, the step from one level of moral awareness to the next is an arduous one. (5) Yet walking with someone through this conversion is a legitimate role for pastoral and secular care. The person who is thus transformed is a new creation. (6) From such a new standpoint, the person can now approach the task of more direct redress with resources of spirit heretofore unavailable to them.

This may appear to be a simple process for a clinician. Unfortunately, without careful thought such action can degenerate into unbridled manipulation of all parties by an underlying desire for clarity and closure. The ones providing care in such situations often find their own values challenged. Healing for perpetrators and victims in the realm of ethics is a process of dialog in which we are invited to stand with one and sometimes both sides of a tortured, tangled relationship. As much as we would like there to be a sterile ethical field upon which to stand, there appears to be only the mud of a crowded No Man's Land. We long for a guide to make completely clear lines of responsibility, guilt, innocence and forgiveness. Such is not possible. We have left both the Garden and Mt. Sinai long ago.

It seems to the author that here the pastor has one distinct advantage. We are outside the rubrics of legal evidence. We deal primarily in the wounded perceptions of persons. Thus our dialog with hurting persons, regardless of their role in the suffering, most often focuses more on restoring the relationship rather than assigning blame. Making this point as clearly as possible, even in the realm of ethics, can free all parties to truly re-examine their values at some future point. This is a particularly powerful process to undertake once the feelings of punishment have been redressed and whatever balance possible has been restored to the relationship.

"This Old Scar From the Tusk Wound I Got!"

Like Odysseus our wounds identify us to both faithful friends and tormenting adversaries. Whether our response to our wounds is to wreak revenge upon our adversaries or determine to allow revenge to come through other long-term consequences is a matter of maturity. Neither response should be automatic nor should either response be necessarily accorded the morally superior position.

When an ethical boundary has been crossed there is a strong desire to 'make things right.' This sense is likely to be strongest when the bulk of an individual's guilt is subjective and results from a perception of personal failure. There is also a corresponding need, again primarily subjective in nature, that another party should 'make things right.' In moral terms this is called a *redress of grievance.* When left unresolved or not addressed, moral grievances can degrade into a life-poisoning affect of resentment. When allowed to fester in this fashion the slights and bumps of ordinary human discourse can quickly become additional examples of the other person's continued animosity. Indeed the subjective need for redress of grievance may result initially from some perceived lack of graciousness, courtesy or respect that the initiating party may be entirely unaware of. This is especially true during adolescence but the emotional maturity that naturally allows someone to place these ordinary slights into wider perspective sometimes needs the assistance of a counselor.

More serious are the areas of grievance where there has been a genuine ethical failure on one individual or institution's part that seems to cry out for some type of justice. With a culture that is ready to sue someone when a cup of coffee is too hot, a therapist may play a crucial relational role in assisting people in gaining enough emotional maturity so they can negotiate their way through a thorny thicket of ethical and relational failure so as to make an informed legal decision. Beyond the therapeutic skills of inquiry and empathy, a counselor or clergy must use wisdom to assist another whether the better course is to adopt an attitude of 'suck it up and get on with the mission' or to 'sue their pants off.' Either course of action does exact a psychological and spiritual cost on all parties.

From a religious viewpoint, ethical guilt is redressed most directly by the rite of confession and the receipt of absolution / reconciliation. Repentance, another key religious concept, is rooted in the behavioral commitment to move in a different direction. Guiding someone through these steps is a legitimate provision of care. Such care is curative in the religious sense since it reconnects the person with God-the object of religious devotion. I have found that even when someone does not come from a religious background, or have a spiritual orientation, they respond to the expression of remorse and regret contained in Psalm 51. Here ethical failure (vs. 1) leads to confession (vs. 3) and is rooted in the recognition that moral renewal restructures the inner person (vs.6). Reconnection with the Divine One leads to "a new and right spirit" (vs.11) that includes both affective renewal (vs. 12) and vocational redirection (vs. 13). This is not cheap grace but is, indeed, a redress of humanity's most fundamental moral flaw-the humble recognition that we have transgressed a divine standard of right and wrong and not merely a socially convenient construct. Most people come to recognize the intensity of their guilt and fear of punishment as a signal that moral standards come from some other source besides a mutually agreed upon social construct.

Conclusion

In summary one should note that clinical awareness of the ethical boundaries within a person's dilemma is important clinical information in the task of naming the individual's pain. The framework of virtues and values around a situation inevitably shape both the perception and outcome of any action. Assessing their presence and strength is thus as crucial to the enterprise of diagnosis as assessing their mood, affect, orientation and thought content of the person(s) who seek our care.

A significant part of guiding the care in any situation includes gaining an awareness of the positive values and virtues that also influence the clinical rhombus. These resources are often obscured by the demoralization that so readily afflicts us when trouble has overstayed its presence on our hearth. Inquiry and empathy will relieve some of this demoralization; the rediscovery of positive values along with regaining the capacity to act in a new way places the person on the path toward forgiveness, reconciliation and perhaps ultimate restoration. The next chapter is devoted to these themes. *Selah!*

Chapter 7: Forgiveness, Reconciliation and Restoration

'Forgiveness' comes just after 'forgery' and just before 'fornication' in the index of the confessional statements used by the Presbyterian Church (USA). Quite providential for a word that's Greek root can means both 'cancellation of a debt' and 'release of prisoners.' (1) This same volume has numerous entries for the topic of 'reconciliation' but none for the state of 'restoration.' Yet the movement through these three conditions and the ethical, psychological and spiritual dimensions of these conditions goes to the core of both naming human pain and providing humane care. In the practice of ministry and in my own life I have lost track of the number of times I have stood at the doorway marked 'the route to forgiveness.' While the necessity of taking these movements in this order never changes, their particularity is always unique and seldom easy.

There are certainly behaviors that must necessarily make up the conduct we recognize as making up this triad of care and healing. But those actions are rooted in the lifetime of values and experiences we bring to any situation where boundaries of the soul and soma have been violated. The individuals and relationships that come to us for care typically feel tension between the varieties of popular notions about these three movements of the human spirit. It is impossible to follow all of the advice contained in these notions: 'forgive and forget,' 'forgive what you did but not forget what you did,' 'trust what you want but verify what you are told,' and the host of other common beliefs about this area.

At their essence these are not simply behaviors one may institute as part of a healing regime. These are values held in varying degrees by both the clinician and the client; virtues to which we may all aspire but conditions that in any given set of circumstance we may employ with serious reservations and over a very lengthy period of time. The struggle to forgive, the decision to move toward another in reconciliation and the desire for some measure of restoration with our fellow creators as well as our Creator occupy the central and deepest aspirations of the human heart.

The neurobiologist may now witness the effect of these attitudes and behaviors through spectrographic images. The psychologist may devise rating scales for freedom from obsession and conciliation. The psychiatrist may prescribe an anti-depressant to knit up care's raveled sleeve and the priest may offer absolution of our desire for revenge. But walking with someone through the nights of their wounding toward the dawn of forgiveness requires of the counselor both ethical clarity and clinical perspicuity to the task of diagnosis.

Forgiveness: The Gift We Give Ourselves

"I want her to hurt just as much as I am hurting right now," he said through clenched teeth. I know this is not what I am supposed to feel. But it is what I feel."

In the task of diagnosis the movement toward forgiveness begins when we can identify the desire for revenge lurking within the experience of punishment and the status of guilt and the stain of shame felt by the person who seeks our aid. Discerning the difference between a desire for justice and the passion for vengeance requires ethical clarity as well as spiritual wisdom. A place of refuge that allows space and time for such discernment is not a new idea; it is a necessary ancient reality.

This is an arduous journey whose length of time and depth required for healing should not be underestimated. Somewhere C. S. Lewis reported it took him over thirty years to forgive an individual. It is very easy for bystanders to say of such a journey 'you ought to . . . . ' until they set out upon the journey themselves. As counselors, pastors and chaplains our task is not to hurry people along toward some destination marked Forgiveness Station. The journey itself is a legitimate destination and calls for our empathy. The individual will be surrounded by voices urging them to 'just get over it!' or 'get a life and move on!' or 'why can't we all just get along?'

Perhaps the individual will resist these urgings out of a desire for revenge. More likely these urgings from bystanders in the person's life will fall on deaf ears because of the depth of the wound. In any event effective care must resist a person's move toward premature forgiveness with as much integrity and skill as we must not encourage them to linger at the altar of their agony.

In an interview for *Science & Theology News* Dr. Everett Worthington makes the point that forgiveness is 'a change in your emotional experience.' He goes on to distinguish 'two basic kinds of forgiveness. One is a decision to control your behavior. The other kind of forgiveness is emotional forgiveness.' (2) We confront the desire for revenge in the behavior-control layer of forgiveness. Sometimes this requires a clinician to encourage their client to seek out a restraining order from a court (to protect themselves from another's vengeance) and at other times this may require we join with a court to help our client find ways to comply with such an order. At the behavior-control layer of forgiveness there is an effort, Dr. Worthington continues, to try to treat the person 'the same as always I did. I'm not going to avoid you.' He then adds with insight, "But you still may hold a grudge and be angry and sick every time you think of this person."

To underscore the corrosive impact of holding a grudge and to highlight the implicit imperative to direct care toward emotional forgiveness, Dr. Worthington cites research that links health symptoms and an individual's general level of forgiveness. "Just getting angry at somebody causes little damage. But it's not really going to make you have physical symptoms. You have to get angry and you have to stay angry and you have to get angry about a lot of things. So that by the time you get to be 65 your body is falling apart." This insight can become a helpful lens through which physicians, nurses and hospital chaplains may view males who present themselves for treatment of any of the 10 most prevalent diseases in men over 50 years of age. (3) While females have a greater history of seeking assistance for relational distress than males, the linkage between physical disease, emotional distress and the difficulty with the task of forgiveness should be explored.

A simple checklist can help a clinician and client assess where an individual stands on the journey of forgiveness. As a part of her doctoral research at Fuller Theological Seminary, Dr Susan Wade Brown developed both a lengthy research instrument as well as a 14-item check-up. Because this check-up is available on-line and provides an individual with immediate feedback on their status, it can be used during a clinical interview. (4) This instrument has five scales that measure forgiveness:

- Desire for Revenge
- Freedom from Obsession
- Ability to Affirm the Person Who Wronged You
- Reaching Beyond Self
- Feelings of Compassion or Acceptance

We see the landmarks as well as the twists in the journey of forgiveness in the titles of these scales, along with the fact they are 5-point Likert Scales. Forgiveness begins as a person focuses on their present life rather than their past wound. This begins to liberate them from the sting of misplaced guilt and inappropriate shame. Because it is both a behavioral stance an individual employs as well as an emotional state an individual can choose, forgiveness is a gift one can afford for themselves whether or not the wounding party is alive, dead, near or far away.

The journey toward a posture of forgiveness does not mean giving permission for the behavior to be repeated. Nor does it mean saying that what was done was acceptable. I find the greatest barrier to an individual starting this journey is their desire to know 'why.' Knowing 'why' is unlikely to lessen the pain; it may make forgiveness unnecessary but this is rare. It is even more rare for the perpetrator to know 'why.' Besides, continuing to ruminate on 'why' places the power of healing in the hands of the perpetrator rather than in the self and fuels both the desire for revenge and the obsession for an explanation.

Here are seven way stations for an individual who undertakes this journey. A counselor or chaplain or pastor can be an invaluable companion at any one of these stations:

- Make a list of what is needed to forgive.
- Acknowledge your part.
- Make a list of what you gained from the relationship.
- Write a letter to the person, acknowledging these things (do not mail the letter).
- Create a ceremony in which you get rid your lists and the letter.
- Visualize the person you are forgiving being blessed by your forgiveness and, as a result, being freed from continuing the behavior that hurt you.
- Do not look back in anger or regret.

This list is singular in its intent and can be found throughout the literature on forgiveness, with slight variations. (5) The fact that it is singular and readily available does not mean that any of these steps are easy. Remember the witness of C. S. Lewis. The literature on forgiveness as well as clinical experience leads me to conclude with this caution: while forgiveness may be the healthiest gift an individual can give themselves, reconciliation is not always possible or even desirable. Reconciliation, which takes two people, also requires careful consideration. It is to a consideration of this stage in both naming the pain and guiding the care that we now turn.

Reconciliation: The Opportunity We Give Another

"You'll be getting an order from the judge," she said with resignation. "Since the Big Creep can't talk to me in a civil fashion on the phone, the judge is ordering our therapists to talk to one another. He wants the two of you to work together to outline a care plan for the children."

"I guess it is something of a blessing he's no longer sitting at the boundary of the property watching you," I said. "But the fifteen e-mails a day and matching voice-mails is just as hostile." Frankly I did not see any way these two individuals could be alone in one another's presence to effectively transfer their children for regular visitations. It was simply too dangerous.

Marriage and family therapists frequently work at the boundary between forgiveness and reconciliation. In a healthy relationship this boundary is permeable; but in a toxic relationship such as the one just ndicated, safety mandates that a wall be built. The courts become involved when there is a total breakdown at this wall and, if the situation is serious enough, there is a great divorce whose animosity appears to endure beyond the grave.

The widespread misunderstanding that conflates reconciliation with forgiveness complicates reconciliation in such settings. Just as there are stages of forgiveness, so there are stages of reconciliation. Thus in the example above the degree of 'reconciliation' may be the uneasy truce of meeting one another across the expanse of a large parking lot with an intermediary accompanying their children across the marital No-Man's Land. All communication, including such basic information as 'Wendy has a soccer game tomorrow at 2:00 p.m.' may have to be channeled through attorneys and therapists. This is far from ideal. But physical assault and emotional abuse are much less ideal.

Clinical experience mandates that safety trumps any move toward reconciliation between individuals where one party remains focused on gaining revenge or maintaining control. Clinical experience also reveals that some individual's disorder is so deep they are drawn to remain in the dangerous dance of vengeance and the resulting dyscontrol despite the mandates of a court and the support of an effective therapist. "But I still *love* her," is the diagnostic signal of someone unable to tolerate the separation that may lead to the behavioral control level of forgiveness. Reconciliation that is nurturing will remain a phantasm for such a relationship.

Frequently the healing work with an individual must begin with undoing the knot that has closely tied 'forgiveness' with 'reconciliation.' The inability to leave childhood or an abusive work setting only intensifies the wounds received during such a time. In such a circumstance the tolerance mandated by an individual's age or financial necessity easily become confused with forgiveness while the endurance mandated by the sheer needs for an income takes on the outward appearance of reconciliation. Naming this peculiar type of pain must come first and typically must maneuver though several layers of statements that minimizes the depth of damage born by the greater demands of survival.

As uncomfortable as it may be for both client and caregiver the road to ultimate reconciliation in such relationships may require going through the passageway of separation. In my experience it is this act of intentional separation that may bring the offender to some recognition of their need for repentance. While repentance is a religious concept, at its core repentance is a behavioral turning away from destructive behavior. While for the perpetrator this means at a bare minimum stopping the abusive behavior, for the victim repentance means either not responding to the cues for the dance of control or not extending an invitation to the dance in the first place. As David Augsburger notes in remarks entitled 'Five Steps to Interpersonal Forgiveness and Restored Relationships,' "I am not my past; I am a person capable of repenting, changing, and turning away from past patterns of behavior. You are not your past; you are equally free to change if you accept the freedom that is within you." (6)

The discovery that an individual has a choice whether or not to offer reconciliation to an abuser is powerful for someone who has been profoundly abused. The counselor or pastor or chaplain must frequently play Devil's

Advocate in such moments, underscoring for the individual the truth that 'not every relationship should be pursued. Not every forgiveness leads to a continuing conversation between the two. Not every healed injury will result in the resumption of the previous relationship.' (7) The challenge for the caregiver is to muster the integrity of diligent caution rather than succumb to the seduction of 'can't we all just get along?' One thing remains certain in the task of reconciliation: there will continue to be failures of both conduct and attitude as individuals walk toward one another. Reconciliation is recognized by the prompt recognition of fault and the rapid offering of an apology; it falls first to the therapist and ultimately to the individuals involved to discern the depth of sincerity involved in such a moment. Genuine reconciliation remains something of a mystery rooted in grace rather than being the mathematical nexus of two souls' moral arcs. (8)

Restoration: The Hope Of A New Life

'I just want my life back' is a frequent plea as people begin efforts toward healing. This is our unstated hope whether the damage to our life comes from human perfidy, dread disease or natural disaster. There is the expectation that taking our punishment, redressing existing grievances, moving through forgiveness and even beginning steps toward true reconciliation will ultimately lead to recovery of the life one feels got lost somewhere in the morass of pain and suffering. While the scent of smoke can be removed from the fires of human loss, life never returns to exactly the same locale. Rare indeed is the person who finds their fortunes restored two-fold after great distress. (9)

The residents of America's Gulf Coast whose homes were devastated by triple hurricanes in 2005 may resettle in the area. They may reopen their business and their marriages may survive the severity of the aftermath. The degree to which they will have a 'new life' whose arc bends toward hope and intersects with joy will be determined by their capacity to relinquish their attachment to the way their life was. This awareness may be fairly obvious in the wake of regional disaster such as this or a national disaster such as the events of September 11th, 2001. Such events come at the top of the emotional and spiritual Richter Scale of suffering.

When it comes to assisting an individual in naming the pain that has come to their heart and home there are other losses which wreak devastation as thorough as a hurricane but whose impact we never see because the local media doesn't show up to anchor the evening news from our doorstep:

- Death of a child or life-long spouse.
- Divorce
- Survival from life-threatening disease
- Chronic pain or genetic abnormality
- Forced termination from work

The list of personal losses is nearly endless. The degree to which an individual regains some sense of hope speaks to their resilience. Thus while helping the individual fully name their pain without apology is the first step of diagnosis, helping them find resources that nurture their resilience is the practical work of guiding their care. While discerning meaning inherent in profound loss will deepen resilience and ultimately determine the degree of restoration, the practical steps one is able to successfully take rebuilds the shattered self-confidence and recreates the fractured self-image. Assisting the individual in acknowledging these steps is practical morality and is guiding the care at its most fundamental level – bricks and mortar, nails and lumber, choosing and then doing the next right thing.

In the period since Christmas 2004 we have seen this dynamic of restoration occur through the humane response to large-scale disasters as well as the rebuilding of two societies making the cultural transition from terrible oppression to the beginnings of democracy. Those of us who show so much patience when helping individuals make the journey of restoration have, unfortunately, too frequently been sideline critics of the restoration rather than recognizing the decades-long timeline necessary to truly recover and move on from any one of these disasters. (10) Therapists, physicians, nurses, construction crews from churches and military personnel who initially responded and who continue to voluntarily donate time and talent to rebuilding these areas are undergoing their own moral transformation. They will be very different human beings in whatever vocational endeavor they pursue for having wept and walked a few feet in these areas devastated miles.

Conclusion

"September 11, 2001, offers a rare opportunity to do research on posttraumatic stress syndrome in adolescents. Since then, I realize that the road to recovery, particularly for adolescents, will be arduous and slow." (11) Whether the devastation comes from massive cultural events or private losses, whether we are adolescents or adults near the end of life's journey, the pathway from loss to restoration includes the way stations of forgiveness, reconciliation and restoration. The pathway for all 'will be arduous and slow' because the human heart desires the stability, security and succor that flower from such efforts.

Those who provide humane care, whether they are religious or secular in their orientation and whether they are professionals or volunteers in their vocation must allow the individual who sits before them the time necessary to fully name their pain even as they rebuild their shattered life. Frequently this is akin to constructing the boat while also steering it through the debris of Chardibys and the continued stages of human development. Patience is the ethically loving and the clinically effective stance toward such efforts. This may not be happy news in our post-modern sound-bite age but it is good news because it is true information.

Some wounds require more than one generation to fully resolve and the memories from some ethical lapses become monuments of hope for future generations. As clinicians and care providers we have the obligation to provide a secure space in which the cornerstones of such monuments may be searched out, excavated and set in place. *Selah!*

Chapter 8: Illustrative Vignettes

Usually when a book of this nature is written the clinical vignettes or case studies are woven throughout the volume to illustrate a particular point. This is effective but has the result of leaving the interested reader wanting to know either more information about the situation or about how the clinician came to arrive at a particular intervention. I am choosing to present these case illustrations in a separate chapter for two reasons.

First, I believe this method allows for a more complete presentation of the situation and thus affords the reader an opportunity to follow my diagnostic thinking in particular clinical settings. This necessitates a fuller presentation of the setting than is helpful when woven into a text. The point of the immediate text gets lost in the presentation of illustrative case.

Second, this volume is written to be helpful to a wide variety of helping professionals. I have tried to reflect this diversity in the types of vignettes as well as through the names of the cases. There are a large number of occupations devoted to officially helping people in their moments of need. There are even more individuals who provide psychological and spiritual assistance as volunteers or simply as friends. Thus while I believe the wisdom that 'a little knowledge can be dangerous,' I believe even more in the wisdom that 'no knowledge can be lethal.' Therefore I hope that the material in this book will prove helpful to a wide audience of people and not languish on the library shelf.

Because the two tasks of diagnosis require wise judgment and discernment as well as the mastery of technical knowledge, these vignettes are illustrative rather than simply clinical descriptions. This first part of the book covers the dimensions of situations that are broadly ethical and laced with themes of guilt. Thus these vignettes will focus on the appraisal and care of these concerns. Since the other two concerns, idolatry along with the feeling of betrayal and dread along with the feeling of defilement, are addressed in subsequent portions of this volume, the vignettes presented in this chapter will be enriched in subsequent chapters by the addition of these other two areas of the diagnostic enterprise. It is my goal that by the end of this volume the reader will see how these three foci are present in a variety of situations that call for diagnosis and how they unfold over time in the provision of effective care.

As I indicated in my first volume, my multi-axial system bears no direct relationship to the DSM-IV categories. I use the term 'axis' simply to facilitate communication between the two communities of humane care: medical – psychiatric and non-medical – religious.

Case # 1 – Depression

"I want to thank you for giving me a new life," said the voice on the telephone. I had listened to Elaine's voice for over a five years. Referred by her minister, her initial presentation was one of absolute stillness. Perfectly dressed since she had come from her work, she sat quite erect in the chair and proffered the opinion that she didn't really know why she came. "My life is actually wonderful," she said. "But I just don't feel like living anymore. I don't sleep at night and I hate my husband. He thinks everything is fine but I'm dying inside from loneliness and I'd rather really end it all than go on living this lie."

I nodded and began working my way through the details of her family history. A rough genogram revealed two children had come from a nearly twenty-year marriage. Her husband dutifully went to work each day and she also worked outside the home in a responsible government position. Her parents were still living and she spoke regularly with her mother. In one-way I felt like Detective Jack Webb, who was gathering 'just the facts, Ma'm' as she dryly responded to my questions. But it was her absolute lack of affect that told me there was more driving this woman's depression and despair than boredom from the good life.

She came regularly for over a year, slowly unpacking the routines of her life. Always prim and professionally dressed, precise in her words yet dissatisfied with life and angry with her husband, she was something of a riddle. An M.M.P.I. revealed both her significant need to present everything in her life as well ordered and her underlying depression. But other facts also emerged: her husband had been through six jobs in twenty years, always in sales and always on commission. He was significantly older than she, so she felt as though she had to provide both the financial stability and the vitality that kept up with their two teenagers.

As a result of this pace in her care, I was factually able to address only what appeared to be a subjective sense of guilt: her perfectionism that life was not somehow even more well-ordered, her children even more well-behaved and her husband more adequately employed. It became increasingly clear she did not receive much affirmation from her mother; rather, her mother regularly made indirect comments that fueled Elaine's belief that somehow her life was a failure and that she had married poorly. Her father's low-keyed acquiescence to his wife's sterility only added to Elaine's belief that marriage was a lifeless contract. Yet to the outside world she appeared to be the picture of physical health, professional competence, and religious piety.

Elaine came to therapy regularly each week. A few conjoint sessions with her husband only confirmed what Elaine had presented: he seemed emotionally flat and spiritually quite conventional. He interpreted Elaine's need for more zest in her life and more support at home as simply a case of 'never being satisfied with herself or anyone around her.' At the end of three years of therapy she had made a bit of progress, showing some more laughter and a bit more assertiveness in asking for help. But the primary ethical concern remained subjective guilt. Until I asked Elaine to do a bit of watercolor drawing in an effort to access her right brain's process and get behind her well-defended probity.

"I did what you asked me to," she said at the beginning of our next session. She handed me the drawing tablet made more substantial by the after effects of her watercolors. She had filled easily a dozen pages with images of physical abuse and sexual abuse at the hands of a faceless figure wearing a clergy collar. "Perhaps I should tell you the whole story," she said after I looked up from the pages. The 'whole story' took another two years for her to unpack. Involved were three different ministers dating back to her adolescence as well as a long-time provision of sexual services to her department's chief. He had purchased her new car and provided her with additional money for clothing that enabled her to dress well beyond her means in exchange for her loyalty and her silent service.

"As you can see, I am an adulteress," she finally said. "I just don't see any way out of this. I cannot quit because I enjoy the extra money but I am a whore. I don't think God will ever forgive me and certainly I cannot go to our internal human resource officer since I could not bear the shame of being exposed and the guilt of ruining everyone's life." So here, finally, was realistic ethical guilt. She was regularly violating a premier tenant of her religious faith as well as providing her superior with sexual favors for which he paid dearly and which extracted a terrible price within her own marriage.

Putting aside these deeper issues for later chapters, the ethical focus of care developed along two lines: what practical steps could she take to begin untangling herself from her on-going exploitation and what spiritual steps could she begin that would place her self-defined identity of 'adulteress and whore' into a different ethical framework? Clearly we had long ago left behind the clinical focus of her depression although a mild anti-depressant began helping her view life more brightly. We had entered this more complex world of bondage that dated back into childhood abuse and continued into her adult life with significant financial rewards. No amount of thought stopping or challenging negative beliefs would reduce her depression if these ethical and spiritual questions remained unaddressed and she remained dependent upon her supervisor for emotional excitement and financial assistance.

Briefly put, the realistic ethical concerns came to a rather abrupt end when, two years later, her husband took a new job that moved them out of state. While this brought an end to her immediate entanglement, it did not end her entrapment in a self-identity rooted in psychological perfectionism and what we came to identify as the sin of greed. Her resulting despair would require the work of a new therapist in her new community. A decade after the move, her telephone call alerted me that this work of this unnamed colleague had been successful. Identifying the ethical legitimacy of returning unopened the supervisor's follow-along mail and quietly placing number blocks on her home phone and cell phone did much was the focus of our final month's work and it set the foundation upon which she re-established her moral clarity and began to see some hope for her marriage.

At this point in the diagnostic enterprise, Elaine's diagnosis would look like this, utilizing both the formal DSM-IV system and my multi-axial system of diagnosis:

DSM-IV Diagnosis:
Axis I – Dysthymic Disorder-300.40
Axis II – Compulsive Personality – 301.40
Axis III – Migraine headaches – 346.90
Axis IV – Marital and vocational problems
Axis V- GAF Current: 55 GAF Last Year: 60

Spiritual / Theological Multi-axial Diagnosis:
Axis I- Guilt – realistic related to violation of marriage vows;
          Subjective related to violation of personal standards of
          performance in work and marriage.

Case # 2 – Adultery

"I brought something for you to listen to,'" Robert said while opening his briefcase. The sound of a telephone being dialed came onto the audiotape. The male voice answering immediately shifted into a soft tone as he heard the woman's voice greet him. "He's left for work," she said. "I'm waiting here for you," he replied. The voices quickly dropped to the conspiratorial level.

He reached over and stopped the tape. The room grew quiet and Robert retrieved the tape, returning it to his briefcase. He looked up, his eyes filled with a mixture of sadness, disbelief, anger and resignation. "What now?" He asked.

"How does this information help you?" I asked.

"Well, now I know I'm not crazy. I would have never have believed she could betray me so thoroughly. I feel so disoriented. This morning she smiled at me, wished me a good day, kissed me goodbye and reminded me that our daughter has to stay after school for band practice," Robert continued. "That means I'll be fixing dinner because Melanie will be picking up our daughter."

"I have hired a detective," he said. "Proving her betrayal will help me regain my sanity and maybe keep me from having to pay so much in spousal support." During the next several weeks he would find out more about his wife of twenty-three years than he wanted to know. "I would have never guessed she could be so devious," he would say again and again. Tears, rage, fear and frustration repeatedly cycled across his face and soul.

While in the end the information developed by the detective provided him with leverage in negotiations, the information also thoroughly destroyed his respect for the woman he had once pledged to love without reservation. To the very end, in spite of very compromising photographs and hotel receipts, she maintained her meetings were entirely innocent and her now-ex-husband a scoundrel for 'spying' on her. Robert struggled to believe his own eyes and ears long after the final decree of divorce was granted.

Digital technology in cell phones and the web-based Internet have given a new dimension to the millennia old betrayal at the heart of adultery. But the ethical, spiritual and existential distress remains the same: trust is compromised, suspicion is heightened and heartache exudes into the next generation. No wonder the Seventh Commandment is an absolute prohibition and is on an equal plane with murder. Regardless of the technology used, adultery places all parties in an ethical and relational hot zone; including the clinician or pastor who is sought out for solace and guidance.

Leaving aside for later chapters the spiritual and existential dimensions of adultery, what are the ethical concerns in counseling when the presenting problem is infidelity and adultery? As is so often the case, simply defining the terms plays an important role in a client's facing realistic and subjective guilt. Frequently the defense of 'we're just friends' is followed up after the divorce with the question, "can't we still be friends?" I have counseled couples and individuals on both sides of this relational minefield, both the one betrayed and the one who does the betraying. The topic of guilt must be fairly and squarely addressed. No amount of legerdemain that 'it is the relationship we're treating' will satisfy each person's deep need to have their moral wound addressed and redressed.

Naming the pain of realistic guilt is a necessary part of bringing healing to a troubled marriage, especially when infidelity or adultery is involved. The person who has broken the marital covenant feels justified in their transgression because of a host of antecedent failures on the part of their spouse. Their spouse must listen to these concerns and the therapist must aid the betraying spouse in expressing them. But in no way do the revisiting of these wounds ultimately justify breaking the inherent trust of the marital promises. The betraying spouse must terminate the affair and submit to a regime of accountability if the marriage has any hope of surviving.

The betrayed partner will initially focus on the very real details of the affair, wanting details that may seem lurid and intrusive. In the best of situations this realistic focus will lay the groundwork for genuine forgiveness. The therapist must assist the one betrayed in gradually shifting this inquiry from one of interrogation to one of interpretation. This occurs once the realistic details are satisfactorily addressed by both parties and they can then begin to look more deeply at the subjective betrayal – both must answer this question: 'how could I have treated you so poorly? What on earth or in heaven was I thinking?'

As a therapist I have seen both clients and colleagues move too quickly away from acknowledging the realistic dimension of guilt when adultery is the presenting concern. Yet because behavioral self-control is the foundation of security, only through an examination of this area can a person adequately assure themselves and their spouse that the relationship is back on firm ground. This examination helps reinstitute both self-control and re-establish central acts of caring within the marriage. Helping couples state their needs clearly, including what they will not tolerate, is an important facet of the couple's rediscovery of their love language and is the only way for them to move into acceptance and ultimately forgiveness.

The subjective side of guilt takes much longer for a couple to truly work through. There is a plethora of popular literature and websites available for this stage of providing care. It is my experience that all of these resources will help people come to terms with the subjective consequences of marital betrayal. The primary issue for the treating clinician and pastor has more to do with selecting the appropriate resource that will match the couple's value system and level of sophistication.

The subjective side of guilt also remains the enduring concern if couple does not reconcile but proceeds to divorce due to adultery. Absent a wholesale admission of moral failure on the part of the offending party, if the person betrayed is to recover they frequently spend years churning over the details of their failures in the marriage. It is the duty of the therapist to guide this soul-felt self-examination in a direction that leads back to greater maturity. Allowing the parishioner or client to remain in the famous Slough of Despond is supremely unhelpful.

At this point in the diagnostic enterprise, Robert's diagnosis would look like this, utilizing both the formal DSM-IV system and my multi-axial system of diagnosis:

> *DSM-IV Diagnosis:*
> *Axis I* – Adjustment Disorder with Mixed Emotional Features – 309.00
> *Axis II* – No Diagnosis on Axis II – V71.90
> *Axis III* – No condition reported
> *Axis IV* – Marital separation
> *Axis V*- GAF Current: 65   GAF Last Year: 65

Spiritual / Theological Multi-axial Diagnosis:
Axis I-Guilt: Realistic guilt over failure of marriage; subjective mood of failure and personal recrimination.

Case # 3 – Developmental Challenges

The first thing I noticed about the eight-year-old boy in the waiting room was his immature appearance. His face still had the round softness typically seen in a younger child. Mother had done her homework, bringing along a two-page list of observations and statements about her son. 'Very few, if any friends' and 'never wants to go into room where all kids stay until time to go into Sunday school class room' were listed side-by-side with more serious observations such as 'has begun saying that he might as well be dead' and 'teacher said he is in another world sometimes.'

I was surprised when she left the room and he began at once demonstrating inquisitiveness about my office. I was also surprised at how easily he made negative statements about himself. He quite readily said 'I am no good at anything' something he repeated consistently throughout subsequent sessions. His father accompanied him to the next several sessions and was quite cooperative with the process of my getting to know his son. But the child's negative self-evaluation continued and he was quite resistant to cognitive challenges or demonstrations of his competence. By the fourth session he said, "I like violence" and demonstrated it by repeatedly trying to strike me. For several moments it felt as though I was back on a locked ward working as an aide.

This experience, along with the primitive quality of the child's drawing convinced me there was more a more basic condition in the child besides depression or either type of guilt. Thus the initial ethical question had more to do with the source of his conduct rather than the consequences of his conduct. There needed to be baseline clarity about his basic neuropsychology or if he was enduring some type of abuse. Since his teacher had noted he 'snarled and glared at a child who offended him even after the child said he was sorry,' I was tending more toward the former rather than the latter explanation.

His parents were quite cooperative about receiving the referral. "We need to rule out whether Philip is having some primary cognitive difficulty or if he is strongly depressed and hyperactive," I said. A thorough neuropsychological evaluation produced the following results:

- Referral Diagnosis of ICD-9 of 294.8 Cognitive Difficulties NOS is supported
- A secondary diagnosis of ICD-9 of 314.00 Attention Deficit Hyperactivity Disorder is supported

- Other diagnosis may be relevant as well, including a possible childhood form of ICD-9 of 29.20 Depression

The recommendations were for a thorough educational assessment as well as continued counseling to focus on increasing his awareness of social cues and continuing to challenge his cognitive distortions.   This approach would hopefully inoculate Philip from receiving the *de rigueur* referral for 'anger management counseling' that many boys receive for standard male conduct while also taking seriously the need for him to learn appropriate social conduct. There was a much more basic condition that needed sustained collaborative attention from parents and professionals.

Providing care for Philip would thus necessitate structuring tasks that were appropriate to his actual abilities. Expecting age-appropriate performance in competitive tasks such as playing soccer or social tasks such as cooperative play would only confirm his negative self-assessment. Care of Philip would also include reinforcing his parents' generally supportive attitude toward their son as they also parented his siblings. Clinically I continued to wonder if Philip was showing early signs of Asperger's Disorder (299.80).

At this point in the diagnostic enterprise, Phillip's diagnosis would look like this, utilizing both the formal DSM-IV system and my multi-axial system of diagnosis:

> *DSM-IV Diagnosis:*
> *Axis I –* Cognitive Difficulties – 294.90
>   Attention Deficit Hyperactivity Disorder – 314.00
>   Childhood Depression – 311.00
> *Axis II –* Asperger's Disorder – 299.80 (rule out)
> *Axis III –* None reported
> *Axis IV –* School difficulties, especially socialization
> *Axis V-* GAF Current: 50 GAF Last Year: 55
>
> *Spiritual / Theological Multi-axial Diagnosis:*
> *Axis I-*   Guilt: no realistic guilt; strong feelings of subjective
>   guilt related to negative self-image.

Case # 4 – End of Life Concerns

It was one of those all-too-common summer tragedies. One moment Steve was a healthy 17-year-old life-of-the-party rising senior at Feitchen's High School. After racing his best friend to the floating dock at Echo Lake, he challenged his pal to a diving context. Before he could be warned, Steve tried to execute a cutaway dive known as the can opener. His head hit the edge of the dock with a sickening crack audible on the shore.

"I just knew it was bad," said his girl friend Jessica as she waited in the hospital's emergency room. "We all screamed. Chelsea ran right away to the house and called 911."

Steve's friend, a trained lifeguard, knew enough to carefully try to stabilize his Steve's neck as he floated limply in the water. "But I really didn't think he was going to make it," he said later to his pastor. "All my training and I couldn't save my friend!"

The hospital chaplain was now meeting with the family. "This has to be your worst nightmare," she said quietly. She stayed with them as the surgeons attempted to relieve the pressure and swelling to his brain.

"This is the most easily damaged part of the brain," the surgeon later explained. It is what makes Steve 'Steve.' Right now his neck is being stabilized." His parents nodded, trying to grasp the unthinkable choice that they would likely have to make.

"Can he get better? Can the doctors save him?" His mother asked later asked after the doctor left.

"We certainly hope for a return to health," the chaplain replied. "But Steve may also retain permanent brain damage or he may die," she continued. "The most difficult choice you will face is if Steve remains alive yet does not recover his former level of health. We do not know at this point what Steve's outcome will be. All of us hope and pray for the best," she concluded.

"Steve sighed the organ donor option on his driver's license," offered his father. "How do we know the doctors...," his voice trailed off into an embarrassed silence.

"Our primary goal is to save Steve's life," said the chaplain. "If you would like to talk about organ donation, it is best to have that conversation once we know more about his medical condition."

"Our pastor should be here any moment," said his mother. "Can he come back here and be with us?"

"Certainly," replied the chaplain. "I'll insure the front desk staff know to bring him back," she said. After excusing herself, she made her way toward the waiting room. On the way her pager indicated a call from surgery. She made her way there after briefly alerting the receptionist to the impending arrival of the family's pastor.

"One look at the surgeon's face told me the news was not good," she later said. The pressure on his brain created by the trauma was significant enough to produce some permanent damage. "The surgeon wasn't sure what the next twenty-four to forty-eight hours would bring. So he was suggesting a family consult in which he would advise continued care. I told him the family's pastor was on the way and he indicated that Steve would be placed in the Instant Care Unit."

". . . .And we ask, O Lord, that Thy healing power would guide this staff and surround Steve in this time of great distress and uncertainty. Amen!" A man obviously their minister was finishing up as the chaplain re-entered the room.

"The family received the update from the surgeon in grim-faced silence," the chaplain would later say. "Their pastor was wonderful and indicated that members of the congregation's Stephen Ministry would be providing a round-the-clock presence with the family in addition to his own periodic visits. We both accompanied the family into Instant Care and had a very brief prayer once the staff had made Steve comfortable," she concluded.

At this point the family's pain is profound and extends across all three diagnostic axis. Yet within the next two days they will likely face a basic practical question that will be the nexus of these three axis: has Steve recovered enough of his life's quality to justify continued care or does the family remove life support and allow his life to end? Their answer to this question will be guided by their religious belief and moral values as much as it will be informed by whatever Steve's medical condition becomes. For now, the diagnostic tasks are ones of supporting this family through this dark passage while they seek to understand the awfulness of fully comprehending their son's pain and finding the voice necessary to name their own pain.

Leaving aside for the moment the examination of this question, a part of the pain in Steve's condition has to do with the awful consequences of his conduct. If Steve recovers full consciousness, there will come some moment when he begins to face the fact that he alone is responsible for his condition. In a similar vein, although it is premature to explore with them, Steve's parents and close friends will not only recognize this but also likely hate themselves for feeling angry toward him for placing everyone in this awful situation. Naming this level of pain and guiding them all through this unfortunate Hellspont will require great sensitivity as well as level-headed directness on the part of the clinician or chaplain who raises the question.

At this point in the diagnostic enterprise, Steve's diagnosis would look like this, utilizing both the formal DSM-IV system and my multi-axial system of diagnosis:

> *DSM-IV Diagnosis:*
> *Axis I –* No Diagnosis – V71.09
> *Axis II –* No Diagnosis- V71. 09
> *Axis III –* Concussion, cerebral – 851.80
> *Axis IV –* Unresponsive to stimuli
> *Axis V-* GAF Current: 0   GAF Last Year: +90

> *Spiritual / Theological Multi-axial Diagnosis:*
> *Axis I*   Guilt: Realistic due to his role in his injury; subjective is
>   unavailable for him but profound for his family.

Case # 5 – Vocational Assessment for Ministry

Hope is a 35-year-old woman who seeks ordination in a mainline Protestant denomination. She holds a Master's degree although not the traditional one in divinity that most mainline denominations require. After demonstrating an initial sense of call to the vocation of ministry in a meeting with her own minister and a review of her activities in the local community by a committee of her church, she was referred to a regional body for further review and psychological assessment. This step included an independent review of her credit and a police background check in addition to completing a battery of psychological tests. The results of this testing was reviewed by an independent pastoral evaluation specialist who conducted a clinical interview with Hope and submitted a report to the regional body's executive.

The initial results of the testing did not bode well for Hope. Like most candidates for the professional ministry, she was sensitive, sympathetic and able to empathize with others. She believes in inherent human goodness. She was academically competent. She will tend to be bold, uninhibited and adventurous. She will have little difficulty meeting strangers. She is forthright to such an extent that she may speak sometimes before carefully considering the impact of her words. "The candidate may feel tension between needing to go out of her way to please others to gain acceptance yet inwardly resent the need to conform to societal rules in order to please people," was how the evaluator put it in her report.

However, Hope's overall response to the testing indicated a tendency to presents herself in a negative manner. She placed herself in an unfavorable light, something rather unusual for an individual applying for a professional position. Hope appeared to be introspective and 'someone who will follow her own moral standards rather than around culturally admired traits such as self-discipline, organization or conventional ideals,' commented the evaluator. Hope appeared to be socially bold to such an extent that she may not pick up on the cues of people's reactions toward her. She will tend to base her decisions about events on her own thoughts and subjective responses rather than on objective facts.

Thus the assessment specialist's initial conclusion was that while Hope had several strengths that would serve well in some helping professions, she would create problems in a local church and bring heartache to herself. Her strengths included an ability to be empathic, to establish new relationships rapidly, to network with other professionals and to think outside of the traditional cultural paradigm. However, based on the testing the evaluator concluded that Hope had a number of liabilities that would inhibit her effectiveness within a religious community. These included difficulty following established cultural norms, a marked tendency to either disregard negative consequences from poor performance or to significantly underestimate the risks in a new situation, and to be dismissive of practical details.

Thus while professional ethics mandated a clinical review of the test results with Hope, the ultimate ethical challenge would remain with Hope and her chosen denomination. Would the results of the clinical interview be enough to offset the obvious deficits indicated by the psychological testing? "Unfortunately, my experience is that most mainline denominations will proceed with a candidate such as this rather than say 'No' to the candidate," said the evaluator to a colleague with whom she sought consultation. The evaluator's consultant advised her to be kind but direct in sharing the test results with Hope as well as documenting Hope's response to the results.

"Your job is to provide an accurate assessment," said the evaluator's consultant. "It is the denomination's responsibility whether or not to proceed with Hope as a candidate. One thing is certain: if you do not provide an accurate report, you and your agency are as liable as the denomination if there is any future failure in Hope's ministry."

Clearly there was pain in Hope that required some degree of identification. Equally clear was the obligation to alert her denomination to the likelihood that her pain could bring significant distress to unsuspecting congregants should they proceed to place Hope in a professional position. In this situation the challenge was not so much to identify the realistic and subjective dimensions of Hope's pain as it was to provide her and her denomination with sufficient effective care so that she was not placed in a vocation for which she appeared to have little genuine aptitude. "How she is living out her baptismal vow is your task to help her and her community discern," concluded the evaluator's supervisor. "Whether or not this should lead to her ordination is not your task," he concluded. Then he added, "I would get Hope's permission to record your session."

At this point in the diagnostic enterprise, Hope's diagnosis would look like this, utilizing both the formal DSM-IV system and my multi-axial system of diagnosis:

>   *DSM-IV Diagnosis:*
>
>   *Axis I* – Depressive Disorder NOS – 311.0
>
>   *Axis II* – Dependent Personality Disorder with
>
>   Narcissistic features – 301.60
>
>   *Axis III* – None Reported
>
>   *Axis IV* – Vocational Difficulties
>
>   *Axis V* – GAF Current: 55   GAF Last Year: 55

Spiritual / Theological Multi-axial Diagnosis:

Axis I- Guilt: Realistic failure of prior efforts at finding work; subjective belief that she is flawless.

Conclusion

The tasks of diagnosis are always secondary responses to the initial encounter between a troubled individual and a person tasked to provide providing care. Thus in each of the above vignettes the counselor, chaplain, evaluation specialist follow a course of action roughly similar to the suffering person and those that are near them: we look to find some explanation for the distress and hope to discern a pathway toward improved well-being.

A necessary part of this all-too-frequently lifelong task is the necessary step of distinguishing between whatever anguish is the legitimate consequence of an individual's conduct and how much of the anguish is an inappropriate subjective response to the situation. It is easy to either dismiss individual responsibility completely for misfortune or for the individual to be crushed under an inordinate amount of guilt and shame. Professional care providers steeped in post-modern ethics are as likely to be uncomfortable with the ethical dimension of diagnosis as are most suffering people to be tempted toward assuming total responsibility for their condition.

These vignettes will be enhanced by additional information and discussion at the conclusion of subsequent parts that address issues of idolatry and defilement. We are now turning toward matters of idolatry. *Selah!*

Part III-Idolatry: the Feeling of Betrayal

Chapter 9: Knocking On Heaven's Door

Depending upon our age, most of us remember not just where we were when significant events occurred; we also hold on to the fundamental sense of shock we felt as the events unfolded. The stock market crash of 1929, the attack on Pearl Harbor, the assassinations of President Kennedy, Robert Kennedy and Martin Luther King, Jr., the triple-assaults of September 11, 2001, the Christmas tsunami of 2004 that overwhelmed Sri Lanka or the multiple hurricanes of 2005 that devastated America's Gulf Shore produced cultural earthquakes that redefined self-understanding as well as national destiny. Other cultures and nations have similar events in their history that alter individuals' belief in their own abilities as well as violate their trust in larger structures to providentially protect them from harm.

Thus in the aftermath of the terrorist attacks of September 11th there was an outcry to first understand and then blame those deemed to have failed for 'not connecting the dots' of discreet clues that might have prevented this devastating surprise attack on American soil. While the intelligence community scrambled to reconstitute itself, even Americans well informed about the difficulties of interdicting a well-planned surprise attack were left with the assessment that to some extent we were betrayed by the very structures we had counted upon to vouchsafe our security. While the most mature post-mortem to any such disaster, whether from natural or human agents, focuses on improving societal safeguards, these improvements rest upon the belief that such safeguards will protect us from future betrayals by Mother Nature's fury and our neighbor's perfidy.

On a much less public but no less devastating consequences this same earthquake in human consciousness occurs when significant personal events shatter our trust in those we had a reasonable expectation of care. Being fired or downsized by an employer, discovering a spouse's adultery, experiencing an assault or rape, suffering abuse by a parent, or finding that your company's pension plan is worthless due to corrupt business practices are but a few examples of such events. Once again there comes with these events both the immediate trauma of loss and the more lengthy loss of faith in those individuals or structures we had come to view as beneficent. As much as we might bravely say that such events add to our resiliency, such statements come long after the events and reflect the wisdom of maturity. None of us willingly chose such betrayals so that our hearts are strengthened and our coping skills enhanced.

Our human trust in imperfect people, limited human institutions and certifiably whimsical natural forces is beneath whatever practical and moral failures lead up to such failures. In religious terms this trust is known as idolatry: placing ultimate trust in something or someone other than God. The most effective parents fail us. The most beneficent leaders prove unworthy or unwise. The most beatific locale reminds us we are no longer in Eden's garden. We may respond to these failures with what we believe to be purely 'secular' resources. But the wisest among us recognize that such betrayals are most fully responded to by the marshalling of spiritual resources of our cardinal virtues and a more fully informed embrace of religion's tenants.

Such failings provide the pain that needs to be named in diagnosis. The search for such resources and learning how to employ them with skill become the provision of care that guides humane treatment. This portion of the volume will focus on this second area of the diagnostic enterprise.

But before turning to this area, one other aspect of idolatry that prompts people to seek professional help needs to be recognized. This aspect is an explicit crisis in religious faith. Most often this crisis comes as a part of an individual's discovery their religious beliefs or spiritual resources are inadequate to succor them in the face of such aforementioned betrayals. This is the age-old issue of theodicy, typically framed as 'why did God allow this to happen?' The thorough naming of this pain may begin with the recognition that an individual's spiritual resources were woefully inadequate for the task of adult living or it may be only that an individual needs to be reminded of the resources inherent in their religious faith. Whatever the level of spiritual maturity or the content of religious faith, adequate and effective naming of human pain and provision of humane treatment must now include an ability to address such concerns or refer people to professionals who can assist them in this task.

Naming the Gods in Diagnosis

The pile on the table is always quite impressive. Keys to a Mercedes Benz may lie beside an archer's shooting glove. A Scofield Reference Bible might repose beside a pitch pipe. Sometimes a bottle of Jack Daniel's or a pack of Marlboro's will join in creating the montage.

"I want you to bring an idol to next week's class," I've instructed them. For those who need a bit more direction, I will add, "make it something you center your life around. Something you might kill or die for. Bring something that has made you the person you are or hope to become."

In the religious literalism of our youth, we may have assumed that because we were not offering our first-born child to Molech we were not worshipping any idols. But any pastor or mental health professional can identify any number of objects and goals to which persons offer themselves, their resources, children and futures. In the broadest religious terms, the diagnostic question is simply "what is the name of your idol?" and not "is there an idol which you worship?" Our violating idols are primarily something, or someone, who's legitimate worth or power has become overly valued or whose true value is suddenly discovered. Some idols have explicitly religious names and recognized ceremonies. But the more insidious ones that drive hurting persons to our doorstep are the implicit principalities, thrones and powers we are absolutely convinced we cannot live without. These form the patterns of our personalities and the rites of our various compulsions.

During my first parish service the tragedy of a mass suicide in Jonestown, Guyana spread across the newspaper's front page in what is typically called Second Coming type. "How awful and incomprehensible," exclaimed a woman in my parish. She spoke for all of us. Here was a situation of clear and explicit idolatry that finally took the lives of over 900 adherents. Learning the details about the tragedy, and the decade of events that preceded it, one could discern the familiar patterns of religious recruitment, individual conversion and gradually increasing isolation of the cult from the mainstream.

But Jonestown is not even the most recent incarnation of a more fundamental process of life-transforming religious violation. What is the difference between the uniform of tennis shoes, black pants and button-down white shirts of the Heaven's Gate cult, the plain clothes worn by a member of Old Order Baptist group who sat in my parish office struggling over continued membership in the "church" and the summary execution of those who convert to another faith besides Islam? So often one community's faithful presentation of God can be wounding and even homicidal to those judged to be heretics or infidels. Sometimes the wounding comes from without our own psyches.

Naming the idol in diagnosis can be a difficult and delicate task. Thus as one practitioner aptly notes, "the task of taking on the gods is at the heart and soul of pastoral counseling." (1) We can suggest three broad categories in which one may search for idols: explicit religion, implicit religion and secular religion. Each area has some recognizable gods. Their violation of our selves and their sacrificial demands gravely affect our well-being. They may even inhabit-and inhibit-our own consulting room and our pulpit. The presence of religious belief in human beings, whether explicit or implicit, is pervasive. The clinician ignores this data at peril to both self and client. It is worth remembering that our calling something an idol does not deprive it of power in the life of a true believer, a family, community or in an entire culture.

Visible Gods of Explicit Religion

Every religious faith has a set of tenants by which it defines itself. We might call these tenants the fundamentals of the faith. These fundamentals are a complex mixture of foundational sacred writings, rites and traditions that interpret these writings in addition to events of the religion's chief promulgators. While all the great religions seek to engender a posture of spiritual devotion toward the universe and moral rectitude toward fellow humans, each religion makes claims about the ultimate nature of reality that in practice are mutually exclusive of one another.

The area of explicit religion contains gods who are supported by a belief system that the worshipper can elucidate. Explicit idols are a perversion of a genuine religious faith, usually reinforced by an identifiable sub-group or cultic community within a major religion although sometimes an individual's misunderstanding of a great religion approaches the status of idolatry. This happens typically when portions of one or more faith groups,' creeds and rites under gird corporate belief or individual piety. An explicit idol can influence religious traditions within a world that are polar opposites, primarily because idols appeal to our more fundamental broken, prideful nature. Because religion by its very nature addresses questions of ultimate meaning, the individual practice of religious belief varies widely within any of the great religions.

For example, within the Christian faith there is a wide range of denominations and fellowships. While these all affirm an explicit Trinitarian understanding of the divine and base their doctrines on the Bible, there is significant difference between Orthodox, Roman Catholic, Reformed and Free Church understandings of their core doctrines. The same is true within Islam, as we see the tensions between the Sunni and Shia as they understand the life of Mohammed and interpret the Koran. Judaism's spread of belief from Orthodox, Conservative and Reformed is yet another example of such diversity within a single religious faith. Idolatry results within a great religion when an individual or group elevates specific aspects of their faith so that it becomes the focus of devotion rather than the mystery of the Deity.

Counselors are likely to see idolatrous religious faith in one of two ways: a crisis of religious belief triggered by an life crisis or chaos in life created by an overly pious practice of a religion's central tenants. The historic way in which contemporary mental health providers have dealt with this topic has been to create the fiction that somehow an individual's problems could be addressed and resolved without reference to their religious belief. While we may be at a point where care providers now take seriously the role of an individual's religion in promoting their mental and physical health, we are not at a point where care providers feel competent to adequately discern what distinguishes a religion's healthy belief and practice from an idolatrous set of beliefs and practices.

One way of helping an individual name the pain inherent within their religious belief is to take them through a spiritual assessment. This is not a theological litmus test of the person's orthodoxy but more of an appraisal of the way in which their religious belief either enhances or degrades the quality of their life. Since no counselor or mental health worker can be an expert on the wide variety of religious traditions even within a single great religion, these open-ended questions formulated by Dr. Howard Clinebell are a helpful framework for assessing the relative health of an individual's religious belief. One can assess to what extent the religious beliefs, attitudes and practices of the individual accomplishes or moves toward the following goals:

- Give them a meaningful philosophy of life that provides trust and hope in facing the inevitable tragedies of life?
- Provide creative values and ethical sensitivities that serve as inner guidelines for behavior that is both personally and socially responsible?
- Provide an integrating, energizing, growing relationship with that loving Spirit that religions call God?
- Inspire an ecological love of nature and reverence for all life?
- Provide for a regular renewal of basic trust by affirming a deep sense of belonging to the universe?
- Bring the inner enrichment and growth that comes from 'peak experiences?
- Offer the person a growth-enabling community   of caring and meaning?
- Build bridges rather than barriers between them and persons of different values and faith systems?
- Enhance love and self-acceptance (rather than fear and guilt) in their inner life?
- Foster self-esteem and the 'owning' and using of their strengths in constructive living?
- Stimulate the growth of their inner freedom and autonomy?
- Help them develop depth relationships committed to mutual growth?
- Encourage the vital energies of sex and assertiveness to be used in affirmative, responsible ways rather than in repressive or people-damaging ways?
- Foster realistic hope by encouraging the acceptance rather than the denial of reality? (2)

This is not an exhaustive list. Use of these queries will assist a clinician in determining whether or not the individual needs referral to someone who can address the way in which the a particular set of religious beliefs is deteriorating their life. It is worth noting that providers of relational and psychological care should develop referral sources for the variety of religious faiths with as much diligence as they develop professionals who are experts at the diagnosis and treatment of specific psychological disorders.

While not idolatry in the narrow sense, an individual who is seeking religious truth often undergoes a period of intense questioning of their childhood religious beliefs. Mature religious leaders and devotees understand that this period of exploration is a necessary step in spiritual growth. However, to the individual and perhaps to their family or community this may appear to be either idolatry or apostasy. In some cases an individual literally takes their life in their own hand when they explore another religious faith (Islam) or they risk being excluded from the community should they choose to leave the fellowship for another expression of spiritual truth (Old Order Baptist). Anyone providing counseling to an individual undergoing such an exploration needs to respect both the intensity and the seriousness of this quest, especially if the counselor's own religious faith is meager or informed by a post-modern viewpoint that tends to minimize the reality of ultimate truth.

Invisible Gods of Implicit Religion

Now let us turn to some idols of implicit religion. They too carry their own structure of belief and piety. They sometimes have their own holy writings, sacred places of gathering and rites of initiation. Their only distinction may be that they are not explicitly tax-exempt and that some of their rites may be illegal. Within the clinical world of the DSM-IV these are the personality disorders, compulsions and addictions. But within the life of the individual and those who surround them, these entrenched patterns acquire a life force every bit as powerful as a religion and they persist down through a family's history by both stories and genetics with as much influence as any spiritual devotion. Understood from a purely clinical viewpoint, personality disorders, compulsions and addictions derive their corrosive power from misplaced attachment and a neurological system hijacked by powerful chemicals. The clinical definition of a personality disorder and the behavioral recognition of a destructive compulsion or addiction reads for all the world like devotion to what the Athenians of St. Paul's day called 'The Unknown God' (3):

> The essential feature of a Personality Disorder is an enduring pattern of inner experience and behavior that deviates markedly from the expectations of the individual's culture and is manifested in at least two of the following areas: cognition, affectivity, interpersonal functioning or impulse control. This enduring pattern is inflexible and pervasive across a broad range of personal and social situations and leads to clinical significant distress or impairment in social, occupational or other important areas of functioning. The pattern is stable and of long duration, and its onset can be traced back at least to adolescence or early adulthood. (4)

The pervasiveness and enduring qualities of these various disorders as well as the havoc they create within the person's life as well as within society are indicative of their life-changing power. Effective diagnosis and care of an individual's personality disorder must include the use of spiritual or religious resources that take seriously the power of idolatry in human affairs.

Wayne Oates noted the essential link between clinical personality disorders and religious sentiment in his classic book *Behind the Masks: Personality Disorders in Religious Behavior.* "These ordinarily are sane people," he wrote, "but they wear their sanity as a mask, not as the outward expression of an inward possession. They are religious, but we are mystified that neither the sacraments of the liturgical churches nor the ordinances and professions of faith of the churches of the revival traditions have changed their obstinate ways of life but have only glossed them over with a veneer of religiosity." (5) His persistent observation that 'such persons have a pseudo self overlying the image of God in them' will resonate with anyone who has sought to maintain a relationship with an individual whose grip on self-destructive character traits approaches the devotion of any true believer, whether the person is overtly religious or not. (6)

While the diagnosis of a personality disorder is ruled out if the character traits appear to come primarily from the 'direct physiological effects of a substance,' frequent substance abuse can be a major factor in the more serious personality disorders as well as a significant disruptor of life's quality in their own right. Like a personality disorder, clinical dependence on a substance also reads much like a religious devotion to a god:

> The essential feature of Substance Dependence is a cluster of cognitive, behavioral and physiological symptoms indicating that the individual continues use of the substance despite significant substance related problems. There is a pattern of repeated self-administration that usually results in tolerance, withdrawal, and compulsive drug-taking behavior. (7)

Like any other religion, maintaining substance dependence and beliefs that maintain a personality disorder meets the criteria for idolatry: they are habits and things we are convinced we cannot live without. People will kill or die for their next hit of a drug; they will maintain their hostility, suspicion, passiveness or avoidant conduct even when facing profound losses up to and including divorce, bankruptcy and prison.

Dionysus, the ancient god of pleasure, has taken on the formidable persona of addictions in our time. (8) Addictions wield significant influence in our culture. Who has looked into the eyes of a baby going through crack withdrawal or listened to the grieving of a mid-life alcoholic and not seen Dionysus' violation? Dionysus offers us salvation by promising to transform our life. This deity has power to violate us from the very moment of our conception, as evidenced by Fetal Alcohol Syndrome. The rites and beliefs of Dionysus infect our family structures and language for generations. Dionysus teaches us the dynamics of denial and rewards deception. The social cost of Dionysian rites can devastate entire neighborhoods more extensively than a Category 4 hurricane. Insofar as the various substances do, indeed, alter our future from what and who we might otherwise have become, Dionysus can be said to deliver what his religion promises.

The various Anonymous programs take the spiritual component of addiction very seriously. They recognize that the addict is facing a crisis in religious belief and not simply a pharmacological problem. Given the pervasiveness of the world's drug supplies, devotees and refugees of Dionysus will be in every worship service, mosque, ashram and consulting room until the end of time. In this sense the worship of Dionysus is eternal. Paradoxically although many worship Dionysus in some form, few readily name him. Dionysian faith may be the best illustration of the ancient belief that to name a god is to finally have power over the god. Perhaps this explains that the first step in any 12-step program is the admission that one's life is in chaos, a tacit recognition that the god one is worshipping has failed.

Peter Tractenberg depicts the essentially spiritual dilemma at the core of addictions of all types eloquently in his study of sexual addiction:

> At the center of every addiction, as at the center of every cyclone, is a vacuum, a still point of emptiness that generates circles of frantic movement at its periphery. It is characterized not just by a feeling of worthlessness, the conviction that one deserves the destiny of a drunk or junkie, but by a blurred and tenuous sense of self – a fundamental uncertainty about one's own existence. (9)

The newly established *Core Competencies for Clergy and Other Pastoral Ministers In Addressing Alcohol and Drug Dependence and the Impact on Family Members* underscores not just the obvious role that religious leaders play in providing first-line intervention to the addicted person, family system and affected children. The fourth Competency prompts pastoral ministers 'to understand that addiction erodes and blocks religious and spiritual development.' It continues, 'and be able to communicate the importance of spirituality and the practice of religion in recovery.' (10) Not only is this competency important for all who treat individuals in the grip of the Dionysian god; its presence as a competency is a tacit recognition that addiction is a spiritual problem of idolatry as much as a neurobiological problem of a disrupted reward cycle.

Venus is the primordial goddess of love and beauty. Mystery and rites of initiation surround her. Like all deities she has the power to bless and curse those devoted to her. Venus is fueled by the fundamental capacity to create life. With the emergence of the HIV virus and other genetically transmitted diseases, the creative sexual act can transmit life and death within a single encounter. The pervasive presence of reproductive energy in all our explicitly religious rites demonstrates the difficulty of discerning life giving from life-shattering power. The ancient fertility gods demonstrate how basic this connection is in our development as creatures. The Biblical prophetic tradition railed against these gods in a way which our age seems to have reduced to a struggle between ma-triarchy and patriarchy. The continuing wreckage of misplaced sexuality indicates there may have been-and may continue to be-something more primary at stake in the prophet's concern than merely preserving male privilege.

One epiphany of Venus is through the masks of Misogyny and Mishomony. As the names imply, Venus can become incarnate through the degradation, brutalization and hatred of a single sex. The physical results of misogyny are grimly visible in any daily newspaper. The fact that the results of Mishomony are seldom reported, and therefore less visible, does not make it less serious. Fractured self-esteem cripples a person and deeply affects their future relationships, regardless of the sex of the recipient of the abuse. Sadism, with its strident paranoia and lust for power fuels these epiphanies of Venus-driven fundamentalism. The growing awareness of the 'war against boys' at least signals that the idol of mishomony is less invisible. (11)

Another epiphany of Venus is through the mask of sexual pleasure. Made incarnate in our culture through easy sexual encounters and the pervasive use of sexuality to sell everything from cars to deodorant, sexual pleasure promises us some facet of a 'better life' if only we follow or purchase whatever is being offered at the moment. The tragedies of AIDS, pregnant teenagers, guilt torn refugees from abortion clinics and the *ennui* of the empty Playboy Mansion speaks of Venus' fundamental barrenness. She is unable to deliver what she promises, although the recognition of her as a stillborn savior comes only once the damage is done.

The primary dilemma in naming the bondage we may feel toward this implicit god is the painful recognition that the very force that creates life is at the core of our destructive actions. It is terrifying to recognize that life and death may be genetically identical realities. It may be easy to describe the *dynamics* of denial but it is very difficult to recognize and leave behind the *behavior* (rites) that causes chronic pain for our self and those we profess to care about.

Secular Gods of Cultural Religion

The term 'cultural religion' most frequently refers to the fusion of a particular world religion with a culture or nation. Thus the cultures of the Middle East may be viewed through the lens of Islam as much as the culture of America may be viewed through the lens of Christianity and the culture of Mexico may be understood through the lens of Roman Catholicism. The tensions between such a major cultural matrix and an individual's specific understanding of themselves as their life unfolds is certainly one area where effective diagnosis requires a dual understanding of both a specific religion and its role within a culture as well as the clinician demonstrating the integrity to enquire how the individual's religious faith may be helping or hampering their response to life's challenges.

Thus while counseling is overwhelmingly focused on the dynamic pains within a single psyche or family, the pressures and themes within a nation can and do weigh upon the individuals who seek relief from heartache. Refugees from religious persecution or political upheaval for example may require counseling for post-traumatic stress disorder, depression, or anxiety. Orphans and the families that adopt them may require a host of resources to overcome the challenges of an attachment disorder. But the transition into a healthy life within a new nation requires coming to terms with the failures or losses inherent in leaving behind one culture and embracing the hopes and opportunities within the new nation. Negotiating through this mountain path requires more of the human spirit than simply the technical challenge of learning a new language.

In addition to this melding of a specific religion with a culture, there are also cultural beliefs or attitudes that, when challenged by events, produce within the individual as much a reappraisal of their values as when the inadequacy of their explicit religion is discovered. The discovery of their idolatry is no less real and the recognition of their idol's failure to deliver the goods is potentially no less or painful than in the other areas discussed in this chapter.

As his son went through the formation of becoming a U. S. Marine, Frank Schaeffer found his heretofore beliefs about America were shattered:

> I discovered a great truth by simply living in America for twenty years, long enough to compare facts to 'prophetic' doom-saying fantasies: the right, religious or otherwise, and the left, academic or otherwise, were wrong 90 percent of the time...It turned out that Ralph Nader and Pat Robertson were both full of shit...When John joined the Marines, I realized something shocking: I loved America. (12)

This shock illustrates what frequently happens as an individual names their pain at an idol's betrayal and moves through the stages of care that lead to greater maturity: they gain a more considered understanding of the culture's core values. These core values carry as much force as any explicit religion or implicit beliefs because of our personality structure. In Mr. Schaeffer's case the idol that crumbled was an amalgam of his father's Calvinistic critique of America as decadent and his peer's humanistic critique of America as a racist hegemony. No nation or culture is flawless. Desiring it to be perfect is as much a remnant of childhood narcissism that is as strong and as idolatrous as the demand that parents be always nurturing or an individual who never seems to develop past the conflict with authority figures that eats up so much of an adolescent's psychological and spiritual energy.

Our various nations invoke founding deities, whether they appear in primal myth or incarnate as historical founders. In times of crisis we appeal to their memory. We mark their birthdays as holy days of special celebration. We enshrine them in public temples of government and our debate over those shrines can be protracted and shrill as our debate over placing F. D. R. in a wheelchair or adding kneeling nurses and standing combat figures to the Vietnam Memorial area amply illustrate. We cast their names upon our boulevards and populate our parks with the their statues. Whether explicit, implicit or purely secular, there is a religious dimension to personal and social practices that shape our hearts and behavior. (13)

These are not necessarily misdirected practices. But as with all other gods, we are often oblivious to their life-shaping power. Or we overemphasize their life-giving contributions. Sometimes the terror these gods evoke is the terror that comes from being an oppressed cultural group. Sometimes the adoration these gods engender is one arising from the gratitude of liberation. More than one society has revolted against the extant gods because they failed to deliver the cargo of life and liberty. Such events never are too far outside of the ethos of a 50-minute clinical hour, the hospital bedside or the challenges around a family's dinner table.

Conclusion

Few individuals enter a counselor's office because they have explicit spiritual or religious concerns. However, the pains that compel them to seek assistance sometimes have a dimension that comes only as the individual refines their Values and embraces virtues that distinguish them from their family of origin or even the nation that gave them birth.

Helping individuals name such terror for what it is constitutes a part of the healing task. So is guiding them in effective ways to express the rage necessary for them to escape the bondage that holds them. Finding a new set of values and reclaiming the spiritual vitality is part of entering a new stage of human maturity. It is to an exploration of this task that we now turn. *Selah!*

Chapter Ten: Feeling Terror and Expressing Rage

We usually reserve the word 'terror' for movies that involve chain saws and aliens. More recently the word has become a descriptor for individuals who intentionally inflict carnage and death on innocent people to further their political ends. This chapter focuses on an individual's spiritual response of terror to the discovery the universe has turned against them and the rage necessary to reconstruct a connection with the Divine as an essential part of the healing enterprise.

Being stalked by a life-threatening disease is not unlike those never-dying monsters in the horror movies. Their claw always seems to come through the wall just when we've relaxed our grip on the theater's soft drink. One may feel a visceral terror as the time for the post-chemotherapy annual x-ray or MRI comes around again. Being attacked by someone you promised initially to 'love and cherish' or having the weather suddenly drop a downspout of destruction onto your home creates a primeval desire to flee to safety (the limbic system's instinctual response to life-threatening circumstances). This is the very response that a terrorist seeks to instill in an opponent's heart so that their victims either submit to their degrading demands or flee in defeat for safety.

We understand the desire to flee from horror. We typically utilize our spiritual resources to stand firm in the face of terror. We are uncomfortable with the expression of rage and marshalling the spiritual resources necessary to fight back against primal failures in our world or our relationships. Yet this response of rage is as necessary for us to name and guide as it is for caregivers to identify and provide compassion for fellow citizens in the grip of some terror. There are many conditions caregivers' encounter where someone's basic trust of another has been betrayed. Divorces, forced retirements, natural disasters and cata-strophic illness certainly provide ready examples of such betrayals. In spite of our best preparations these events can be terrifying. We desire our world to be predictable and safe for ourselves and for those we care about. This is more than a desire. We believe this is our *entitlement*. We do not *deserve* to get AIDS. We do not *deserve* to find our wife in the arms of another. We do not *deserve* to have the river wash away our home. It is not *fair* to watch the flag-draped casket of our son disembark from a military transport, carried by six comrades.

Try as we might to calm the post-disaster nightmares, the memories may echo whenever we hear the wind whistle or the boss clear her throat. Somehow the mantra 'I know that life isn't fair' fails to express our rage or help us reclaim the Holy. We long for the Greatest Grandfather to tell us about the good old days or for the Wisest Grandmother to hold us secure against the night.

Our feelings of terror have their roots in the ancient formulas of blessings and curses that under girds every religion. Gods demand followers who adore them. Believers who express the appropriate adoration and faithfulness are promised the blessings of prosperity and health (cargo). Gods may destroy followers who leave them for other gods, spread nasty rumors about them or who are generally disobedient. Thus to leave a god is to run the terrifying risk of being on the receiving end of a curse. Ancient myths are full of such stories and our nightmares give urgent power to such terrors in spite of our 21st century postmodern sophistication.

Yet our various gods fail us! We feel abandoned or singled out for special tragedy. When these failings occur we can find a way initially to explain their failure through a system of theodicy. But if a god's failures are persistent or their blessings are unsatisfying, we may finally feel compelled to abandon the god. Abandoning a god who has failed a believer inevitably involves destroying the deity. Thus iconoclastic rage becomes the converted backside of devotion to the icon. Conversions and new vocations may ultimately blossom from such a firestorm. But first comes the dark night of the soul. Reformations and the pronouncements of great church councils may be the ultimate institutional result of such demythologizing and restructuring. But their elder siblings are Ghost Dances and Inquisitions.

The immediate implications for both religious and secular clinician are that these dynamics of terror and rage may likely be present whenever there is a situation of betrayal or isolation. Our presence may evoke these deep feelings, seemingly unbidden by our action but more by our representative (countertransferential) status. If we have the presence of mind and grace of spirit to remain secure in the face of such terror and soothing in the swirling firestorm that destroys the idol, then we offer the opportunity for the person to reclaim the Holy. These are the continuing tasks for individuals as they slug their way through the mire of significant trauma as well as others for whom the distortion of early attachments have hardened into a mask of sanity behind which there is terror and out of which comes life-sapping rage.

"I Am Terrified at His Presence!"

The story of Job is one of a righteous man whose blessings are summarily removed by enduring unmerited suffering. As he struggles with three friends to express his anguish and understand the recent turn of events in his life, he comes to this fundamental expression of terror. (1) Whether an individual is explicitly Jewish or Christian, or comes for counsel from a purely secular background they are likely to be at least vaguely familiar with the story of Job.

We assume our life will unfold in an orderly pattern. If our childhood has been one of trust and appropriate nurture, we develop the resilience that is able to face the momentary terror of catastrophe, endure the suffering inherent in dread disease and discover new resources of belief and conduct for coping with the new life we have been given. But if our childhood has been one of distrust and we have not developed an appropriate sense of initiative and industry, then we come to expect life to be a negative venture of unending disappointment and distress. Our response to this corrosive turn of life's path typically shows itself in one of the many personality disorders found on the DSM-IV's second axis.

In his exploration of personality disorders, Wayne E. Oates aptly describes the underlying idolatry such individuals maintain. Whether caught in a dependent way of life deficient in personal initiative, living out the dramatic excitement of a histrionic personality or the darker hostilities of an anti-social personality that flouts the conventions of shared living, people cling to destructive patterns of life with a devotion worthy of a god. Oates lays the core flaw in these disorders as a longing for orderliness in life, even if that orderliness causes untold grief in others and chronic chaos for the individual. (2) Terror looks different in the various disorders and Oates does an exceptional job of providing any clinician with a compendium of ordinary-language depictions of how this idol-induced terror gets expressed.

Such terror, whether expressed through personality traits or embedded in a fully formed personality disorder, rob an individual of life's vitality and obstructs the peace of those who live with them. To cite just one example, Oates adds the characteristic of 'ignoring the foresight called for in planning' and a passive refusal to accept the instruction, discipline and sacrifice involved in earning credentials for getting ahead' to the passive-aggressive personality traits of 'procrastination, dawdling, stubbornness, intentional inefficiency and forgetfulness.' (3) Oates identifies this as a familial and cultural pattern as well as an individual trait. This is an approach to life genuinely fearful of divine wrath.

So is the lifestyle of the compulsive individual and the person whose detachment from life nevertheless prompts them to expect abuse from the world around them. The compulsive individual seeks to forestall divine wrath by taking for themselves the role of being God's attorney generals. The hyper vigilance and sensitivity to injustice of the avoidant personality also seeks to avoid the abuse and rejection from those near them to such an extent that they hold a fundamental belief that the divine has nothing better to do than to inflict additional suffering upon their life.

Effective diagnosis certainly begins with a thorough appraisal of the individual's family history and childhood; the roots of such terror are inevitably found there. Yet to fully comprehend the person's anxiety or negativism that resists fundamental transformation a clinician or minister must recognize the individual has come to believe reality is fundamentally terrifying in the way life is structured. For some individuals just naming this level of distress is the healing challenge. For others, the challenge is assisting them in getting beyond this deeply entrenched belief. In either case this is a lengthy process.

Standing alongside someone terrified at the prospect of leaving an inadequate god may be difficult but it does reimburse the counselor's efforts with a feeling of benign power. It is satisfying to be protective of another person. It is much more problematic to withstand the rage of someone whose projective identification may view the care provider as a primary source of their anguish. This virulent rage seems to boil up without warning from the very depth of a private Hell. For a period of time the caregiver as the person they know themselves to be *ceases to exist* in the psyche of the counselee. In "our" place the individual or couple "sees," incarnate, the very one who has produced the primary disruption in his or her life.

The major personality disorders and the results of chronic drug dependence are the primary categories where the pastor should be alert for such strong eruptions. It is important to remember that the person is trying to destroy a *god* even if the deity is manifested only through the epiphany of alcohol, the natural response of a frustrated employer or the client's misperception of a long-suffering spouse.

Sometimes the "god" that is left behind is an enmeshing parent or social structure. This de-structuring causes great anxiety for all concerned. In writing about this process within Jewish families, Howard Cooper notes, "the over-enmeshment of Jewish families can mean that parents, while consciously wishing for their children's success and independence, may unconsciously fear or resent or envy that same independence. Feelings of emptiness or rejection or anger can be hard to acknowledge when one is supposed to want all the best for them." (4) Obviously the counselor will need to position himself in such a way as to avoid replicating this anxiety within the family, whether the client is the parent or the separating member of the next generation. The linkage between this rather natural process and clinical realities is underscored by Cooper, for he notes, "sometimes the anger at the smothering expectations of parents becomes directed by the child . . . .against themselves. This leads to depressions, the eating problems and disorders, the use and abuse of tranquillizers, alcohol or drugs and the psychosomatic complaints that have become so prevalent in Anglo-Jewry." (5) It is more than fair to say this pattern is not limited to Anglo-Jewry.

Individuals with deeply engrained personality disorders come to counseling as a result of some social catastrophe or personal trauma. The temptation is for the clinician to repeat what other benevolent authority figures and social structures have attempted to accomplish with the person: support them through the crisis and assist them to adapt to life's present insult. This is not an entirely ineffective strategy, especially if the clinician can maintain an effective degree of empathy that provides for optimal frustration. Such a professional posture creates the bond necessary for the individual to lose some of their edgy terror while still challenging the person to address their own role in maintaining a dysfunctional life pattern.

One barrier to success with this therapeutic posture is likely to be the financial cost to the individual of remaining in therapy long enough for this terror to be fully recognized and resolved. Then there is the emotional cost such basic change requires as well as the necessity of confronting the fundamental resistance of individuals with this level of distress to accept counsel or guidance from some new authority, even if that authority is benevolent. It is easier for both the person and the caregiver to become sidetracked into a moibius band-like recitation of life's latest insult rather than addressing the core dynamic of terror.

Another barrier to naming the pain of terror is the overall reductionism by which the system of managed care imposes upon care providers. The image we have made is visible in any managed care's outpatient treatment plan. Check-off boxes from "mild to severe" cover a range of symptoms. More boxes from "none to high" cover "risk assessment" and there's even a pre-packaged list of interventions that I need only circle to indicate my treatment approach. I can choose from psychodynamic to experimental to psychopharmacology to strategic interventions.

Now while this is a helpful schema, the idolatry comes in when I begin to believe that in checking the appropriate boxes I have adequately described the person who has sought my care or, even more depraved, that I have actually delivered care through the act of checking off these boxes! This idol is the antithesis of the multidisciplinary approach advocated by Paul Pruyser for patient assessment, for it elevates the strictures of one profession's language and leaves no space for any competing language that might also enrich our understanding of either naming the pain or guiding the care of the person who seeks help. (6) Just try finding a space in which to describe a person's dilemma from a religious viewpoint on any of these forms, let alone discussing it with the case manager. Managed care's hostility to extended "talk therapy" is well known, documented even in the popular press. (7) Not only do we *feel* uncomfortable with the strictures and paperwork of this idol, our *thinking* about our clientele is likewise affected. From the language of diagnosis and the formulation of treatment plans to the mountains of paperwork now required to provide care, our *practice* of care and our *perception* of those who receive care is twisted in ways sometimes at great odds with humane care. Like any idol, managed care imposes a monistic solution upon a pluralistic reality. The clinician must guard against embracing this idol even as they provide assistance to the individual who struggles within the bonds of their own idol.

We make idols because we recognize our vulnerability in the universe. We believe that at some level if we follow the prescription of the god behind the idol we will be protected and blessed. Our crops will flourish, our children will be above average, our work will succeed and we won't need others to care for us. The god fashioned in the image of our heart will keep her promises! Our clients will have their depression lifted in six sessions; their anxiety-ridden compulsions will be redirected in positive avenues. The word salad and poor self-care of schizophrenia somehow isn't dealt with very well in managed care, but we don't often talk about this failure.

But this idol is not life giving. The sad but realistic truth is this: the idol of managed care is "globally insensitive to the psyches of patients, whatever the infirmities of their bodies." (8) The very thing we constructed to save our clinical practice by increasing efficiency or salve our souls by helping us cope with difficult people now contributes to our own professional deconstructing.

Any clinician or physician who has delivered care within the managed care environment can see the parallels. What is pernicious is the near-religious zeal with which treatment strictures are enforced and the stranglehold that managed care now appears to have over care delivery. Belonging to a managed care network is nearly a precondition to providing professional care. But this belonging comes without the satisfaction of being attached to a community of care; rather, there is a pervasive sense among physicians and counselors of all disciplines that 'their occupation became different from what they signed up for.' (9)

This idol has its roots in a genuine crisis in health care. Resources are limited. Provider costs were spiraling in a nearly geometric fashion. In the medical field, the cost of equipment, tests and staff salaries were exploding. Consumers' ability to pay, however, was hardly able to keep pace with these costs. In the counseling disciplines, provider fees have gone to nearly a $150 per hour average. Remember, this is for *conversation and relationship*. These tools may be healing but at their core pulses the mystery of human speech and the warmth of human relationship to relieve spiritual pain and untangle psychological anguish. Few people can afford such conversation indefinitely. In fact, the most recent survey of the usage of mental health services suggests that most of us who use the services do so in fewer than eight sessions.

Clearly something had to be done to contain costs to the consumer and also to contain the expenses of the providers. The need that gave rise to the idol is quite genuine. Unfortunately the god that we crafted and who's saving arrival some cheered may be more damaging than the cure that we cried out for. What appears to be missing is the very thing that is lacking from any monistic solution: flexibility.

In fairness to managed care it must also be said that not all networks are equally difficult to negotiate or rigid in their policies. There are certainly a number of networks that put both patient and clinician through a numbing maze of authorization forms and protocols that must be followed precisely before, during and after care is provided. Obviously such networks compound a person's anguish. While it may be fortunate that in a consumer-driven society these networks will not survive, they do cause unnecessary suffering as long as they remain in control of a person or company's healthcare. It is more difficult, but not impossible, to locate a care network that is capable of allowing for individual flexibility in understanding a person's pain and guiding their care. This flexibility primarily turns upon the individual judgment of a case manager or their supervisor.

"Today My Complaint is Bitter and Rebellious!"

Naming the idol requires illuminating the individual's sense of betrayal. The bitterness and terror is frequently rooted in a fundamental sense of betrayal. The unfolding tragedy exposes the implicit belief that either life will be only full of blessings or that the Divine owes me an explanation for why life has taken such an awful turn. Thus while Job appears ready to receive bad at the hand of God, much of his discourse with his friends devolves into his bitterness that God is silent in the face of his suffering. (10)

The search for an explanation of suffering and a desire of the soul to be cleansed from bitterness will prompt people to seek wise counsel. I recall being approached by a rather large man after being the guest at a congregation's mission dinner. When he stood close to me there was an immediate sense of physical power. Seventy-seven years lined his face yet his eyes still carried the fire which was placed there as a young man.

"I was one of the suiciders," he said. "They told us we could handle seven men, with a knife or our hands."

There was a pause. I had the feeling that the after dinner conversation had taken a decidedly serious turn.

"I've talked to pastors and counselors before, but no one has been able to tell me why I am *still* this way?" He persisted. *This way* meant his awareness that he could still find that place of grim power within his heart and act violently without a moment's warning. "I wasn't *this way* before the training," he concluded. "I was glad to serve, but I have never been the same." It didn't take a combat veteran to hear this man's core of despair. For just a moment his eyes hinted at the softness of his seventeenth summer. Yet he felt fundamentally betrayed and violated as a result of giving assent to receive special training. He was well able to name his pain.

The financial success and enhanced social status of many of his fellow veterans from World War II only heightened this man's recognition that his life had not progressed along a successful arc. No one had yet found a way to help this man name the uncomfortably inconvenient truth: individuals with chronic post-trauma adjustment difficulties frequently enter military service with deficient resiliency or complicate their post-deployment recovery with alcoholism. The man standing beside me in the church's fellowship hall was no less a visible incarnation of an invisible god's betrayal than if I had been approached by an overly self-revealing teenage girl or monopolized by a self-righteous raconteur of any political or theological persuasion. Bitter pain and rebellion frequently appears in deceptively wrapped packages.

In the religious literalism of our youth, we may have assumed that because we were not offering our first-born child to Molech we were not worshipping any idols. But a pastor can identify any number of objects and goals to which persons offer themselves, their resources, children and futures. In the broadest religious terms, the diagnostic question is simply "what is the name of your idol?" and not "is there an idol which you worship?" Our violating idols are primarily something or someone who's legitimate worth or power has become overly valued. Some idols have explicitly religious names and recognized ceremonies. But the more insidious ones that drive hurting persons to our doorstep are the implicit principalities, thrones and powers we are absolutely convinced we cannot live without.

The area of explicit religion contains gods who are supported by a belief system that the worshipper can elucidate. Explicit idols are a perversion of genuine religious faith. They typically use portions of one or more faith groups, creeds and rites to under gird their belief and piety. An explicit idol can influence religious traditions that are polar opposites, primarily because they appeal to our more fundamental broken, prideful nature. An implicit idol can be a deeply rooted personal habit or group practice that overwhelms the self. Addictions and the various sexual perversions take up residence here. Secular idols reveal themselves through the overwhelming press of cultural values. The various "isms" and fads of our age live here. The most notorious ones are those we cannot see except in the shadows of our perceived personal and national enemies.

For example, the god of fundamentalism makes an appearance in every age and in every faith group. Regardless of the cause for which one enters this god's service, its chief signature is the *demand that there is only one right way or viewpoint* on any matter. This god appeals to our primary desire for an unchanging center within a dynamic world. We long for a singular lens through which all reality will assume an unmistakable clarity. This god supplies such clarity as well as the motivations for extreme self-sacrifice. It is also the one in whose name we slay or excommunicate our perceived enemies. In religious areas this god has an appeal that spans the theological spectrum. The inerrancy-testing conservative is no more vulnerable to this god's sway than the coercive, politically correct liberal or the hallelujah shouting Pentecostal. (11)

The litmus test of this god comes at the crossroads where one must choose to hold on to the world as interpreted by this god or accepting a new interpretation as witnessed to by one's neighbor. Fundamentalism's appeal is particularly seductive to established religions where the fault lines between faithful belief and heresy carry eternal consequences. My experience has led me to conclude it is as just as violating to be in the presence of a liberal fundamentalist as it is easy to be a conservative fundamentalist. Fundamentalism frequently surfaces as a response when too much social or theological change has occurred too rapidly or evokes the fear that change is 'going too far.'

With individuals who have an explicit religious faith the clinician can guide people toward a more mature or nuanced understanding of their beliefs. This transformation may involve leaving behind a magical view of the Deity and gaining a more conventional level of religious belief. Or it may involve the transition from a conventional level of faith to an integrative level of belief.

Typically this process involves the individual in a cognitive reassessment of their religious belief as much as it involves them in an emotional expression of their discontent.

The doorway to this transition is typically made with an expression of lament. A true lament begins with an explicit expression of rage or terror – or both! God has failed! A healthy psyche with a well-informed spiritual life will eventually arrive at a new understanding of God's providence in the midst of their suffering. This is the pattern of Job and we are helped by the fact that it takes Job thirty-nine chapters and the ministrations of four outsiders before he begins to receive some relief. But with a troubled psyche or with someone who does not have an adequate spiritual grounding, this transition may never arrive. The chronic bitterness of many people after suffering a profound betrayal is ample evidence of this reality.

"Do Not Let Dread of You Terrify Me!"

Job's expression of his suffering is vivid and unrelenting. It is helpful to read some of his words as a way of giving someone the words they frequently fear to use. Like Job, the only way through this time of suffering is for the individual to 'not restrain' their mouth. Helping them 'speak in the anguish of my spirit' and complain in the bitterness of my soul' is a necessary prelude to any genuine relief. (12) Journaling, drawing with the non-dominant hand and an adolescent's love of head-banging hard rock are helpful ways of expressing this rage. The more self-destructive expressions of rage, such as anorexia, self-mutilation and drug dependence are the darker avenues of rage's expression.

Job expresses his terror of God in equally graphic terms. Aware of his newly minted vulnerability, he describes himself as a 'windblown leaf' and 'dry chaff.' He accuses God of writing 'bitter things against me' and he experiences his suffering as a direct consequence of some yet-unrecognized flaw. "You put my feet in the stocks and watch all my paths," he says. "You set a bond to the souls of my feet." This is the depressive side of rage, ending in a despondent recognition that he is 'wasting away like a rotten thing, like a garment that is moth-eaten.' (13)

The task of making such confessions is a primary step in any recovery program. The crafting of such laments is a necessary prelude to the birth of hope. It is to these tasks that we now turn our attention. *Selah!*

Chapter 11: Confession, Lament, and Hope

A confession is an admission of personal fault and an acceptance of personal responsibility. Usually accompanied by a plea for forgiveness and a desire for reconciliation, confession is generally described as being 'good for the soul.' The classic example of such a confession is Psalm 51. Imagine not just admitting your worst personal sin in public and then also having it witnessed by millennial generations of anyone who reads this Psalm. It is introduced with the explanation, "A Psalm of David, when the prophet Nathan came to him, after he had gone in to Bathsheba." It is the recognition of that relief and ultimately restoration comes from such honesty that is at the core of naming the pain on this axis.

A lament is a legal complaint against God. While most laments begin with an exposition of the individual's suffering, the core of the lament is this: God has not kept promises made to the person yet has continued to bless others whose lives are much less righteous. The classic illustration of such a lament is Jeremiah's complaint against God.(1) What makes this lament so helpful for our diagnostic purpose is not just the form of Jeremiah's complaint and its graphic language; God also replies to Jeremiah. It is the desire of such a reply that drives the provision of care along this axis.

Living in constant alienation from one's deepest values, closest relationships and ultimate source of meaning is a description of Hell. When that alienation is expressed first through terror and then through rage, an individual loses hope that they will ever restore those vital connections. The very demeanor of the caregiver through empathy as well as a clear treatment plan provides the initial relief so necessary for hope to take root once again in the human soul. "Perhaps I am not such a lost cause after all," the individual says. Usually confession, lament and hope happen as part of the tangled fabric of diagnosis and care that occurs within the opening sessions of counseling. But sometimes care proceeds most effectively when they are separated and identified for the individual in pain. For our purpose here I have separated them in order to explore each dynamic in some detail.

"Have Mercy On Me, O God!"

The most well known formal example of confession in the process of caring for the human condition are the fourth, fifth steps and sixth steps of Alcoholics Anonymous. These steps prescribe making a 'thorough and fearless moral inventory' in which one acknowledges to God 'as I understand Him, myself and one other human being the exact nature of my wrong ways.' What follows hard upon this step are others indicating a person's willingness to have their character flaws removed and finally willingness to make whatever amends are necessary 'except where doing so would cause more harm.'

Few individuals who come for counseling go through such a formal process. Suffice it to say that genuine confession does not begin until an individual or couple arrives at the posture of taking responsibility for their role in their own condition. The therapist must help the person balance honest recognition of their role in whatever pain they bear against the sober estimation of where their responsibility ends and the responsibility of others begins. Some individuals are too wracked by guilt and shame to recognize the role that others have played in the pain they bear; others lack the maturity to see themselves as responsible in any way for their situation.

More typically the dynamic of confession comes out piecemeal as the person recounts their anguish. Blame, recrimination, insight and confusion pour out of the human heart in a maelstrom of pain that sometimes lasts for months or even years. Just as frequently confession is intermingled with the dynamic of lament explored below. But for the moment, the clinician must remember that in confession there is not just an admission of fault and responsibility; there is also a plea for mercy and a hope for restoration.

I always begin with the assumption that the individual's presence in a counseling relationship is the sign of this plea; unfortunately this is not always the case. In some instances an individual comes to a counselor in order to justify their own righteousness. This is especially true in couple's counseling. It takes great courage for individuals in couple's counseling or an individual whose marriage is crumbling to get beyond the pro forma admission of fault to a genuine exploration of how their character and conduct contributed to the failure of their most intimate relationship.

While the wisdom of the age's points to the cleansing necessity of such an honest step, the corruption of our moral and spiritual language renders this something of a challenge for both clinician and client. The professional must avoid reinforcing the natural tendency of a genuine victim to blame themselves and the contemporary sensibility that views the universe as a disinterested party in human affairs. This is where the religious or spiritual counselor can play a significant role. The chief insight of all religions is that the Deity is an interested Third Person in human conduct whose mercy is released through humanity's honest confession of moral fault or through the Deity's unilateral will.

This is a theological or metaphysical insight and not merely an ethical statement. Whether or not the person receiving care openly acknowledges a religious belief in God, their pain is a prima facia recognition that the world is operating on some other system of principles besides the ones they were expecting. In secular language a person may simply say, "My life isn't working out" or "Life just doesn't seem to be going my way" or "I keep screwing things up and I don't know why." Even for a religious person it is rare for them to explicitly simply say, "I need God's mercy." Yet the deep wisdom of all the healing arts suggests that this is one place to begin:

> "Merciful God my home is crumbling
> And the hopes of my heart are dashing
> Upon the rocks of my many failings,
> You alone know the depth of my sin
> And the responsibility born on my soul
> For this unfolding tragedy."

These are not easy words to write or speak. But the effective therapist or physician must be ready to tease them out from behind or within the person's anguish, anger, and anxiety.

Arriving at this internal posture is not an easy or simple task although it is a singular task in the process of diagnosis. Whether the diagnostic conversation is primarily religious in nature as illustrated above or primarily behavioral in nature through the use of assessment instruments, the naming of an individual's pain ultimately comes down not just to an acknowledgement of one's own role but may include the individual or couple or family's reorientation to an entirely new worldview. In secular language sometimes the unfolding distortion of our human condition challenges our fundamental sense of entitlement – we must face either our unmerited good fortune or our uninvited tragedy.

We survive a terrible accident with minimal injury or recognize the necessity of now keeping the foxhole promise we made with God one fire-drenched night. So we alter our life's course in the dim light of this grace. Or we finally face the reality that our child will not become the next Tiger Woods or that the corner office is not ours to possess by birthright. So we alter our conduct with our child and co-workers. Whatever route sprouts from such confessions, our path now leads toward a destination whose character is as ontologically different from our heart's starting point as life at the bottom of the Marianna's Trench is different from life in the Amazon's rain forest.

Terror is the primary affective state of affairs as an individual contemplates such a primary change in their worldview. The conflicted couple is not just learning a new skill set for communication, they are also leaving behind the unexpressed but very powerful assumptions about one another that heretofore lived in an unexamined state behind their overt expressions of affection and fidelity. The avoidant person is slowly reaching out toward a world that past experience had imprinted as a place full of threat. The addict is not just leaving behind the life-altering god of alcohol or cocaine; they are slowly transforming the neurological structure of their brain.

The clinician must recognize this level of terror that is inherent in the process of care as treatment proceeds. This is why it is necessary to maintain a steady holding environment and a consistent therapeutic demeanor throughout the course of care. Having followed a life-course built on assumptions that produced significant pain, most of us are reluctant to undertake a new life-course with untried assumptions unless we see some tangible hope we can move toward and not just a terrifying reality we are intent to leave behind.

"Let Me Put My Case Before You!"

The terror that lives on the cusp of spiritual transformation sometimes transmutes into rage. This rage flows from the insight that one has been betrayed by an ineffective or insufficient god. Sometimes this insight is objectively true when the god is one of the ancient deities of Venus or Dionysus or Mars. Their promises of instantaneous transformation through unquestioning devotion ultimately lead only to heartache and the denaturing doorway to Hell. But just as frequently this rage, while directed at God, is more truly a realistic grappling with the tenants of religious faith.

At other times there is true spiritual transformation at work through the dynamic of conversion. In this case while there is likely to be some degree of terror as one works through the transition, the period of lament and rage in this case more frequently transmutes rather quickly into hope and joy of which I will say more in a moment. But typically as an individual or couple leaves behind the idolatry of destructive patterns, it becomes necessary to effectively and thoroughly break with the beliefs and patterns that has enslaved the mind and heart.

Rage is relieved through an explicit, affective expression of distress. The appropriate religious avenue that relieves god-destroying rage is the lament. A lament is not merely whining before God that life isn't really fair. A lament is nothing short of a behavioral bill of particulars and theological indictment against the Almighty. It is an explicit statement that God hasn't kept His part of the bargain that a faithful person felt they had. This is not an easy type of prayer for a person to utter. Thus part of the task of care may be for the clinician or clergy to utter such a lament. But it is ultimately the only type of petition that is likely to help the person or couples grow through their rage to a more mature spirituality of hope. The lament retains their connection with God all the while also expressing their subjective feelings of utter contempt and dismay toward God.

A lament that expresses god-shattering rage is a profound act of faith. The lament is a cry of the heart for the resumption of a nurturing, satisfying, comforting, protecting, just and righteous experience of God in the face of a shattering life experience that is the very antithesis of these positive elements of religious faith. For example, the results of battle that includes the loss of comrades and perceiving the cruelty of humanity is more than enough to shatter a soldier's faith in all of the positive elements he has been taught about God and life. The same is true when marital vows have been breached, catastrophic weather has snatched loved ones from the earth or a dread disease has caused a grave to be dug too early.

It is also true that when one leaves behind the implicit gods of addiction and promiscuity anyone may feel so repulsed by their former life (and the self-deception upon which their life was based) that a lament can assist them in naming their pain and beginning the road toward recovery. The phrase in most Twelve Step programs is that one commits life to a higher power 'as I understand Him.' Part of the recovery process is reaching a new understanding of the self through self-directed rage expressed as 'How could I have been so selfish?' and lament expressed as 'create in me a clean heart, O God, and put a right spirit within me.'(2)

Let me be absolutely clear: this rage is healing and leads to transformation only if it is directed against the idolatrous belief structure of an individual and leads to a change in behavior. Rage in and of itself is not healing. Sometimes in marital or family counseling there is an effort to be 'totally honest' with others by saying whatever one feels or thinks in an effort to have 'open communication.' This type of communication is seldom helpful or healing. Rather, it is more akin to guerrilla warfare brought into a home in which hostility is now masked through the guise of 'openness.' Communication in a couple or family that leads to transformation only happens as each individual examines their own role in the current distress, expresses regret and apology to those they have wounded, makes whatever amends are possible and then sets about *editing* their words in a way that most effectively communicates the needs they have to those around them.

So how does a clinician help someone express this rage through an effective lament? The first step is to help the person achieve as exact an expression of the breached covenant as possible. 'I thought my daughter would never develop leukemia' or 'It never occurred to me that I might be dismissed from a company I had devoted two decades of my life to' or yet again 'How could God allow someone so corrupt to gain control over our church?' might be among the betrayed agreements the person might express. This is the easiest step.

The more difficult step is to help the person unravel the exact nature of how they came to hold this belief. It is more healing if the person clearly says 'what' it is they believed than 'why' they came to embrace such a belief. Thus 'I believed that no one in our family would get sick because I provided them with nutritious meals' is more helpful than 'my daughter doesn't deserve to get sick' although the latter statement is also a lament of the heart. The statement 'I believed my company would reward my loyalty and hard work' is more healing than 'I don't deserve to be dismissed to make way for a younger worker' even though this second statement certainly expresses a deep betrayal. Helping the individual explore and express the content of their beliefs brings to light the sense of entitlement that fueled their now-broken covenant and assists them in placing their rage into a framework that allows the healing process to begin.

Some individual's broken covenant is rooted in a sense of positive entitlement. Most of us are familiar with this because their sentences typically begin with the phrase 'I don't deserve.' But other individual's idolatry is fueled by a sense of negative entitlement. This is much harder to understand and unravel. Negative entitlement is the belief that one does *not* deserve decent treatment and thus views reality and the Author of reality locked in a permanent posture of threat toward them. These folks have built an altar to their own abuse where their only entitlement is abuse. In either case it is likely to take more than one year for an individual to make this adjustment in their belief structure, especially because an individual whose heart feels only negative entitlement frequently suffers with chronic depression while the person whose lament is against a god who has failed to deliver the good life continues to long for the 'fleshpots of Egypt.' (3)

It is not uncommon for a spiritual disorder of this depth to produce a clinical personality disorder. Thus the whole enterprise of guiding care in this area must take seriously the highly resistant nature of personality disorders. While individuals with a high sense of positive entitlement bring with them the obnoxious personalities of narcissism or histrionic, the individuals with strong beliefs in their own negative entitlement just as frequently are bedeviled by the reclusive personalities of schizoid, dependent or avoidant. The most dangerous personality disorders of paranoia and anti-social will be addressed in following chapters.

"Put On the Hope of Salvation for a Helmet!"

Childish belief in ineffective gods endures long into adulthood under the guise of complaining that life isn't fair. Child-like terror and the rage of betrayal are symptoms that we are losing our childish innocence about the universe. Thus crafting the lament, whether via art or via spoken words exchanged in counseling is an exercise in gaining maturity. "Life isn't fair," we lament. "So get a helmet," replies the adult providing care. Whether said gruffly by the counselor in learning center for conduct-disordered adolescents or embodied kindly by a minister walking through the rubble of a parishioner's failed dreams, part of the healing from idolatry is the rediscovery of hope through a more adequate structure of belief.

Because individuals have different levels of maturity in their spiritual development, it is important to properly assess the level of faith development that is being challenged – and the level of maturity toward which events are propelling them. James Fowler describes the stage at which most adults come to rest as that of *Synthetic-Conventional Faith*. His description of the angst at this stage as the individual is challenged by life's circumstances aptly describes the process of leaving behind a failing god for a more adequate belief structure:

> This stage demands a complex pattern of socialization and integration, and faith is an inseparable factor in the ordering of one's world. It is a stage characterized by conformity, where one finds one's identity by aligning oneself with a certain perspective, and lives directly through this perception with little opportunity to reflect on it critically. One has an ideology at this point, but may not be aware that one has it. Those who differ in opinion are seen as "the Other," as different "kinds" of people. Authority derives from the top down, and is invested with power by majority opinion. Dangers in this stage include the internalization of symbolic systems (power, "goodness," "badness") to such a degree that objective evaluation is impossible. Furthermore, while one can at this stage enter into an intimate relationship with the divine, one's life situations may drive one into despair (the threshold to the next stage). Such situations may include contradictions between authorities, the revelation of authoritarian hypocrisy, and lived experiences that contradict one's convictions. (4)

Making the transition from the earlier *Mythic-Literal Stage* into this more conventional level of maturity demands one come to terms with one's lack of ability to be perfect. Making the transition from conventional faith into the next stage, what Fowler calls the *Individuative-Reflective Stage,* requires the individual to embrace the imperfection of the universe and the ambiguity of received orthodoxy. Fowler's notion that this latter step in faith development most frequently affects individuals as they enter their mid-thirties to mid-forties suggests that the bulk of people who seek counseling will likely be facing these types of questions and struggles.

Some type of bibliotherapy that encourages the individual to gain a better cognitive understanding of their religious faith can be especially helpful at this juncture. This intervention calls for wisdom on the part of the clinician. Most clinicians will be tempted to quietly urge the individual toward the belief structure with which we are most comfortable. Indeed it is questionable whether or not a clinician or religious professional can truly guide someone to a level of faith development that exceeds one's own level of maturity.

The clinician must exercise caution at this point to not unconsciously impose their own religious belief onto clients' quest for a more adequate spirituality. Let me be clear at this point: the fact that a clinician has an explicit religious faith does not automatically qualify them to make recommendations here. The wisest course of treatment is for clinicians to develop referral sources within their community's religious professionals to whom they can either refer with confidence or to whom they can turn for guidance regarding a client's religious or spiritual dilemmas.

Having sounded this cautionary note let me also make the following observation that continues to be born out by longitudinal research: people gravitate toward counselors who share their values, especially their religious values. This provides both the client and the clinician a place to start in the journey toward health. This also underscores a fact of spiritual development – growth or change in this area occurs over a long period of time, typically taking years rather than months to fully integrate whatever new insight may sprout from a tragic event. A counselor or religious professional who can walk with an individual as they discover the new helmet of hope to wear during the next stage of their life performs a genuine service. This discovery will be greatly assisted if the professional can direct the person toward a community of faith that can afford the individual or family a variety of living examples of maturity in their newly found level of faith. Thus I would reinforce the fact that professional counselors of all theoretical persuasions have the obligation to maintain connections with colleagues within their community's religious professionals. We also have the obligation to continue our own spiritual growth in the same way that we continue our own theoretical growth and physical health.

Conclusion

It is rare that the human soul leaves behind a primary but deeply flawed view of themselves quickly or easily. Beliefs forged within a decade's long developmental process do not give way easily to either new realities or the suasions of even the most skilled therapist. This is especially true when the patterns of destructive conduct are under girded by either addictions or strong secondary gains. All too frequently most people prefer to live with the devil they know than embrace the savior they do not know.

A first-century description of this level of distress may be found in Luke's gospel. (5) Today we would call the person going through such an experience as 'relapsing' or being 'out of compliance with treatment protocols.' By whatever name we choose to describe the terror and rage of such a state, the individual in the grasp of such an experience is in profound distress and feels hopeless. The length of time and amount of effort required on the part of both the individual and the clinician is noted elsewhere in the Bible and continues to be born out by clinical experience.(6)

Yet individuals do pass through this Hellespont of transformation and gain a new vision of themselves and the world around. Whether they enter the stage three of James Fowler's *Synthetic-Conventional* faith where the individual is now able to enter into a personal relationship with the divine, the *Individuative-Reflective* stage where one 'leaves behind the agnostic rationality of Stage Four' or the level of *Conjunctive* Faith where one now lives on 'the cusp of paradox,' world is once again filled with hope. (7) The individual also experiences a new measure of social competence and vocational clarity.

In the next chapter we will revisit the illustrative vignettes of chapter eight. These vignettes will be enlarged to illustrate this dynamic of confession, lament, and hope so that the reader may see how this process unfolds in actual cases. *Selah!*

Chapter 12: Illustrative Vignettes Resumed

As noted in Chapter 8, while themes of idolatry along with the feeling of betrayal and dread along with the feeling of defilement may be hinted at during the initial evaluation, it is rare for the full details of these concerns to be fully evident at the outset of treatment. More generally the depth of these concerns surface once a relationship of trust has been firmly developed and the more pressing concerns of daily life have been somewhat addressed. This does not suggest that such concerns are not factors in the issues that bring people into counseling. They are inevitably the etiology of an individual's anguish. But providing care for these themes takes a lengthy period of time and patience to address.

Thus in this chapter I will present a brief summary of each case from Chapter 8 so that the reader does not have to read this chapter with their finger in a prior chapter. I will then either describe the moment in the clinical vignette when the theme of idolatry and betrayal surfaced or simply note in what way the individual's religious or spiritual resources helped them address the matter of guilt. Concerns related to dread and defilement as well as their interplay with idolatry and guilt will be addressed in a subsequent chapter in a similar manner.

Like all primary attachments in life the acquisition of an ultimate attachment is a process and not an event. So too is the matter of providing care for individuals who find they must leave behind one ultimate concern and grasp the brass ring of another supreme belief and its accompanying style of life. Thus in these cases and in the chapters that lie ahead the reader will recognize a much greater emphasis upon care and a reduced emphasis upon cure. Even when one undergoes a religious conversion (which is the spiritual equivalent of 'cure'), the transition into a new belief structure with its accompanying interior theology and social piety requires the good soil, proper climate and adequate nutrients of an entire community to truly produce an abundant life. The only thing in nature and in the soul that grows fast is a noxious weed. (1)

Case #1 – Depression: Greed and Faith Development

The reader will remember the precise moment when the root of Elaine's depression was explicitly named. She was regularly violating a premier tenant of her religious faith as well as providing her superior with sexual favors for which

127

he paid dearly and which extracted a terrible price within her own marriage. She saw herself as a moral agent in this tableau rather than as a victim. She understood her conduct in a strict religious sense as an offense against God as well as her marital vows that she made 'in the presence of God and these witnesses.' The revelation of these watercolors and what they signaled was her true confession.

Here is a signal example of the mythic-literal level of faith development. In spite of Elaine's surface sophistication in her bearing and advanced education, her interior perfectionism and belief in her own irredeemability are one hallmark of this rather early stage of faith. While the therapist would necessarily bring a more sophisticated and forgiving understanding of how the earlier predations and betrayals of covenants of trust by others would precondition her to live out such a life, the core of Elaine's depression was kept alive by her basic mythos of being a sinner in the hands of an angry god whose agents delivered some material goods but who, in the end, would judge her harshly and eternally for enjoying the benefits of those goods.

Elaine's workaholic devotion to her family and church could now be seen for what it was: an attempt to earn the favor of this demanding god. In spite of her attending a church that preached the forgiving grace of God through Christ, the ears of her heart did not believe this proclamation. The theological term for such an ideology is works-righteousness. But no amount of proof text references to the grace of God apart from our own righteousness would be effective in either relieving her guilt or providing her with the courage to step on the bridge to a more mature synthetic-conventional faith.

The strength of the synthetic-conventional level of faith development is the person's capacity to separate the Deity from the hypocritical authorities who represent the Deity. This initial tolerance for ambiguity allows the individual to begin allowing the ambiguity of grace to take root in their soul. In Elaine's case the consistent presence of two successive male therapists over the period of her therapy provided the consistent integrity that stimulated her hope enough so that she began to address her terror.

Elaine had produced the terrified watercolors in a single weekend when her husband was away on a business trip. She did not want them at her home where either he or their children might discover them. So I kept them locked in her file. For approximately two months we would review them, taking one or two each session. This exercise became her time of lament. For the first time in decades she wept tightly controlled tears. Then, just as suddenly as she had opened up her heart, she announced she was 'done crying' and indicated she did not want to see her watercolors anymore. "Now what do we do?" she asked. She was still primarily operating at a very literal level of faith development. This rather dependent level of faith looks to the religious authority to tell her what to do next.

The hope that Elaine needed to rediscover would come only as she began to 'hear' the good news in a new voice – in her voice. What developed was a month-long exercise of her reading the Biblical story of *Jesus and the Woman of Samaria* aloud (John 4:1-42). I split the passage into four parts and instructed her to read the section aloud each morning and evening as a part of her daily devotional exercise. This proved to be mildly beneficial and I continued to assign her other readings from the gospels that emphasized Christ's empathic and forgiving posture or readings from the Old Testament that portrayed God's mercy and patience with people. I had to remind her to read these passages aloud, something she at first found distastefully embarrassing but as time progressed she grew more comfortable hearing her own voice.

Elaine was still a very wounded woman. Her days of depression began to be less intense and her perfectionism began to erode, albeit very slowly. The remaining work of addressing her dread would ultimately have to be left for another therapist, although we made some headway in this area over the next two years before her move. This will be addressed in a subsequent chapter.

At this point in the diagnostic enterprise, Elaine's diagnosis would look like this, utilizing both the formal DSM-IV system and my multi-axial system of diagnosis:

DSM-IV Diagnosis:
Axis I – Dysthymic Disorder-300.40
Axis II – Compulsive Personality – 301.40
Axis III – Migraine headaches – 346.90
Axis IV – Marital and vocational problems
Axis V- GAF Current: 55 GAF Last Year: 60

Spiritual / Theological Multi-axial Diagnosis:
Axis I-   Guilt – Realistic related to violation of marriage vows; Subjective related to violation of personal standards of performance in work and marriage.
*Axis II-*Idolatry – Describes herself as a 'sinner' and believes her sin places her outside of divine grace. Cannot conceive herself as being forgiven.

Case # 2 – Adultery: Idolatry and Virtue

Robert's discovery of Melanie's torrid and enduring adultery brought him to the edge of despair. "I worshipped the ground she walks on," he said more than once during the two years of weekly therapy. "I wish you knew her before all this," he would regularly say, as though she had suddenly succumbed to some dread disease or alien visitation.

"I'm going to give you some advice as we start this journey," I had said at the end of our first session. "In the months ahead you will find your wife to have been a very different person – someone you will not recognize. You will find hidden credit cards, lingerie you have not seen before, and friends you thought were shared will become co-conspirators with her out of a warped sense of loyalty to her finding her own 'truth.' I hope I am absolutely wrong," I concluded. "But prepare yourself to be utterly confounded by the person you will soon meet."

As the months turned into the second year of negotiations, Robert would refer to this initial conversation. "It looks like this has gone on for years," he would wonder half-aloud. "I know we didn't have a close marriage; we both worked and we hadn't been intimate for several years because she would say she was 'tired.' Now I wonder if she was tired or being satisfied elsewhere?"

Robert's feeling of betrayal and terror were not merely emotional or spiritual states. They were financial and relational realities. A significant early facet to his terror and then rage came as he discovered a separate set of account books. In what he would come to see as utter naiveté he had literally turned his earnings over to Melanie and never gave the family's finances a second thought. He would eventually discover in excess of $50,000 of uncovered credit card debt, IRS refunds that had disappeared and arrears notices on their mortgage.

It took him months of interior wrestling with these cold hard facts before he could take the steps necessary to protect himself financially. The ground gained in a therapy session as he struggled to destroy the idol he had made of Melanie's probity would quickly crumble whenever he heard her voice on his phone or he would try to have a factual conversation with her about new debts. He was absolutely enchanted by her. He continued to have lengthy conversations with her about his legal strategy in ways that brought his attorney very close to firing him as a client. "The Melanie I knew would never have done these things," he kept saying.

This became the theme of Robert's lament for his dying god. Even two years after the divorce was finalized there were still echoes of this lament in his conversation, although he would quickly interrupt himself and say, "I was blinded by what I wanted her to be rather than who she truly was."

What helped Robert find new hope? Surprisingly it was his immersion in the raising of his teenage daughter and the shouldering of responsibility for his aging mother. Growing initially out of his desire to protect his daughter from her mother's flameout, Robert realized he had to provide her with positive values. Simply shielding her and saying 'don't be like your mother' would only increase her curiosity for the Bad Boys that now drew her mother's attention. Coming to terms with his mother's increasing dementia renewed his connection with a woman of genuine virtue.

Thus Robert rediscovered both innocence and wisdom in the face of his wife's spiritual flaws and moral failure. To his eternal credit, Robert maintained a steady presence with his daughter, redirecting her questions about her mother's conduct back upon her mother. "You'll have to ask your mother about that," became a standard refrain as his daughter queried him about her mother's sudden interest in NASCAR and horse racing, the missed school events and the changes in her mother's wardrobe. Only when his daughter's response to a missed birthday was 'I don't know who mom is anymore' did Robert say, "Neither do I. Perhaps it is time for me to tell you a bit of who she has become."

Regaining regular connection with his religious community started as a part of Robert's effort to demonstrate he was 'the better parent.' But as Melanie's betrayal deepened and his lament grew more intense, Robert grew hungry for the nurturing of his religious community. He had to shift from the traditional service that felt so familiar to him toward the more contemporary service in order to keep his daughter and two boys interested in attending church with him. While the more lively music and lack of vestments initially bothered him, he came to experience the Holy that still pulsed behind these outward changes in appearance. This recognition began his movement from a stage of conventional religious faith toward a more reflective level of insight.

Caring for his mother, living again in his boyhood home and managing her financial affairs reminded him of his core values. He rediscovered a tenderness that years in the business world had blunted. He also noticed he suddenly had more time. This wasn't simply because he became more efficient. "It's like I suddenly have 'more' time," he mused. "I don't think I'm more efficient. Somehow there literally seems to now be 27 hours in the day." This latter awareness signaled Robert's initial entry into the numinous, one of the qualities of Fowler's Individuative-Reflective stage of religious development. Thus as his mother's time with him grew increasingly shorter, he marveled that he seemed to be gaining time. His affect softened, his pace slowed and his heart was redirected away from Melanie's detective-style mystery and on to the mystery of Real Presence.

At this point in the diagnostic enterprise, Robert's diagnosis would look like this, utilizing both the formal DSM-IV system and my multi-axial system of diagnosis:

DSM-IV Diagnosis:
Axis I – Adjustment Disorder with Mixed Emotional Features – 309.00
Axis II – No Diagnosis on Axis II – V71.90
Axis III – No condition reported
Axis IV – Marital separation
Axis V- GAF Current: 65   GAF Last Year: 65

Spiritual / Theological Multi-axial Diagnosis:
Axis I-Guilt: Realistic guilt over failure of marriage; subjective
          mood of failure and personal recrimination.

Axis II – Idolatry: Betrayal by spouse fuels his rage and signals his misplaced worship; terror results current alienation from religious tradition of his youth.

Case # 3 – Developmental Challenges: Education and Socialization

"C'mon Philip, let's go for a walk outside," I said as I entered the waiting room.
"I don't want to," he responded automatically.
"It will do you some good. Besides, it will blow some of the stink off of you," I replied playfully while heading toward the door. He followed obediently. Once outside he quickly matched my pace.

Philip then began playfully bumping into my shoulder as we walked and I queried him about his day at school and his week with his family. The negative statements about him self had been gone about six weeks. Indeed, they had been replaced by comments that he liked coming to my office and that he thought I was 'cool.'

What factors contributed to this change and does it have anything to do with the dynamics of spirituality or religious faith? What changed his primitive aggression into boyish playfulness?

Based on Philip's neuropsychological assessment I was convinced he was an active child who needed behavioral guidance in socialization and plenty of cognitive challenges to his negative self-assessment. If he responded quickly to social cues it would rule out the Asperger's Syndrome that I wondered about.

So right away I began agreeing with him. "You're the world's biggest complainer," I commented. I made up a certificate on my office computer. With him in the room I conducted a Google search for "World's Greatest Complainer."

"Ooops! You're not trying hard enough, Philip," I commented as the search results came up. "Someone else has already claimed the title!" I had alerted his parents that I would be taking this paradoxical approach. Philip protested me mightily, as I knew he would. His parents did a great job of expressing their encouragement for Philip to complain more so that he could win the award.

It took about three sessions to reduce his complaining to an age-appropriate level. I had been working with him four months at the point of the bumping-walk. It was the first time in weeks that he had been this physical with me and it absolutely lacked the hostility that had characterized his initial sessions.

Certainly the increased time with his Dad, robust involvement in organized sports and periodic reminders that 'Dr. Denton is still evaluating you for the award of World's Greatest Complainer' played a role in reducing his negative comments and conduct. The affirmation from his Sunday school teacher, his academic success and the applause of his academic peers who labeled him 'unique' all combined to alter Philip's negative self-assessment.

The diagnostic task with children primarily focuses on religious or spiritual formation rather than transformation. A child is drawing fundamental spiritual conclusions from their life's unfolding experience because of their inherent vulnerability. Thus it is important for a counselor to gently raise spiritual questions with children. This calls for a respectful attentiveness to the family's religious tradition. If the counselor is uncertain about that tradition the professional avenue of inquiry is better initially explored with the parents and only secondarily with the child.

In Philip's case he was a direct referral to our agency because of our pastoral orientation. He had expressed his iconoclastic 'I like violence' and 'I think I'll kill myself' statements during a Sunday school class. So when he began making these statements in our counseling hours, I asked him directly about them.

"I'll bet Jesus really thinks it's cool that you like violence," I said one day. "You're probably a real star in the Sunday School class."

"Noooooo!" he complained. "Jesus wouldn't like it at all," he said with the exasperated tone of an eight-year-old expert who was correcting an obviously stupid adult. "Jesus is peaceful!" he maintained.

"So I'm confused," I persisted. "If you go to church to learn about Jesus, who is a peaceful guy, why would you keep saying you like violence in Sunday school class where you learn about him?"

"Aaargh!" was his only reply and then a period of silence. "I do not like to *be* violent," he finally concluded. "I like *watching* violence," he clarified. This would be a topic that we came back to in the ensuing months of his counseling. But Philip was learning an important social boundary as much as a religious truth: telling people you like violence doesn't win you many friends. Philip learned the same lesson about other shocking statements that he was wont to utter.

Religious education and the socialization that necessarily accompanies such task thus played a central role in deflating his childish preoccupation with evil and gore. Reinforcing the religious values beneath positive conduct as well as the religious prohibition against negative conduct and comments were thus as much a natural part of our weekly meetings as any other more secular 'social education.' (2) Learning that saying 'I'm sorry' to a peer he had clumsily lurched into or growled at was an important thing for a follower of Jesus to say was a much more important positive adjunct to the basic social prohibition of 'we don't talk like that.' The religious education Philip received provided additional positive social rewards he received for his change in attitude and conduct

At this point in the diagnostic enterprise, Phillip's diagnosis would look like this, utilizing both the formal DSM-IV system and my multi-axial system of diagnosis:

<u>*DSM-IV Diagnosis:*</u>

Axis I –   Cognitive Difficulties – 294.90

          Attention Deficit Hyperactivity Disorder – 314.00

          Childhood Depression – 311.00

Axis II – Asperger's Disorder – 299.80 (rule out)

Axis III – None reported

Axis IV – School difficulties, especially socialization

Axis V- GAF Current: 50 GAF Last Year: 55

<u>*Spiritual / Theological Multi-axial Diagnosis:*</u>

Axis I-   Guilt: No realistic guilt; strong feelings of subjective

          guilt related to negative self-image.

Axis II – Idolatry: No genuine idolatry; making age-appropriate

          developmental transition between intuitive-projective faith and

          mythic-literal faith.

Case # 4 – End of Life Concerns: A Decision Full of Faith

Steve's family had a deep traditional religious faith. Thus they brought to this tragedy the recognition that terrible events such as this happen in everyone's life. They did not feel that their son had been singled out for punishment by some angry deity. Rather, they viewed his signature on his driver's license donor card as an expression of his religion's affirmation of eternal life and his sense of responsibility to enhance the lives of those around him.

"I remember when Steve got his driver's license," his mother told the chaplain. "We talked about his decision to sign the donor card. It was his first really adult decision."

The task of diagnosis is not merely a discovery of what is broken or wrong or amiss in an individual, couple or family. While this is certainly the initial concern due to the press of time and the intensity of trauma, it must not be the only concern. This is especially true in the second task of diagnosis, guiding the care. In the arena where ethical values, religious sentiment and existential vocation intersect the clinician must become cognizant of whatever strengths inhere in the person's life and context that are available as resources. Restoration, hope and joy will most likely come from these pools of awareness, whether the clinician points them out or the client is grasped by these assets.

This was the case with Steve and his family. "As I got to know his family it became obvious that they were people of deep traditional faith. They were grateful to God and generally felt God had blessed them. But they didn't wear their religious sentiment on their sleeves," commented the chaplain in a later case consultation.

"What do you mean?" asked a fellow chaplain.

"They don't go around saying 'praise the Lord' or 'I'm so blessed.' They don't have to wear 'What Would Jesus Do?' bracelets to remind them of their faith or announce to others that 'Jeeeeesus' is the guiding light of their conduct and conscience," she replied.

"So when their pastor said simply 'the church is praying for Steve' I took him at his word. He didn't need to elaborate. But there wasn't any doubt that an entire community had focused their entire spiritual resources on this young man and his family," she continued. "I could tell those resources were considerable."

Over the next day and a half, a routine emerged. One of Steve's parents remained in the waiting room while the other went home for sleep. Their pattern was sporadic, based more on their own restlessness than any outward schedule. Two members of the congregation's Stephen Ministry sat with them, having set up a vigil in the Instant Care waiting room. Another pair of lay ministers replaced them every four hours. A similar rotating quartet sat in the hospital's chapel. "There were other pairs who were visiting with Steve's girl friend's family," related the chaplain. "I don't think I ever saw anything as thorough and as automatic," said the chaplain. "It had the rhythm of a regular expectation. Nobody got dramatic or looked inconvenienced. I really felt like I was witnessing an organic community embracing one of its members. I've never seen this kind of care from a church happen before or since," she concluded. "I would be wonderful if more churches did this."

At about thirty-seven hours into this ordeal the nurse noticed Steve had opened his eyes. She began the protocols necessary to assess his neurological functions. She also paged the staff neurologist and chaplain on call. Steve's condition would need careful medical assessment. Given the significant ongoing religious ministry taking place it would be essential to accurately interpret any change in Steve's status. "The physician will meet with family as soon as the neurologist has a clear picture of Steve's status," said the chaplain at their morning staff meeting.

As the morning progressed the medical picture became clear. Steve's body was coming back on-line. The next medical hurdle would be assessing just how much of 'Steve' would be available to work with. "So while there appears to be some measure of healing, it isn't initially apparent whether this is 'happy news' or just 'true information,'" Steve's minister said to the chaplain?

"This is one small but important step in Steve's recovery," she replied. The pastor nodded.

At this point in the diagnostic enterprise, Steve's diagnosis would look like this, utilizing both the formal DSM-IV system and my multi-axial system of diagnosis:

DSM-IV Diagnosis:
Axis I – No Diagnosis – V71.09
Axis II – No Diagnosis- V71. 09

Axis III – Concussion, cerebral – 851.80
Axis IV – Unresponsive to stimuli
Axis V- GAF Current: 0   GAF Last Year: +90

<u>*Spiritual / Theological Multi-axial Diagnosis:*</u>
Axis I - Guilt: Realistic due to his role in his injury; subjective is
            unavailable for him but profound for his family.
Axis II – Idolatry: Age-appropriate synthetic-conventional faith that
            will come to terms with end-of-life concerns

Case # 5 – Vocational Assessment for Ministry when the Answer is 'No'

Hope's clinical interview did not go well. While she appeared poised and well dressed in the center's waiting room, she quickly fell apart at the first hint that the report was not a glowing tribute to her gifts for ministry. The evaluator stayed gentle but firm, "these are the statements you made about yourself," the evaluator reminded her while reading some of the critical items from the psychological testing. "What did you have in mind when you marked these answers?" she inquired.

Lest the reader believe at this point that the testing items were obscure, they were straightforward indicators of significant psychological or relational distress. Among them were items such as replying 'True' to statements such as 'evil spirits possess me at times,' 'I have had days, weeks or months when I couldn't seem to get going,' and 'I believe I am being plotted against.' While Hope had used complimentary adjectives to described herself on another instrument, she also described herself as 'greedy, cynical, argumentative and touchy.' Thus the evaluator's questions asking Hope to elaborate on her answers were entirely appropriate.

"How do you think it will affect your ministry when you have a month that you 'just can't get going?' the evaluator inquired.

"I don't know. God will help me. God always helps me," Hope replied. She then dissolved into tears. "I know God wants me to be a minister," she eventually stated firmly.

The evaluator's report described what happened during the interview. Having received an instruction from a denominational official to make no explicit recommendation on any of their candidates, she simply laid out Hope's deterioration during the interview in response to her requests for elaboration. The immediate diagnostic challenge for the evaluator lay in determining whether or not Hope would be sufficiently recovered to drive home. "I guess this underscores the problem she would have in any church," the evaluator later said in a debriefing.

Unfortunately for Hope, and perhaps for her denomination, this was not the end of the story. Hope wrote a lengthy description of the interview to several denominational regional officials. A flurry of telephone calls and ultimately a face-to-face consultation resulted between the evaluator, her supervisor and a sub-committee of the regional judicatory. "I hope I'm not the sacrificial lamb," commented the evaluator as she rode over to the meeting with her supervisor.

The judicatory officials were worried. "Hope and her parents have retained a lawyer. They're considering a suit for employment prejudice and an abusive candidacy process," the denomination's staff member indicated. "I t was not the best way to begin a meeting," the evaluator would later remark.

"It is a matter of practice that we record evaluative sessions when we anticipate a troubled candidate," began the evaluator's supervisor. "While you review the full scope of Hope's psychological testing, let us listen to the full recording of the session." With that said, her supervisor started the audiotape.

For the next hour the committee listened intently to the recording. Some took notes directly on their copy of Hope's psychological assessment report. At the conclusion of the hour, the supervisor looked at the denominational official and said, "Is Hope someone you would want leading a church?" The room was very quiet.

The attorney broke the silence. "You have the right to determine your own standards for vocational fitness. Those standards include emotional stability," he said calmly. "The psychological testing indicates instability, the report reflects her instability in a balanced way and the tape certainly demonstrates the conclusion of the report. I don't think this will go to court. I recommend that you stand firm with Hope through a brief letter reaffirming your decision to not allow her to proceed further."

As tempting as it is to speculate on a psychological diagnosis for Hope, such a designator is actually outside the scope of a vocational assessment. Clearly her distress over not being allowed to proceed was profound and appears to be rooted in a more basic disorder of the self that includes distorted thinking. Simply put, she fits the characterization of having a mask of sanity that quickly crumbles when challenged by life's circumstances.

Certainly Hope's condition made it impractical for her to have a responsible position leading adults in their quest for spiritual or religious growth. But what about her own spiritual growth? She clearly complied with all of the formal requirements for education. She was obviously bright. She also demonstrated the persistence of a religious call by continuing to appeal to a successions of denominational bodies.

Hope's primary disorder projected her interior need to be supremely special onto God. She had enough education to recognize that a corporate body such as a diocese or presbytery or synod has a role to play in confirming a call to religious life. But her education was an intellectual veneer over a more primary idolatry of the self and thus insufficient to carry her through the experience of rejection.

At this point in the diagnostic enterprise, Hope's diagnosis would look like this, utilizing both the formal DSM-IV system and my multi-axial system of diagnosis:

> *DSM-IV Diagnosis:*
>
> *Axis I* – Depressive Disorder NOS – 311.0
>
> *Axis II* – Dependent Personality Disorder with
>
>   Narcissistic features – 301.60
>
> *Axis III* – None Reported
>
> *Axis IV* – Vocational Difficulties
>
> *Axis V* – GAF Current: 55   GAF Last Year: 55
>
> *Spiritual / Theological Multi-axial Diagnosis:*
>
> *Axis I-* Guilt: Realistic failure of prior efforts at finding work; subjective belief that she is flawless.
>
> *Axis II* – Idolatry: Mythic-literal level of faith with high need to see self as special agent of God. No tolerance for ambiguity of divine purpose.

Conclusion

The notion of idolatry may offend the sensibilities of the sophisticated reader. When such is the case, the discomfort is diagnostic of the reader's lack of exposure to the depths of the human condition. Entire cultures are willing to sacrifice themselves for a variety of gods, as recent events all too clearly illustrate. Just as significantly, individuals will both inflict and endure extreme discomfort to maintain engrained patterns of behavior. They will justify their conduct with a belief structure that has all the elements of a religious system: a sacred place, a community of like-minded believers, sacraments, rites, holy seasons and a defining myth.

In the best of conditions care in this arena of the soul involves a spiritual transformation. This can include the acquisition of new religious insight, recovery from an addiction, recommitment to marital vows or a significant change in political philosophy. Such a transformation typically requires both the loss of naiveté and the acquisition of a second naiveté. Such transformations occurs naturally as one matures across the lifespan at significant developmental junctions as well as pushing through what the Melancholy Dane described as 'the slings and arrows of outrageous fortune.' (3) It is imperative that the provider of humane care allow both time and space for the soul to ripen through such mountainous passes of adversity as well as for the mind to grasp what life now requires and for the human body to marshal its ample powers of restoration.

We will return to these vignettes one more time in chapter sixteen. This chapter will be followed by an examination of special diagnostic cases that illustrate the way these three themes appear when working with children, substance abuse, significant stress disorders and mass bereavement. For now, we leave behind the distress that comes when penultimate concerns become the focus of our soul and turn our attention to the condition of dread and the feeling of defilement. *Selah!*

Part IV-Dread: the Feeling of Defilement

Chapter 13

Waking up In Gomorrah

The story of Sodom and Gomorrah continues to inform the consciousness and conscience of even non-religious people. It is an ancient story of grace and judgment as well as an exemplar of how perversion in a community ultimately affects a family system as well as leading to the destruction of an entire region. It is a symbol of corruption and defilement as recent as the collapse of levees in New Orleans and the rumors that swept through the media about the conduct of people abandoned to their own fears. The dread of defilement underlies the cultural tensions within the United States as well as the way the theocratic Middle East views the democratic West. But the focus of this part of the diagnostic enterprise will be much more limited.

One thing must be said clearly at the outset. I am using the symbolism of Gomorrah solely as a marker for the presence of a seemingly indelible stain on a human soul that results from some type of fundamental failure in genetic endowment, failure of care, societal collapse or natural catastrophe. A small percentage of humanity is born with a catastrophic genetic failure that creates unspeakable heartache and challenge for themselves and those who love them. A much larger percentage of our fellow creatures endure unspeakably devastating trauma whose effects alter the course of their life. Even if their post-trauma life brings great blessings to many, the 'memories of it are still vivid sixty years later' as more than one survivor of such events will tell you. (1) For the caregivers of our most gravely damaged fellow creatures and for our companions whose memories include a repository of indescribable horror there is a sense of living in or near a place where the price of admission was an eternal stain on the soul. The symbolic name of such a place is 'Gomorrah' although the actual address may be that of someone's childhood home.

The feeling of guilt pushes the soul toward washing. The feeling of terror prompts a person to flee or fight. The feeling of dread and the state of defilement initially roots one in place. Pastors and counselors periodically have the opportunity to sit with others whose brain and soul appear to be broken apart. It is not that all of these persons are intellectually marred or socially isolated. But their inward emotional experiences appear to set them apart. Some hold responsible social positions. Others are able to remain only marginally employed. Most do

143

not seem to do exceptionally well in intimate relationships, whether in marriage or work. There appears to be an air of detachment about them which others find mildly to significantly troubling.

It is as though there is a coating of broken glass upon their life. Sometimes when the sunlight strikes the glass there is a refraction of light into a rainbow. But just as often the glass of their inner experience simply cuts upon those who draw close to them. More important for diagnostic purposes, such individuals seem to symbolize God in ways which depict an experience which is at once overwhelming and yet alienating, unreachable and yet persistently at hand, fundamentally confirming while at the same time evoking feelings of their being utterly damned. They give every appearance of attempting to hold life together through a bewildering series of disruptions that they seek to explain through a painful array of paradoxes.

For some of these individuals a psychiatric diagnosis of 'paranoid schizophrenia' or 'schizotypal personality' appears to be behaviorally descriptive. Yet for many others there is not a clear psychiatric nosology. We do not have a consistent religious way of assessing these individuals' religious life, gauging the pain which they bear or which we perceive ourselves to be bearing if we were in their condition. Hearing their anguish and bringing some order to their pain is difficult for even skilled clinicians, regardless of theoretical orientation. Guiding the religious care of such a person is even more problematic, especially if the person is otherwise healthy and not in a hospital setting. They appear to move through life not merely to the fabled different drummer; they appear to be at once aliens from a strange land yet living among us with no effort being made to assimilate into what we view as normal or typical.

One other truth should be recalled at every turn in our care of individuals and families with this fundamental shattering of human neurology and psyche: our most powerful medications and best intentions still provide only relief of symptoms. The language of 'cure' is a phantasm; only the language of 'care' and 'control of symptoms' is appropriate here. The dread we experience as we face these disorders comes from the awareness that we have reached the limit of our science and our sensitivities. Here the line between 'cure' and 'care' becomes Hadrian's Wall .

Primary Failures in Attachment

I recall a man who was a periodic visitor to a church in Chicago. Since the church was routinely open, he would enter, sit at the piano and play for hours. You could hear the piano playing inside the church from outside the large, red double doors. Its chords penetrated the traffic noise. When I entered the sanctuary I recognized the muscular form bent over the keys. Although the music was not a song, it was a tuneful rendition of his inner world. Rhythmic. Forceful. Chaotic. Phrases of tenderness were followed hard by passages of violent urgency. I sat in the rear of the sanctuary. This was holy ground.

When his prayer was over, he rose and walked toward the rear of the sanctuary. His way of greeting was to ask me if I had seen one of the church members who was an attorney. "I'm going to sue the builders of the John Hancock Building and the Sears Tower," he said simply. "They heard my prophecy on North Avenue Beach and used it to plan their buildings. Now there are rich people living in the buildings I designed while I'm sleeping on the street."

Through the years he would sometimes rise during the middle of worship to ask a question. When he remembered to take his thioridazine he enjoyed periods of lucidness. When he did not maintain himself in this way the need for hospitalization and psychiatric care would quickly overtake him. He seemed unaware of his effect on others, although he was perceptive about another person's ability to help or harm him. The details of his psychiatric and social history did not seem to matter nearly as much as his current experience of isolation and the court's demand for continued vigilance on the part of those around him. This case is severe and most outpatient clinicians and pastoral caregivers will not encounter this level of disruption in an individual's psyche. Nonetheless although this signals a profound disintegration in a person's neurology, the consequent social and spiritual chaos is not limited to the individual. Family members and society bear a cost and anguish that cannot be counted.

This is an extreme example of what happens when the human need to receive nurturing attachment combines with genetic predisposition and marginal social conditions. We do not yet thoroughly understand the origins of severe mental disorders such as schizophrenia. Recognizing the roots of profound mental retardation and providing for long-term care of individuals who bear with this affliction likewise creates profound hardship on the families whose name they bear as well as the armada of caregivers who seek to relieve their suffering and support their families. An entire cadre of institutions and providers becomes focused on the physical, social, emotional and spiritual distress associated with these conditions. Social planners may quietly thank God this profound distress is not more common even as their families walk a life-long path of self-blame, discouragement, resentment, financial hardship, social isolation and emotional exhaustion.

"You learn early not to constantly ask yourself 'why?'" more than one parent has said to me. "At least consciously," they frequently confide. But it only takes one poorly timed view of a 'normal' family to bring more than a twinge of sadness to their eye and heart. Some marriages and families cope well with such catastrophic distress; others do not. But even divorce does not remove from the heart, mind and pocketbook the burdens of guilt, the rage at betrayal by the universe and the life-changing stain of being genetically linked to someone with a profound mental disorder.

Of course it is easier for caregivers to focus on providing support and succor to the families of individuals with profound mental distress. But this is only so because in them we have individuals with whom we can empathize. We can place ourselves in the position of a parent or sibling who lives with or who has birthed someone with significant mental handicap. We can sooth ourselves with neologisms that their relative is 'differently-abled' or 'challenged.' The families themselves may eventually come to speak of their child as a special gift from God who has allowed them to find a depth in themselves they would have never known. True enough; but it is doubtful on the front-end that any of us would make such a *request* of the universe. Such is the stuff of quiet heroism for which there must certainly be great reward in another life or place.

Fortunately with the advances in neurological imagery and genetic understanding a parent no longer needs to hold themselves responsible in quite the same way as in past millennia. Indeed we now have just enough knowledge of these areas to heighten the pre-birth ethical quandaries for parents of some individuals who are birthed with or who have an increased risk of developing profound mental or physical disorders. To provide the reader with a bit of history, one of my earliest pastoral counseling supervisors was on his hospital's first efforts to provide such genetically informed counseling. From a spiritual standpoint these advances in our knowledge adds a profound dimension to the awareness that we have lost our ethical and spiritual innocence eons ago. (2) The primary 'failures of attachment' thus appear to be at the level of neural pathways and genes rather than in the misplaced touch of a hand or the poorly chosen word of praise.

The primary task of spiritual care for the afflicted individual initially focuses on the caregiver or counselor gaining an appropriate level of knowledge about the specific developmental condition. I remember learning about a young intern whose assignment was to shadow a severely autistic child and assist the treatment staff where he could. One day he happened to bring his clarinet into the treatment facility to play. It appeared to calm the child. This pleased the intern and he began bringing the instrument regularly. When the child one day reached out his hands as if to ask to see the instrument, the intern thought he had made some type of break-through. As he extended the clarinet toward the child, the child grabbed his hand and bit him severely enough to require stitches. Such are the challenges of providing humane care and having competent understanding of such profound disconnections within the deep recesses of the brain. The enduring scar on his left hand is a permanent reminder to all who know the story of this moment of revelatory staining.

Catastrophic Fractures in Affection

The photographs of abandoned children inevitably tug at our heart. Whether we are going on a video tour of an orphanage in one of the 'former republics of the Soviet Union' where there are hundreds of abandoned children or a single child whose care has been neglected by a meth-addicted mother, we instinctively reach out toward such children. This impulse says a great deal about who we are as creatures as well as about most peoples' primary values.

Once adopted and placed within a normally caring environment, many of these children recover and thrive. Some have enduring physical health problems from years of neglect but the resilience of the human body and advanced medical treatments available in Western nations appear to work magic. But the child is an emotional and spiritual time bomb. The son or daughter who initially greeted new parents with gratitude and affection quite rapidly appears to slide into an entirely different child. The normal stormy passage of puberty becomes a raging tornado of destruction of physical violence typically toward one parent coupled with psychological manipulation, academic problems and severe oppositional behavior. These marked shifts in mood and conduct replace the innocent child brought home from the adoption agency.

Somewhat less severe but no less troubling are children whose suffer significant abuse at the hands of one or both parents. Children of divorced parents who maintain a guerrilla war with one another likewise exhibit some of the same symptoms. A certain percentage of the host of oppositional-defiant disorders, learning disorders, conduct disorders and other adolescent mood disorders appear to have their roots in a primary failure of attachment to one or both parents. In working with these children what may surface is the troubled attachment of one parent to their own parents; other times there appears to be no clear genetic or behavioral antecedent by which to understand the root cause of the young person's behavioral and emotional distress.

One thing is clear in such situations. The nosology of the DSM-IV-TR hardly does justice to the anguish of all concerned with such situations. This includes the frustration of caregivers whose primary impulse to bring relief to suffering hearts and fractured relationships is thwarted by the limitations of neurology and physiology. But these are not the only conditions of failed attachment that stain the heart and profoundly affect an entire family or community's destiny.

I recall a client who began her work with me by recalling how the sharp stench of gasoline shook her awake! It was still dark in the box canyon where her attackers had brought her more than six hours ago. Her broken arm, ripped clothing and numerous wounds caused by the knives bore mute testimony to the violence of their assault.

"We're gonna burn you like the garbage you are," snarled one of the men. Under the deep starlight of an Arizona sky she prepared to die.

Later she would confide, "I don't know why they didn't kill me. I don't know what stopped them. But they argued among themselves for a while and then left. I fainted again. Later I found a creek and washed myself in the water. Somehow I made it back to a main road and help."

"I feel so utterly unclean. I wonder who would ever want me. I hold myself at night and try to cry. But my tears are dry."

"I haven't been back to church. I feel so unworthy to be there. And I keep wondering. In that hell of a canyon, *where was God?!*"

Her words were a confession of abandonment and defilement.   Her query is echoed by multitudes of people whose suffering we, the sheltered, can hardly comprehend. Yet many of these who have suffered so grievously sit, walk and work among us. They are our wives, parents, brothers and bosses. In a previous generation we could identify some who had known such horrors, for they bore the tattoo of the Holocaust upon a forearm. Today the names of the tormentors differ. But the wounds they have left upon the human heart are well known by those called to be healers.

Whether etched upon the psyche a single slice at a time or impressed into the marrow during the grim Sarajevo winter, humans who undergo such deep suffering report a feeling of abandonment and defilement for which there are few words. Some people describe the inner awareness of a creature inside of them, seeming to utter a continuous low wail. Others report being aware of a deep inner darkness that they "see" as a visual background to every waking moment.

I remember speaking with one veteran of the 1st Marine Division's retrograde march out from the Chosin Reservoir in Korea. He could not talk in detail of those awful days. But this comment was telling in its sparseness, "You know, I have *never* been able to get warm. Even right now, I feel cold," he confided one magnolia scented Richmond afternoon.

At other times the distress occurs at birth or appears to spring fully formed at the bidding of a genetic calendar. As religious counselors, pastors and clinicians we stand here at the very boundary between genius and madness, between the true prophet and the person whom the gods have set out to destroy. The torture and joy of the inner life appears through the word salad of schizophrenese or the complexity of James Joyce's *Ulysses*. Those who seem to bear the burden of retardation have a religious joy many of us may envy. Yet the sheer marginality of their life may make us recoil. To struggle with the deterioration of aging or a life-concluding disease may be enough to completely erase a lifetime of hopefulness. All clinicians are confronted by the sheer 'un-redemptiveness' of some human suffering in the course of a professional career.

What matters most here is not so much the content of the experience as the profundity of the experience itself. (3) In each instance a human soul is attempting to express what is ineffable, trying to point toward that which is beyond eyesight but not beyond human vision. They, no less than we, long to connect in some satisfying way with a Being 'that than which a Greater cannot exist.' (4) A Reality that is at once immanent and transcendent. Yet the core reality that these separate individuals all grope to express is one that, apparently, is utterly debasing. They truly believe they are beyond the reach of the Almighty One. It is as though in some way they have been inducted into a secret fellowship of suffering from which all others have been excluded. Including God.

For such persons the language of defilement seems to evoke the most self-awareness. The cry of abandonment seems to resonate most deeply within their experience. It is the fundamental recognition that one has been in an unholy place, seen or done unholy acts, heard unholy words and crossed the boundary that separates their living soul from what they know is more traditionally spoken human experience. In our religious and clinical rush to soothe every ache and pronounce grace upon every sin, we may be sorely tempted to gloss over a person's report of such primitive feelings. In particular, our modern church music and liturgies soft-pedal this element in religious life. In attempting to be non-offensive we may offend what is most Holy in both the person and in the universe. If we do not speak the language of defilement or acknowledge the depth of abandonment to which the human soul can sink, then we have no genuine good news to offer those for whom this has become their primary experience.

Defilement and the Symbolism of Stain

Stains come in various ways but they remind us that something is fundamentally flawed. Whether it is our shirt's visible memory of a hurried cup of coffee or a sidewalk's memory of a murder, stains symbolize an event that was vital. Stains are snapshots of the past that haunts or at least linger into the present. We may joke about the hunting jacket that gets its oil changed every decade whether it needs it or not. But the real jacket is a visual statement in the present of the owner's past activity. While it is a badge of honor among hunters there are many places where such a visual and vital statement would make people recoil. We do not feel neutral about stains. Stains symbolize our uncleanness. Stains picture our flaws. Stains are not only left *upon* us they are tangible memories of things we have *done upon* the world-our world. Stains symbolize "a 'something' that infects, a dread that anticipates the unleashing of the avenging wrath of the interdiction" for the taboo which the stain symbolizes. (5)

Stains shock us. Several years ago a young woman who described herself as a Performance Artist drew the outline of a body on the sidewalks where a rape had occurred. The public outcry was immediate and intense! Imagine! In *Richmond!* Someone leaving a mark on an *historic* sidewalk! People were much more upset by the "stain" left by her white paint than the human stain left by the rapes. For those of us who lived or worked in the neighborhood, her staining art was a sobering reminder of our shared vulnerability, our impotence and our guilty lack of outrage.

Religious consciousness is filled with the symbolism of stain. One of the most ancient Biblical stories carries the image of a stain or mark left upon Cain. While the function of the mark was to protect him from revenge, its presence functioned as a continual reminder of his homicide. (6) Significantly this story speaks of both the soil and the person bearing a stain as a permanent mark of defilement. One of the dominant images of absolution is that of cleansing a stain, a reality reinforced by our Psalms of penitence such as Psalm 51 and hymnody such as *Love Lifted Me:*

> I was sinking, deep in sin / Far from the peaceful shore,
> Very deeply stained within / Sinking to rise no more,
> But the Master of the Sea / Heard my despairing cry,
> From the waters lifted me / Now safe am I, (7)

Stains upon the heart are more than powerful metaphor. Stains typically have their antecedent in real fluids that are present as an integral part of the defiling action. It can be as fundamental as the discoloration of a woman's birth water which signals major infant distress. Indeed the monthly cycle of menstruation has been, perhaps unfairly but nonetheless realistically remains a continuing symbol for feminine weakness. Semen spilled during a rape or molestation, bloody tubercular phlegm, vomit encrusted clothing from alcohol poisoning, bandages upon a wound and our deep dread of blood carrying the AIDS virus are genuine substances which imprint real scars upon both body and soul. Our obsession with soaps and scents for home and self reveals how deeply we desire to avoid being, or at least showing, our stains to one another. We avoid people and places that are stained. They are unholy and profane. Although Ricoeur argues that 'defilement was never literally a stain; impurity was never literally filthiness, dirtiness,' clinicians may find that inquiry into the exact nature of a person's distress does, indeed, lodge within the memory of a literal stain. (8)

Our secular culture tells stories of unholy stains and longs for rites to cleanse stains no less than our religious communities. The most potent stories are ones that symbolize the utter transformation and damnation of people who have contact with the blood of another. These are the myths of vampires and werewolves. These stories do more than scare small children around campfires. We may walk out of the movie theater's darkness saying, "It deserved the two thumbs up Siskle and Ebert gave it!" But in the darkness of the theater our pulse raced because we were truly fearful. Our hair stood on end and our skin crawled because we recoiled in genuine dread. Our science may tell us such creatures and unholy transformations do not occur. But our unconscious that comes from the dawn of our existence remains unconvinced. We react with revulsion.

The impact of such fundamental brokenness upon a life is difficult to gauge. For a majority of persons the dynamics of their stains and the feeling of dread do not incapacitate them. Most of us can wall off or repress such memories. We continue with our lives in what we believe to be a pathway unaffected by such fundamental tragedy. But there are others among us whose flaws are so overwhelming that the barriers of repression and impulse control are over-whelmed. A few of these persons will seek the care of a pastor, the hope embodied in a religious community or the relative sanctuary of a psychiatric facility. Many more will not. We will instead perceive glimpses of their stain upon the pages of our society's daily record. Ricoeur's comment that "primitive dread deserves to be interrogated as our oldest memory" may be fruitful advice for clinicians, whether their orientation is secular or religious. (9)

Defilement and the Saving Sacrifice

Her dreams were always vivid. They have plagued her sleep for years, because their violent and bloody content is so at odds with her serene and fastidious appearance. Sometimes Rose is fleeing in horror from a faceless man who wields a knife. Other times she is in a junk yard watching a man drag a woman into a bedroom. Often she is sheltering a group of children. Her cries often wake her up.

"I fear I am losing my mind," she said. "My life is not this horrible." As our work progressed through the first year of conversation, another image began appearing alongside of the bloody violence: water. Sometimes there was a tile bathroom shower or a nearby river. In other dreams the setting is a seaside cabin or she watches rain wash the grime from a darkened city street through the glass wall of an urban apartment.

Then one day Rose said, "We're not going to get anywhere unless I tell you what really has happened." So in a voice nearly devoid of emotion she recounted being tied up on her wedding night. She has remembered three minis-ters, so far, who have assaulted her while also telling her she "was helping God's work." She remembered her mother's long-standing frailty, along with the cryptic instructions that she and her husband would "work out an arrangement."

The events behind this woman's dread and stain continued to surface. But like her mother before her, she did not leave her abusive husband. She did not transfer to a job where her boss was not predatory. She had made a decision to endure continued staining and humiliation for the sake of the safety of others. Rose soothes the dread and tames her emerging rage with medication.

Sacrifice is one of the basic ways that we cope with the profound abandonment of such assaults upon our being. Whether it is the parent who interposes themselves between a child and danger or, just as likely, a child who decides to offer a portion of their self for family stability, the dynamic element in the event is one of partial self-slaughter. There always comes the heroic moment when a living soul chooses the unknown depths of abandonment in a desperate gamble to forestall the known horror which confronts them. We give medals to soldiers who make such a sacrifice. But many more people make similar offerings of the self and go on living as though nothing has happened. Thus the counselor may live and work for years beside another who is deeply stained by some prior sacrifice of psyche and soma yet be unaware of the events that have so profoundly shaped the person's current life.

There are a number of clinical profiles that have such saving sacrifice at their root. Multiple Personality Disorder, Anorexia and Bulimia come readily to mind. But even where there is not such profound disturbance in the outer life there can be a staining sacrifice. Depression which robs one of hope, anxiety that disrupts one's peace, repetitive unemployment as well as pervasive drug dependence and cyclic infidelity may all have a core memory of a stain whose outline we can see only through repetitive behavior. The clinical description of 'personality traits that are inflexible and maladaptive and cause significant functional impairment or subjective distress' begins to approach this area of religious interest. (10) While religious diagnosis lacks the specificity of Schizoid Personality Disorder (301.20) with full-blown differential diagnostic options, the existential dimension of human experience is no less genuine and the language of stain no less descriptive of the person's dilemma.

Conclusion

Religious sensitivity in general and the theological training of pastors specifically equips them to understand the profound connection symbols have upon the human soul. Symbols obtain their numinosity precisely because they participate in the awesome, dread acts to which they point us. Thus the mute anguish of many people is a religious awareness of the ineffableness of the staining acts to which they have been a party. Our spiritual awareness of such connections embody the hope of healing for others, for we may understand more than many that new life and resurrection awaits us. But resurrection comes only after one faces the dread abandonment of an *Old Rugged Cross,* has been touched by the *Balm in Gilead* and has drunk deeply from the Cup of Transformational Suffering. Only the religiously attuned counselor can use the healing story of Jacob's Well, listening there to another thirsty person's confusion and reminding them of the Spirit's living water . (11) *Selah!*

Chapter 14

Feeling Abandoned and Receiving Cleansing

The letter usually arrives sometime between Thanksgiving and Christmas. Another one arrives sometime between the Fourth of July and Memorial Day. Or at least they used to.

In barely legible printing I can make out the return address of one of Virginia's state prisons. His writing has deteriorated over the years, especially once he was transferred to one of the hospital units within the prison system and confined to a wheel chair.

He sent me his Bible and two mathematics textbooks when he left the facility where I met him. For several years I had made a bi-weekly trip to lead a therapy group for incarcerated veterans and it was always well attended.

There are many more people whose interior experience, family life, and social position place them behind bars. As more than one inmate said to me during the years I made that trip, "At least here we know where the bars are and why we're here. The people on the outside don't admit there are bars and locks in their life."

There are millions of people in the world whose daily experience is one of being abandoned. They are the elderly who live out their days in extended care facilities or the psychologically troubled whose sleep is on the steam grates in major cities. They are the orphaned children who form their own families around older children or the refugees who trade the violence of their homeland for the instability of a United Nation's camp somewhere near the a contested border.

For these millions it is cold comfort to know where the bars are. Very few of these individuals will ever come into a counseling center or church for even emergency care. But millions more throughout the world have the experience of feeling abandoned while having around them the appearance of family, community, social status and even abundance in its many recognizable forms. They are the survivors of rape who nevertheless shoulder the challenge of marriage. They are the men and women whose write alternative chapters to a life begun with childhood poverty or maternal alcoholism or paternal suicide. They are men and women who come home from war and find ways to quietly soldier on with their life, building a tabernacle from whatever carnage they saw rather than 'bringing the war home' to their community and family through replicated violence.

The list of individuals who feel abandoned at some point in their life exceeds those whose physical circumstance is literally one of abandonment. While this masks the extensive emotional and spiritual cost, it also obscures the interactive creativity of the Divine and human spirit. Multitudes among us discover a measure of cleansing from this primal stain and go on to make significant contributions to the human family. Sometimes the healers among us are privileged to be midwifes to this transformation. More frequently the transformation happens in the quiet of individual souls and the benefit is initially an unintended consequence of their quiet individual courage.

Identifying the Primal Stain

Somewhere in the corpus of cases from Sherlock Holmes, the world's most famous detective, he shares with his companion Dr. Watson the secret of his extraordinary success at solving the most mysterious and complex of cases. Along with the profound powers of observation that are available only to characters in a novel, Holmes says in effect that one rules out all other causes and the remainder, however inconceivable, is the solution to the crime.

We have available to us in this century forensic and medical tools inconceivable to Mr. Holmes. They essentially work magic on what would heretofore be cold cases of the most heinous kind. But the tools available to the average clinician remain the same as those utilized by Holmes and Watson: the well-tuned ear, the observant eye, the informed mind, the open heart, and the warmth of appropriate touch. They are virtually unchanged as the tools used by the earliest healers. What is different is our understanding of the depth to which certain experiences shape the neuronal structures of the brain and thus influence an individual's life for decades if not for all eternity.

For the clinician there is a period of academic training and clinical supervision that launches them toward licensure or some other official certification. Continuing education and regular consultation reinforce and enrich this initial period of formal preparation. But this instruction still relies on the hurting individual's ability to somehow disclose their primary brokenness to a well-prepared care provider. As most clinicians soon discover, few people disclose such basic distress during their initial hours of counseling. As most clinicians also soon discover the stain they most readily identify is more than just an echo of their own earliest wounds.

Thus the most effective healers, utilizing whatever theoretical discipline available, learn to pay attention to what is formally called 'counter-transference.' A statistically significant portion of effective physicians, nurses, social workers and ministers have had an encounter with the death of someone close to them by the time they reach age eighteen. Or they have undergone the loss of some cardinal virtue or individual by virtue of a parental divorce or some other primary parental failure. (1), (2)

There are some visceral and thematic indicators of such a primal stain that clinicians learn to pay attention to. Thematically any event in the personal history that entails contact with a staining bodily fluid such as blood, urine, semen, phlegm, or cranial fluid. Contact with toxic chemicals such as dioxin or biologic agents such as anthrax or other virus under conditions of duress appear to produce in the psyche similar effects in the person's long-term development More viscerally the seasoned therapist or physician learns to listen carefully for the sudden thickening in the voice or to notice the subtle tearing around the rim of the eye as the person relates seemingly innocuous events. Making the inquiry, 'do you know what your tears are about?' so that such wound begins to be seen in the light of day requires both appropriate empathy and exquisite timing.

Most significantly, effective healing results as the clinician pays attention to their own visceral and intuitive reactions to the person and their story. The clinician must learn through effective supervision how to utilize these counter-transferential responses to frame both their diagnostic understanding of the person and their posture of care. Sometimes the naming of the pain occurs through a deeply shared silence that grows over years of gradual exposure.

At other times the stain can be explicitly named and a regime of care begun that brings a measure of relief. Use of a spiritual injury questionnaire, such as that developed by a chaplain at the White Cloud Veterans' Administration Medical Center, can help identify both the nature and intensity of this primal stain. The inventory asks individuals to 'report if they never, sometimes, often or very often experienced such spiritual injuries as guilt, shame, rage, grief, unfair treatment by God or life and other injuries of the soul.' (3) This instrument may be effective when used explicitly as an intake or in the midst of treatment as an additional assessment document.

This instrument asks individuals typical items such as 'do you feel that life has no meaning or purpose?' or 'do you feel disappointed or betrayed by others?' Items such as these clearly identify the long-term consequences of a staining experience. In this regard the instrument assists the client in naming their pain. Just as importantly for the provision of care, the instrument asks 'do you have membership in or participate in any local church / synagogue / mosque or other organized expression of religion?' and 'do you have a personal / private spiritual practice?' The response to such items can become the basis for inquiry by even non-religious care providers since the best practice of care in such situations includes encouraging the individual to develop spiritual practices.

Most significantly for the purposes of diagnosis, the form follows up on this last query with these two items and includes room for the person to elaborate:

'What is your spiritual practice?' and "If you are not religious and you do not have a spiritual practice, how do you cope with life's cares and what gives you a sense of purpose or meaning in life?' These are clearly the 'big questions of life' that uniformly require an appeal to spiritual or religious resources. Although in the history of psychotherapy this area has been generally regarded as off-limits by clinicians, the more recent research of David Larson (4) now buttresses what many humanistic theoreticians have long held: "as Jungian, existential, transpersonal and humanistic psychologies have argued, attending to the big questions might make other facets of life fall into place." (5) Thus even though it has been argued by several psychologists of religion that 'every therapy entails spiritual matters,' addressing such primary human stains without utilizing spiritual or religious resources certainly borders on ineffective diagnosis and treatment. (6) While some theorists argue persuasively 'unless therapists have pastoral credentials, they court violation of professional ethics when they delve into religion and theology, as such' these concerns are stumbled upon in the practical delivery of care as it unfolds. (7) In my earlier treatment of this topic I urged secular clinicians to develop consultative relationships with pastoral theologians or pastoral counselors who can enrich if not guide them through this thicket without the cumbersome necessity of the client having to start over with a new therapist. It is a view I still hold. (8)

Thus far we have looked at the symptoms of such a primary stain upon the human heart. Psychologically resolving the stain and cleansing the stain through the use of spiritual or religious resources bear directly on the delivery of care. This primal stain is the common wound and its aftermath that runs through all catastrophic events and failures of care in the same way that spirituality is rightly understood as 'a common human core that runs through all religions and cultures and might be expressed in theist terms.' (9)

Resolving the Primal Stain

I am indebted to the work of Daniel A. Helminiak's explication of the nature of the human spirit for providing a quartet of directions in which psychological resolution of primal stain may be pursued. In his manuscript "Treating Spiritual Issues in Secular Psychotherapy" he notes that the human spirit is our capacity for self-transcendence, he then outlines four areas by which this transcendence can be expressed:

> Human spirit is self-transcending in that its spontaneity leads one to continually to move beyond one's former self and into Ever broader experience. It is dynamic in that it is a relentless movement that would rest content only in some ideal fulfillment of knowing everything about everything and loving all that is loveable. It is structured in that it expresses itself in four shifting and interacting foci. (10)

So here we have the first clue to how this stain may be resolved: our deepest inner process seeks always to move toward what is healthy and good. Helminiak's description of these four directions outlines the ways in which a therapist may assist an individual whose therapeutic desire remains motivated toward resolution of a primal stain:

> It is empirical in that we are open to experience, aware and also aware of our awareness. It is intelligent in that we question for understanding, arrive at insight, and formulate understandings as ideas, hypotheses, or theories. It is rational in that we assess the sufficiency of the evidence for our understandings and, thus, make judgments, arrive at facts, and thus know reality. And it is existential in that we deliberate and decide about choices to be made and values to be embraced in our everyday living. (11)

Thus therapy may proceed in one of these four directions: empirical awareness of the surrounding world and its possibilities, intelligent understanding aimed at generating insight of the self within the world, a rational exploration of evidence for beliefs about the self and world and finally assisting the client in making more healthy choices for everyday living in the world as one comes to know the world and the self based upon new awareness, insight and evidence.

When these four directions are utilized as a posture of diagnostic they can be framed into four imperatives that a therapist may use to guide a wide variety of psychodynamic, cognitive, behavioral or existential interventions. Citing Bernard Lonergan, Dr. Helminiak frames these four imperatives as: be attentive, be intelligent, be reasonable and be responsible. (12) A somewhat humorous yet ironic way of offering this guidance to a client comes by reminding them of the statement 'do what you've always done and you'll get what you've always gotten.' A much darker way of underscoring the imperative nature of these paths was in a cross-stitch plaque one of my early supervisors had positioned in his office: "Sometimes you have to shoot your own dog. Don't farm it out. It only makes it worse." Such imperatives remind one and all that effective therapy involves matters of life-and-death, not just helping someone emote warm feelings or rehash old grievances one more time.

These four imperatives are transcendental in character and thus speak precisely to the primal nature of these stains. These four imperatives also acknowledge the route to resolution is through self-transcendence. With such stains one grows throughout the lifespan but one does not outgrow the stain. One's soul and mind and body learn to find a style of life that is ever more authentic to the self while at the same time being more responsible to the greater community and the highest values birthed through the interplay of the human-divine spirit

These four imperatives apply equally to the work of the therapist. It is the task of the therapist / caregiver to assist in this process of self-transcendence. The task of guiding the care of the individual, couple or family burdened with such a stain is sometimes done through silence, sometimes through confrontation, sometimes through suggesting an appropriate book or medication, sometimes through taking a walk and sometimes by prayer.

We too must be attentive, intelligent, reasonable and responsible. Clinical training, codes of ethics and continued attention to best practices sets the caregiver on the right path of personal self-transcendence. But only a personalcommitment by the caregiver to continued personal growth will equip us to remain authentic and effective as diagnosticians and care providers.

These four imperatives require one additional change for the therapeutic provider of humane care: a theoretical shift in how the human being is understood. Traditionally the scientific model has been a dualistic mind-body or 'ghost-in-the-machine' understanding of humanity. Our contemporary interest in spirituality has now brought us to conceptualize human growth professionally as a trinity of body-mind-spirit. Within the mental health disciplines guided by the medical model we have tended to think diagnostically along the lines of a biopsychosocial schema of understanding. But if we are to fully name an individual's pain and guide their care in a way that includes resolving such primary stains as described here, we must now view the human person as a biopsychosocial*spiritual* entity.

The challenge for the person and the provider of humane care is to preserve some core psychological stability even as one encourages social change, adapts to physical limitations and hopes for spiritual growth. Reliving an individual's primal stain may be seen as a precondition for the integration of these four dimensions of human experience in a way that promotes continued self-transcendence. While one may approach this goal from a purely humanistic viewpoint, I would argue that since the traditional social expression of spirituality is some form of organized religion, whether theist or non-theist, a full regime of responsible care must include the religious belief structure of the person who has come for healing.

Cleansing the Primal Stain

The vast majority of the human race is not born with profoundly disabling conditions nor develops chronic syndromes that are the consequences of catastrophic trauma. Given the harsh conditions under which some humans live and the genetic roll of the dice that occurs each time one of us is conceived, this may seem miraculous. This is a tribute to human resilience. Our neurological structure, social diversity, individual creativity and cussedness combine with that evanescent quality we describe as 'grace' to move the preponderance of humanity toward a greater measure of health and stability than toward disease and instability.

One the front end of life there are profoundly disabling conditions that challenge the resources of parents, extended families and entire communities to reach some measure of reasonable understanding and provide humane care. The entire autism spectrum, Downs Syndrome, Williams-Beuren Syndrome, and Hurler's Syndrome, comprise a very short list of such disorders indeed. Yet throughout the millennia our human tendency has been to not only marshal the most humane care available at the time, we also find ourselves gaining greater compassion toward infants and children who are afflicted with profound genetic maladies. We no longer routinely abandon children on the sides of mountains or chain them in dark closets. Organized religion has been one of the primary engines of such transformation of humanity's consciousness and conscience in this area.

As life progresses some disorders appear during adolescence. The schizophrenic and paranoid thought disorders are among the most well known. Their eruption produces severe personal and familial consequences. The beginnings of substance abuse disorders in adolescence and their long-term costs are sometimes reversible to a greater or lesser degree. At other times the biopsychosocialspiritual consequences of substance abuse results in death either in early adulthood or ultimately in a shortened life. The interplay of severe biological compromises with the familial and societal consequences of substance abuse underscores the primary nature of this stain and is why they will be addressed in a separate chapter later in this volume.

In mid-life and toward the conclusion of a normal lifespan other chronic conditions develop that once again challenge our human resiliency in all four quadrants of human choice. Multiple Sclerosis, Parkinson's Disease, Hodgkin's Disease, dementia and cancer in all of their various manifestations, along with the side effects from the treatment of numerous medical conditions makes up a veritable steeple chase of challenges as we age. We approach these adversaries with the skills and resources developed over our lifetime as well as find new avenues through which to endure what the Bard of Avon through the voice of *Hamlet* rightly called 'the slings and arrows of outrageous fortune.' (13) These are not mental disorders in the precise sense of the term. Nevertheless these conditions create mental anguish or have associated with them alterations in human consciousness that makes us and those around us say quietly 'she is not herself today.'

Depending upon the resources of body, mind and spirit developed prior to the age of onset, such states initially create the sense of being a defective member of the human family, the target of a malevolent turn of destiny and perhaps even someone abandoned by the Creator to a greater or lesser extent. In the midst of these inheritable disorders and syndromes that are the exigencies created by trauma, we may come ultimately to a posture where we wish with the Biblical Job that we had the indictment of our adversary written large so that we could not just understand the exact nature of our distress but also resolve and cleanse our condition and return to full health and sanity. (14)

Major traumatic events occur across the lifespan. A tsunami devastates an area of Sri Lanka. Three hurricanes in a single year overwhelm the resources of America's Gulf Coast region. The Horsemen of the Apocalypse routinely ride across the planet's face inflicting their psychological and spiritual stains on human consciousness as well as the social realities of war, famine, plague and pestilence. More individual tragedies of murder, assault, rape, join with the private degradations of family violence and broken promises to wound the spirit as well as mind and body. I will address the diagnosis and treatment of these concerns in a future chapter. Yet their presence is so pervasive in human experience that one study concluded that just within the USA some ten percent of women and twenty percent of men experience post-traumatic stress disorder at some point in their life. (15)

Suffice it to say at this point that in addition to the application of psychological interventions and the balm of medications to the immediate effects of trauma, the long-term stains on human consciousness and societies of such events necessarily includes the use of spiritual and religious resources. While such resources appear to be 'supportive' to the outside observer, these rituals exert a powerful curative influence over the arc of human consciousness. Some wounds to the public spirit are so great that ceremonies of remembrance endure long after the debris have been cleared away, treaties have been signed, and more gracious winds and gentle rains have restored fertility to the soil.

Conclusion

There is within the realm of spiritual life the intuition that some events are so profoundly heinous they stain the very ground upon which the event occurs. When we know of such events or locales the human impulse is to either build a memorial to such an event or in some other way declare the space as an unholy wasteland to be eternally avoided. Our knowledge of forensics and the way traces of trauma linger long after human memory has healed now discloses the physical component to such spiritual sensitivities: stains upon the earth do indeed 'cry out' to those who have ears to hear. (16)

So too do the stains of profound distress remain upon the paths of memory and the synapses of our soul. Thus our impulse to assist another in the naming of their pain, hoping to provide them with a mark that provides them some measure of comfort is as old as our species most ancient myths. Yet not all people and places desire to disclose their primal distress. Some individuals literally go to their graves and take others with them rather than relinquish the dark power such stains exert upon psyche, soma and polis. The killing fields of Cambodia and the mass graves of Iraq as well as the societal dynamics that gave them birth will remain long after the last living participant in this age has vanished from the earth.

The discipline of theology calls such primal brokenness 'original sin..' Despite more recent voices that wish us to recall humanity's original blessing, the practice of diagnosis and the care of human souls must ever take account of this dragon lurking in the cave of humanity's collective unconscious if we are to bring any measure of genuine liberation to either the person in our consulting room or the culture within which we live. *Selah!*

Chapter 15

Communion, Vocation and Joy

Elie Wiessel is one of the world's best-known advocates of human rights. Simon Weisenthal was, at the time of his death, the world's pre-eminent hunter of former Nazi's hiding after outside of Germany in the aftermath of World War II. Both men went through an experience of feeling dreadfully abandoned and receiving on their forearm the staining tattoo of all who entered one of those camps. Both men drew the inspiration for their life's work from the hellish experience of German death camps. Both men found a new community and life's work among those who survived those camps and who vowed that never again would they permit such organized horror to stalk the earth.

These two individuals transformed their dread into joy. In doing so they not only transcended their former selves they also enabled the world to take another step along the moral arc of the universe. Elizabeth Kubler-Ross and Mother Theresa have likewise exerted a similar world wide culture-spanning and era-transcending influence that grew out of their own personal self-transcendence.

Throughout human history in every field of human endeavor a nameless multitude of humanity has undergone a similar transformation of their excruciating pain into an exultant purpose. Founders of religious orders, self-help groups, not-for-profit organizations, special interest groups and now thousands of blogs and websites illustrate this basic dynamic of healing through self-transcendence. How far the influence of an individual's self-transcendence and transformation extends may be difficult to fully determine, especially given what we have now begun to know about the plasticity of the brain and human genetics.

But the question of how far beyond the individual such self-transcendence extends is very secondary to the provision of humane care and the resulting maturation of a single soul. For the overwhelming majority of us who have endured some type of personal fiery forge of dreadful abandonment the change is quite private and known only to those who live closely with us.

The story of this transformation is the story of salvation. Its soundtrack is as soulful as *Amazing Grace*. Its story line is as triumphant as *Superman Returns*. It is also a story written in blood, sweat and tears more expensive than whatever co-pay exchanges hands at the conclusion of the clinical hour.

The majority of us find succor in this journey through the discovery or rediscovery of traditional religious values and inspiration from one of their founders. In the words of Sam Shoemaker's immortal poem *I Stand By the Door,* we find 'the door to God' with the 'latch that only clicks and opens to the person's own touch.' Some of us go on to help others find their way to this door, as did the individuals named above. Multitudes more are content to simply get inside the door and continue the journey. (1)

What waits on the other side of that door is a dynamic communal mystery capable of transforming the sacrifice of the self into the salvation of the self. A portion of the journey on the other side of this door is the discovery of a call to service that transcends mere work. Remaining on the journey long enough leads one out of a land where, in the words of C. S. Lewis, 'it is always winter but never Christmas' into terrain where joy comes with the morning. It is to an exploration of these transcendent dynamics that we now turn.

Communion as Transformation of the Sacrifice to Salvation

Throughout the course of clinical experience I have encountered many heroes. Many have been warriors whose *bona fides* quietly display themselves on the small ribbons worn on their best suit. Many more heroes are people who made – or who continue to make – some type of saving sacrifice of their identity in order to prevent a greater evil from afflicting their spouse, sibling or entire family. These are not individuals who responded to some variation of a Storm Trooper's knock on the door some rainy night with the question, "Are you hiding Jews in the basement?"

These are people whose assessment of life within their own family drew them to the conclusion they must sacrifice some portion of their own identity in order to preserve the stability of their marriage or family. Thus the older brother who endures the beatings of an enraged parent by lying about who really broke the lamp rather than allows the younger sibling to receive crippling punishment is one such sacrificial hero. The sister or brother who allows a predatory parent to sexually molest them and keep the secret in the belief that others will not receive the same treatment is yet another such hero. The stay-at-home mother and the no-promotion father who places family stability and security over personal career satisfaction are other such sacrificial heroes.

So too can be the precocious children or the super-achiever adults whose public performance compensates for a private flaw. At times academic brilliance, financial abundance, community service, or other sterling triumph accomplishes an important secondary gain: it somehow compensates for some significant interior wound. At times the truly great success comes from drawing the outer world's attention away from some private wound that must never see the light of day or, so the person believes, the dawn of redemption. We do not think of these individuals as having made a 'sacrifice' for we are blinded by their external success. The truth is they desire us to be misdirected in just such a fashion.

The first step in diagnosis is for the clinician to recognize such misdirection or compensation. While this may be a straightforward task it is seldom an easy task. An even more difficult task is helping or guiding the person toward a view of themselves as a sacrificial hero. The primary reason for this difficulty comes from the length of time invested in the sacrificial identity by the time they are able to gain any reasonable or more wholesome view of events that were absolutely formative for their core identity and overwhelmingly extreme for the ordinary resources available to them at the time. Thus adults whose childhood includes the Great Depression and Pearl Harbor formed a communal bond around those primal sacrifices that neither the prosperity of their post-war life nor the losses of later life compels the majority of them to relinquish either their emotional reserve or their independence, even when these admirable traits produce difficulties. So too can be adults who enter the work of being first-responders or the plethora of other vocations or hobbies whose activity includes work with a close-knit team.

The children who lived through the triple hurricanes that devastated America's Gulf Coast region in 2005 or who survived the tsunami that obliterated a portion of Sri Lanka or those who have grown up in any one of the world's terror-scarred neighborhoods have as much of an opportunity to devote their adult life to such redeeming conduct. This vocational direction depends to a large extent upon the follow-up spiritual and moral virtues that grow up in their base community rather than the prescient insight of a consulting room clinician. Thus values transmitted by the religious community, educational enterprise and other voluntary organizations play an essential role in communicating positive values and redemptive conduct to all who go through such life-altering events. Unfortunately not everyone has an opportunity to be immersed in a life-giving community of positive virtue. Equally unfortunate are the demagogic groups who thrive on interpreting such personal or corporate catastrophes not as an opportunity for redemption but as an excuse for retaliation.

The community of care-giving professionals interprets this dynamic under the heading of 'secondary gains.' This is a helpful lens for the clinician in that it triggers our desire to identify the core value or virtue the person is acting out underneath what appears to the world as a single-minded quest or a rather self-limiting if not self-defeating pattern of conduct and structure of belief. But such a title does not do justice to the depth of the individual's often-unconscious spiritual connection with the invisible community of fellow travelers throughout the human community who have made rather similar sacrifices for some perceived greater good or to redress even some century-old insult to tribe, clan, sect or nation.

This underscores the imperative necessity of guiding the care for individuals who endure personal trauma or corporate disaster. The framework of meaning through which the event is perceived and which grows out of the terrifying circumstances must proceed toward positive values. So too the crucial role that professionals can play in providing this guidance through post-event activities and public ceremonies of memory. While there will be an increasing number of people in society too young to recall the formative catastrophe, formal public ceremonies of recognition and memory assist in the crucial activity of assisting both the individual and the society in the crucial task of making meaning out of events that are otherwise overwhelming, horrific, and perhaps pivotal in the destiny of both individuals and the society as a whole.

These ceremonies create the public recognition of the communion and thus the sacrifices that grew out of otherwise mute horror. Such ceremonies may touch on the flaws that led to the horror (*we still recall the losses at Gettysburg)* and the rage that such disasters may have initially produced (*we still recall December 7th as a 'day of infamy')*. But if the ceremony is to be healing and truly help individuals move forward in their life, the focus must ultimately turn toward whatever good sprouted from the ashes of tragedy. Americans who gather at Gettysburg no longer curse those who fired the first shots. In another generation the words of President Roosevelt will likewise lose some of their passion in our communal memory.

Vocation as the Transformation of Work to Service

Sigmund Freud proposed love and work as the two engines that drive human endeavor. A generation later Frederick Buechner opined that one's vocation may be discovered at the intersection of the world's deep itch and the individual's deep joy. The ancient myth of Hercules links a dreadful horror with great redemptive effort. The apostles Paul (2) and James (3) link work with the activity of faith and the consequence of salvation. In this case 'faith' is a verb (what we do as a result of what we experience and believe) rather than a noun (the content of what we believe as a result of our education and background).

Thus while ortho*doxy* and ortho*praxis* are linked, when responding to a dreadful stain it is the event itself that provides the content for the belief while the cleansing of the stain that provides the fuel for the new vocation. Individuals who emerge from such a fiery forge not only undergo a personal transformation, they frequently become agents of change either within the institutions and communities where they already work and live or they create new institutions or communities of cleansing intention that embody their newly found vocation.

The story of one individual recently appointed executive director of Bon Secours Spiritual Center illustrates this two-fold process:

Diagnosed with cancer a year ago, Dr. Thomas Little was faced with a life crisis and a decision. Now in remission, Dr. Little speaks of his experience as a time that has led him to re-evaluate what he was doing and how he was doing it. 'When you are looking down the barrel and facing death, you appreciate how precious life really is,' says Tom. 'I asked myself how am I truly helping people come to healing and appreciate what they have? When the opportunity to serve as executive director of the spiritual center arose, I felt it was a natural step given my background in learning and creating change. It was my chance to use my skills and experience to help others take very seriously the opportunities that life affords them. (4)

In this man's life he already had prepared himself to be an agent of institutional change before the diagnosis of cancer and its consequential treatment. The article goes on to cite his extensive academic training and life experience. Without knowing anything besides what this article depicts a therapist or shepherd of the heart may reasonably postulate that some type of earlier encounter with deep dread may have started him on this path of life-long service to others. Be this as it may, coming face-to-face with one's mortality underscores the realization that this life is not a dress rehearsal. One must make each day count, even if there is no life beyond this one in which every great religion maintains the Creator will weigh our lives and found to be either wanting or rewarding.

For others the cleansing of a dreadful stain propels them gain additional training or to reunite with an institution or community of value. For others still their encounter with catastrophe compels them to leave the community, work and sometimes even the family in which they have spent much of their life. This type of transformation of a person's life frequently creates additional disruption, especially for those nearby who may not fully comprehend the depth of meaning from which the individual is acting and toward which the individual desires to move.

This process of vocational change speaks directly to the two tasks of diagnosis. The individual must frequently find a new language to name the pain to which they are responding. They must also search for a new word to describe the voice or vision to which they feel compelled to travel. Those around them likewise need assistance to understand and support the individual as they undergo this transformation. All too often a part of the transformation involves the individual having to go through the obstacles created by the very ones to which they might reasonably have expected help in taking such a life-changing step.

In terms of effective care, mentoring, coaching or additional professional education are much more effective than weekly therapy in guiding the person through this step. Mentors, coaches and educators are frequently more familiar with the kinds of resources an individual needs than therapists. Moreover, they are more adept at providing the practical advice and having the personal relationships that are essential for vocational growth. Clinicians are too often loathe to provide such practical counsel out of concern for their own liability or because they work from a theoretical perspective that insists the client must 'find their own answers' to life's persistent questions. What this perspective overlooks is this: a person making a major vocational change shifts from those 'persistent questions' to asking very 'practical questions' once they commit their will to the steps of making the change. At this juncture practical advice rather than more self-exploration is the caring necessity.

Joy as the Transformation of Winter to Christmas

I am indebted to C. S. Lewis for this descriptive phrase. In the mythical land of Narnia it was 'always winter but never Christmas.' This story and description lends much to the two tasks of diagnosis generally and to the effort to transform the sacrifice at the core of a dreadful stain into the salvation necessary for new life. Lewis captures in a single sentence the despair that shadows every heart stained by life's deepest tragedies, a description immediately confirmed by all who bear such a stain once they hear it. To paraphrase another great writer, the contrast in diagnosis of Lewis' phrase rather than the DSM-IV-TR is like the contrast between 'lightning and lightning bug.' (5)

Lewis' phrase and the story of Narnia are instructive for this final step in the transformation of the soul's deepest anguish. In this story there are all the elements that contribute to such a deep stain – the deceptive abuse of power by a powerful entity who is at once personal yet eternal, the savage entrapment of living souls through that power and their transformation into figures of stone, and the utter rapaciousness at the core of such a twisted eternal dynamic. There is salvation and transformation in this story, as there is with all great myths. But it comes only at the conclusion of both a great battle and the use of 'deeper magic.' Homer's *Iliad* and *Odyssey* and every other great myth right down to the writings of Tolkein, George Lucas and J. K. Rowling speak a similar language to the heart. So too does every great religion.

As adults we may smile at this story. As professionals writing treatment plans in a well-appointed office we may never speak of Aslan's sacrifice and the battle with the Snow Queen. But when we sit with another suffering human being who fears the journey of healing that lies ahead of them, and we tell them the path ahead will be a treacherous struggle for their soul, they instinctively comprehend we are speaking the truth. In addition, when with our words we signal to them that we will journey with them as a companion who is not entirely safe but nevertheless good, we have as adequately laid out for them the course of their healing as if we were to say, "the healing of this wound will take several years. There will be many set backs and you will feel like giving up. We will use medication and meditation. You will discover skills in yourself you never knew you had. You will have to leave behind patterns of thought and behavior that right now contribute to your failure at effective living."

Put another way, here is what we must tell those who come to our offices to relieve the suffering that lies at the core of their sacrifice. They must grasp for the life their best angels desire. They must slowly but ultimately be grasped by this eternal truth: success in life is not a lottery that we win but a goal that we again. The culture's opinion-makers only portray young men who aspire to be the next American Idol or young women who hope to be the next Hilary Duff. As noted above, all the great myths speak this eternal truth we find on the lips of Jesus. If we want to save our life and gain new life, we must relinquish our death hold on the life we have. This is why genuine heroes don't look especially handsome – their faces reflect the struggles of loss, their hands disclose the wrinkles of hard labor and their eyes reflect the fire of having endured a costly battle.

It is the task of diagnosis to articulate this course of treatment to the person in language they can understand. For some it will be the language of the great myths or religions. For others it will be the language of medicine. For others still it will be the language of a Twelve Step program. Simply stated, those who desire this joy of winter turning into Christmas come to see life in this new way, hopefully sooner rather than later. But ultimately each of us recognizes that if they desire what a joyful person has they must do what a joyful person does. In spiritual terms, one must set aside the debate over the authorship of the religious texts and embrace the authority of the text as a guide to life. One must set aside time for private prayer so that they can distinguish the voice of the Master from the speech of the multitude. They must learn to call down God's blessings on their adversaries so that their heart is not consumed with revenge. They must pay attention to the logs in their own eye and the flaws in their own conduct before seeking to remove the splinter from others eyes or correct the actions of their neighbors. This may not be rocket science but it is as costly as an interplanetary trip. It also happens to be the good news of the Gospel.

Conclusion

The transformation of a soul's profound stain takes decades. The echoes of the initial wound and the habits that allowed one to survive that initial staining never completely go away. This is not happy news to people who want their life back. But it is good information for those who want a new life. The new life is costly to obtain. For most who enter this new land of the soul there yet remains a deep awareness of how close at hand lies the doorway to that other land where it is still winter and never Christmas.

It is because these who have been transformed by their suffering *remember* the transformation of their past they frequently find a way in their transformed present to provide an opportunity to relieve the present suffering of another. Thus in the week before Christmas 2006 as I write these words my table is graced by the words of another from our shared past urging an effort to support current Americans deployed in harm's way 'to make this Christmas more memorable as a holiday, rather than just another memory of a war zone.' I offer a lengthy excerpt of his words as a concluding meditation on the task of both naming the pain and guiding the care of the transformation of the soul's most grievous wounds:

> You would think that I would have remembered eating anything Other than C-rations during the Christmas holiday season of 1967, but I don't. For those of us in the infantry, holidays were just like any other day. In fact, the Christmas holidays were sometimes worse than any other day, because we would declare a 'holiday truce' that gave us a false sense of security, and our enemy would immediately take advantage of the situation. I think we should all remember our own experiences during Christmas or other holidays in a combat zone, and make an effort To send a card or care package to a young American serving overseas. (6)

Selah!

Chapter 16

Illustrative Vignettes Concluded

Sometimes the journey toward wholeness begins with questions of defilement and stain. As shocking as such situations may be, the obvious presentation of the wound makes the initial tasks of diagnosis and treatment fairly straightforward. Not simple but singular, at least initially. I will address these situations in an up-coming chapter.

More generally these existential concerns, and certainly matters of joy and vocational transformation, rise to the foreground only after much trust has been built and many hours logged on the treadmill of restoration. Building enough trust between therapist and client, salving if not solving the pressing concerns of daily life, and maintaining the growth already achieved make this final pain elusive to name and resistant to relief. Perhaps the most challenging situations come with individuals whose clinical diagnosis of an Axis II personality disorder points at once toward these primary distresses but the individual is nowhere near tolerating any exploration or exposition of such a wound. Great patience is required of the caregiver to wait until the proper moment of receptivity before crossing this final boundary of the soul.

The reason for this complexity of care is singular if not simple: so many life-skills and assumptions are based upon and surround this wound that the individual intuitively grasps the costly nature of such a profound change. Whether we call this intuitive insight 'resistance' or 'addiction' or 'selfishness' or 'original sin' depends more upon the diagnostic framework of the clinician or the primary value system of the client than the interior process that requires healing. We now know that the brain is the fundamental broken organ. We also now know, thanks to thermal imagery, just how delicate and longstanding are the neural pathways that carry the impulses of our most self-defeating and self-salving actions.

As in Chapter Twelve I will update the reader about each vignette. In some cases the existential concern was evident at the outset of treatment and I had to wait for that moment of *kairos* when their ego could withstand the probing query of their primary wound. In other cases the wound gradually became evident only as trust built and nothing else was left to account for the person's distress and dread. In many situations there either is no existential dread or the individual makes clear in some manner they do not wish to address this core concern at this time. In all cases the diagnostic and treatment focus must be guided by the client's concerns. The matter of vocational change frequently requires consultation with other professionals, educational resources, religious communities and perhaps even geographic relocation.

Case #1 – Depression: Repetition and Restoration

Elaine's use of watercolors to draw out her dreadful terror and guilt exemplifies the symbol of the stain and its saving sacrifice. I am still touched by the power of her drawings to communicate her utter sense of despair as well as the shock when she first exposed these drawings. The remaining two years of therapeutic work illustrates the delicate nature of care required at this depth of distress. Because she was a bright woman, she could intuitively grasp the connection between her current predicament and her earliest violations. Because she was a practical individual, she also knew that simply mounting a sexual harassment suit against her politically powerful 'sponsor' would bring her only more heartache, end a stable but loveless marriage and pour shame on her children.

There were other concerns that periodically dominated these two years. Her children were growing into adolescence. Her parents continued to age. Holidays came and went. Weekly church services for which she had to rehearse the choir and then perform at the organ brought its own challenges. There were interruptions in the regime of weekly therapy due to vacations, children's schedules, the need for other appointments and finally the necessity of simply her taking a short respite. In the pristine world of theory, all of these things could be read as 'resistance' to treatment. I preferred to view them as the necessary rest one instinctively takes when hiking across arduous terrain. The destination is never in question; but the destination is reached only if one adequately manages the resources of body, mind and soul.

During this time I had a few sessions with her husband, no more than five. He was absolutely in love with Elaine, worried about her and suspected there was something else – or someone else-that troubled her. What I saw most clearly was the man's passivity. He was safe and good but not very well defined. Thus he wasn't a brutal predator but he also didn't inspire much confidence in others. He was stable but rather uninteresting. I could see why Elaine would be vulnerable to – or even encouraging – of a male whose 'bad boy' interior was masked by social prominence. They had been one another's ticket out of their small mountain town. Now didn't know what to really do with one another.

The standard theoretical suggestion would be for her husband to take more initiative in their relationship. The challenge would be to motivate someone who was quite content being passive to become more assertive. She would likely mount objections to any effort he made for just the two of them to get away, an intuition he confirmed when I 'wondered' about this in about the third session. "She usually gets a headache or the kids have something scheduled," he commented. It was as if he was saying 'buddy, I've been dealing with this problem a lot longer than you have and I've about run out of ideas. So if you've got some really helpful idea, let me know. But don't tell me to do the obvious.' He made this point nicely and quietly but nevertheless I knew I'd been put in my place.

So I began talking with him about the one thing a man can safely talk about with another man: his work. I learned that he'd been at his present level for a long time, waiting for the boss to promote him. Of course that wasn't going to happen and he now was slowly figuring that out. "Where would you like to go and what would you like to do?" I asked him.

"I'd like to get into management in my final years," he replied.

"Then if you make those steps with a job coach, I'll make a deal with you," I said. "I'll keep helping Elaine chip away at her depression long enough for you to make this happen." A few months later, Elaine was surprised by his announcement they were moving to a new town in another state. He'd be promoted, effective the following year and contingent on his completing the company's management training program.

"I guess I'll have to do all the work of getting us moved,," she complained. But the move marked an important change in their marriage and ultimately her life. The stain would always be in her soul; but it had begun to fade with this move. It would be the work of a future therapist who would help her rediscover a sense of joy.

At this point in the diagnostic enterprise, Elaine's diagnosis would look like this, utilizing both the formal DSM-IV system and my multi-axial system of diagnosis:

DSM-IV Diagnosis:
Axis I – Dysthymic Disorder-300.40
Axis II – Compulsive Personality – 301.40
Axis III – Migraine headaches – 346.90
Axis IV – Marital and vocational problems
Axis V - GAF Current: 55 GAF Last Year: 60

Spiritual / Theological Multi-axial Diagnosis:
Axis I -   Guilt – Realistic related to violation of marriage vows;
       Subjective related to violation of personal standards of
       performance in work and marriage.
Axis II-Idolatry – Describes herself as a 'sinner' and believes her
       sin places her outside of divine grace. Cannot conceive
       herself as being forgiven.

Axis III – Dread – Repetitive sexual molestations in adolescence.

Case # 2 – Adultery: Vocation and Venture

"Somehow I never talk about what I intended to but I always leave here feeling better," Robert would often comment. "Something different happens once I get to your office. I guess I talk about the things that I need to rather than the things I want to."

As his therapy passed the eighteen-month mark and his divorce wound its inexorable way through the court system, Robert gradually left behind his obsession with the details of Melanie's unfaithfulness. The emphasis should be on the word 'gradually.' His soul was much like piece of porcelain cookware that had been left in the oven too long. Even after the shards of whatever had been the meal is scraped away through repeated washings, the stain of that miscalculated casserole remains indelible in the porcelain. So too with the soul's deepest stains. Her forgeries would be a legal fact. The forgeries would eventually cease to be an emotional imprint on Robert's immediate consciousness.

Thus even in what became his final session, he would briefly return to look at the duplicity that forever changed his life. After over two years he no longer expressed his anger nor his heart nearly as flamboyantly. But if his life continues on his recently begun more joyful arc, it may be that in a decade he will no longer feel the burning sting of this discovery.

Robert's journey had, indeed, just begun although he could begin to see the outline of his new vocation. When he passed his first Christmas while separated, he was only able to recall how he had decorated their home. At the second Christmas, he looked forward to attending an evening worship on December 24. In the intervening year he had begun to recognize values and virtues long made dormant by his loveless marriage and his substitute deity, productivity.

Robert had begun to recognize a different way of being productive as his pace slowed to match his mother's deteriorating condition. As her present memory failed and her long-term memory became more active, Robert was reminded of impulses that pushed him into government employment once his bones ached too much after the semi-pro football games. His sharp mind led him into management and his early egress from sports allowed his vitality to remain. The early counseling sessions were often punctuated by his ringing cell-phones.

"I have three more years before I can retire," he would comment. "I'm still reasonably healthy and by that time the kids will be starting college. Mom will need even more help, even if I place her in a sheltered facility. Perhaps there will be a need for me to do something in fund raising for long-range care of people who have Alzheimer's disease."

Robert's pattern will be one familiar to Christian people: finding purpose and joy through remembering the past so one can also remember the future. Robert's memory of his past included his mother's tenderness when he was a child, something the intervening years of the failure to make it into the NFL, two failed marriages, working 75 hours a week and raising children had all but erased. Now that his mother truly needed his attention, he wisely began attending to her personally rather than writing yet another monthly check for her to receive professional live-in care and then working even more hours to afford her care.

Yet he rediscovered that his care of his mother and his hope for her future was rooted in another memory: the belief in a life beyond this one. "I know nobody really knows what happens after death," he said one morning. "But you're a minister. What's your best guess? Tell me what you believe in your heart – not just what you're supposed to say at the funeral."

I could have said 'Sounds like you're wrestling with the ultimate meaning of life' or 'I wonder what prompts you to inquire about my belief when you have questions about your own belief.' But neither of these nor a dozen other non-directive responses would *guide* his care.

Responsible care isn't just letting someone come up with their own answers and then baptizing it as 'truth.' There are times in counseling when the heart will not endure 'teachable moment' until the mind is filled with information. This was one of those moments when a straightforward request for information is the heart of the matter and thus bears directly on providing effective care.

"I believe our soul survives in a recognizable manner," I began. "Thus your mother will recognize her husband (your father) shortly before the moment of her last breath on this side of that great divide. Indeed, she will experience him and maybe others as waiting to welcome her."

"Funny you should say that," he replied. "Mom's already saying she talks to Dad all of the time. Is she crazy?"

I chuckled. "It all depends on what they're talking about. If the conversation is really a continuation of the kind of repartee they would have when he was alive, then I tend to think it is okay, especially if it isn't constant. If Dad starts to say things 'I want you to join me, go buy a gun' or 'sell the stock portfolio to Rev. Jimmy's Healing Ministry and Used Car Emporium' or starts berating her, then it's time to have a psychiatric consult."

He nodded. "That sounds better than what her new pastor told her. He said 'nobody knows.' Mom got angry with her and asked her to leave!"

"Your mother has more good sense than she does," I replied. "She can still spot a professional's desire to avoid uncomfortable questions by giving a quick answer. You can tell your mother yourself what you believe," I added. I also suggested some verses of Scripture that he could share with his mother. "Talk these over between you," I urged him, knowing that it would deepen their relationship in addition to giving them a starting point in common.

Robert's venture thus will be not only the rediscovery of his mother and perhaps a new vocation upon retirement. Robert's venture will also include a rediscovery of his childhood religious faith with the eternal questions that only a thrice-wounded adult can truly ask. The answers he finds will increase his joy even as they may continue to puzzle his mind.

At this point in the diagnostic enterprise, Robert's diagnosis would look like this, utilizing both the formal DSM-IV system and my multi-axial system of diagnosis:

DSM-IV Diagnosis:
Axis I – Adjustment Disorder with Mixed Emotional Features – 309.00
Axis II – No Diagnosis on Axis II – V71.90
Axis III – No condition reported
Axis IV – Marital separation
Axis V- GAF Current: 65   GAF Last Year: 65

Spiritual / Theological Multi-axial Diagnosis:
Axis I-Guilt: Realistic guilt over failure of marriage; subjective
          mood of failure and personal recrimination.
Axis II – Idolatry: Betrayal by spouse fuels his rage and signals
          his misplaced worship; terror results current alienation
          from religious tradition of his youth.
Axis III – Dread: Failure to 'make the team' produced alienation
          from community of faith.

Case # 3 – Developmental Challenges: Collaboration and Progress

"We're considering a second opinion," commented Philip's father at the end of a session. Philip had already bounded out of the office, shoeless but relatively happy. "We just worry about the level of medication. His grades are great and the level of whining has decreased. I guess we just aren't sure about having someone so young on such a large dose of medicine," he concluded.

It had been months since Philip had said he wanted to kill himself or upset the Sunday school teacher with his expressions of liking gore and violence. He kept his shoes on at school now rather than taking them off in the middle of the day. He only removed them when he was home or in a place he felt comfortable. He still needed constant reminding about appropriate social behavior in my office. He now responded to this with obedience rather than complaints.

"There's one other thing we're concerned about," his father continued. "It's hard to get him out of the house, especially on good days. He's fearful of dogs. We're considering getting a puppy or gradually taking him to the animal shelter and letting him approach dogs that are caged. What do you think?" he asked.

"I think taking him to any place where the dogs outnumber him ten-to-one and making lots of noise is a mistake," was my immediate reply. "I think finding someone he knows whose dog has puppies, and just taking him there to see them is more likely to be successful. Has he asked for a puppy?"

"No, he hasn't," was Dad's reply. "But we don't want him to grow up so that he goes through life afraid."

Dad's concerns are perfectly normal and understandable: parents want their children to be both normal and traditional. 'Normal' here means not having any major developmental challenges. 'Traditional' here means generally following the same path in life that the parents followed as they were growing up. Phillip was fortunate to have a set of parents who were rather relaxed about his developmental delay – their patience and enthusiasm about him were assets that offset their disappointment about his physical awkwardness, odd social habits and now the surfacing of his fear. They were fortunate insofar as Phillip's delays were not more serious – he did very well in school, had real skill in soccer and was genuinely caring toward his younger brother and sister.

Phillip's father bonded very strongly with him. I never sensed in all of our meetings that this Dad was anything but positive about his son. He seemed to take whatever frustrations Phillip created for him in stride. Indeed in one session he remarked, "Phillip reminds me a lot of myself when I was his age." This raised a significant diagnostic question: how does a clinician respond to such family history in a way that helps the child and parent? The first goal here must always be to maintain a strong alliance with both parent and child rather than the therapists positioning themselves as intrusive experts whose first task is to simply get the appropriate label for a child by blaming the parent's genetics or honest lapses in parenting skills. No parent is automatically equipped to raise a child with a developmental challenge or leaves behind their own limitations once children appear on the scene.

Many parents are fearful of sharing such important information with clinicians or educators out of a well-founded belief that an intrusive social service network will suddenly appear knocking at their door. Phillip's father was expressing both his hope for his son and making an observation about his own childhood out of a sense of collaborating with me and other professionals. As my work with Phillip progressed, it would be important to maintain this man's trust and build on it in a way that helped him and his wife be effective parents to Phillip.

Here it is important to restate the goal of therapy with a child: to assist both the parents and the child so that the child can become as fully functioning adult as possible. Absent the evidence of gross parental abuse, profound parental mismanagement, or obvious impairment in the child, I make this assumption about parents. This doesn't mean there are no toxic parents or children who are absolute monsters despite the best efforts of numerous adults. But this is not usually a helpful place to begin, despite whatever immediate frustrations parents and child bring to therapy.

It would be important to conduct the care of Philip and his parents in a way that built a long-term relationship. Philip reminded me of many of the youngsters who go through the Scouting program: only two out of one hundred make the rank of Eagle Scout. But thousands of men look back on the socialization skills and comradeship built in Scouting throughout their life. Thus it would likely be for Philip. Helping him gain the life skills necessary to maximize his strengths will allow him to go much farther than he can presently see.

At this point in the diagnostic enterprise, Phillip's diagnosis would look like this, utilizing both the formal DSM-IV system and my multi-axial system of diagnosis:

> *DSM-IV Diagnosis:*
> *Axis I* – Cognitive Difficulties – 294.90
>   Attention Deficit Hyperactivity Disorder – 314.00
>   Childhood Depression – 311.00
> *Axis II* – Asperger's Disorder – 299.80 (rule out)
> *Axis III* – None reported
> *Axis IV* – School difficulties, especially socialization
> *Axis V*- GAF Current: 50 GAF Last Year: 55

> *Spiritual / Theological Multi-axial Diagnosis:*
> *Axis I*- Guilt: No realistic guilt; strong feelings of subjective
>   guilt related to negative self-image.
> *Axis II* – Idolatry: No genuine idolatry; making age-appropriate
>   Developmental transition between intuitive-projective faith
>   and mythic-literal faith.
> *Axis III* – Dread: no diagnosis.

Case # 4 – End of Life Concerns: Facing 'Death in Life'

By mid-afternoon of the second day it was apparent the medical staff had the body of a pretty healthy 17 year old fighting for survival. All of the physical signs of restoration were giving evidence of returning. Pulse, blood pressure, and respiration were within normal limits, thanks to the respirator. It was apparent Steve's own organs were under the control of the one organ on which everything else depended: his brain.

"It just isn't clear yet how much of 'Steve' is available to us," the neurologist informed the chaplain. "I don't want to remove him from life support just yet. The indicators are that his organs healthy; neurologically it is another matter. It is still early, " he said cautiously.

The neurologist updated the family on Steve's condition, balancing the physical hope with the neurological uncertainty.

In a later conversation with the hospital chaplain, Steve's mother confided, "The last thing Steve would want is a situation like that girl in Florida went through. We talked about it at length, especially since we're of the same faith as she. Steve said he would never want to live in that condition or put us through that kind of suffering." The chaplain nodded.

Steve's condition remained unchanged throughout the rest of the day and into the evening. 'Both parents soberly assessing their son's medical and neurological condition,' she wrote in her follow-up call log.

At morning report the Instant Care nursing staff began discussing whether to move Steve to Critical Care. "This reflects his physical stability," commented his nurse. The neurologist agreed; the nurse and neurologist also quietly asked for an ethical consultation on Steve's medical prognosis. "He is still unresponsive to external stimuli," she reported. "Aren't we going to have to consult with the family before we insert a feeding tube?" she asked.

At this point in the diagnostic enterprise, Steve's diagnosis would look like this, utilizing both the formal DSM-IV system and my multi-axial system of diagnosis:

> *DSM-IV Diagnosis:*
> *Axis I –* No Diagnosis – V71.09
> *Axis II –* No Diagnosis- V71. 09
> *Axis III –* Concussion, cerebral – 851.80
> *Axis IV –* Unresponsive to stimuli
> *Axis V-* GAF Current: 0 GAF Last Year: +90

> *Spiritual / Theological Multi-axial Diagnosis:*
> *Axis I -* Guilt: Realistic due to his role in his injury; subjective is
> unavailable for him but profound for his family.
> *Axis II –* Idolatry: Age-appropriate synthetic-conventional faith that
> will come to terms with end-of-life concerns.
> *Axis III –* Dread: diagnosis deferred pending survival

Case # 5 – Vocational Assessment for Ministry when Systems Collude

"Unfortunately, these denominational systems eventually give in if someone is persistent in desiring ordination," commented the clinician's supervisor as they left the interview. "This denomination looks like they will support your conclusions. But it is likely that at some point Hope will find some group that will give her the title and authority she seeks."

"You mean she'll come back to us through another denomination?" ask the assessment specialist.

"Perhaps, though it isn't likely," replied the supervisor. "What is more likely is she will find some religious body that is not connectional in nature, impress them with her brightness and beauty, and then repeat the cycle of ingratiating herself into the congregation who has the authority to hire her if not grant her ordination."

The evaluator shook her head in disbelief. "Why does the church have such a hard time saying 'No' to someone who is obviously broken but not to some of the candidates who have good pastoral skills but who need non-traditional educational preparation?"

The clinicians continued their conversation over several days. Not surprisingly, the evaluator received a personal phone call from Hope eight months later. She apologized for breaking down in the office. "I've found a new church," she confided to the evaluator, "and they like me." The evaluator made a notation of the conversation and placed it into Hope's now extensive file.

There is a peculiar kind of pain in a case such as Hope's. We typically presume that 'pain' involves some type of loss or horror or trauma. In this case the 'pain' is the result of never being subjected to the imposition of healthy limits. Hope's family system apparently worshipped her, burnishing her self-image so much that her self-concept became as distorted and one-dimensional as if they had locked her in a closet. Never experiencing the limits necessary to produce genuine maturity can be as destructive of the self as never experiencing the freedom necessary to empower authentic independence.

Perhaps her parents believed they were providing effective care for a precocious child, a trans-generational distortion given Hope's realistic abilities. The evaluator and her supervisor could only wonder since by this point in Hope's journey she and her parents had invested significant emotional, spiritual and financial resources in shoring up their belief in her divine vocation. "The supermarket tabloids are filled with beautiful people whose resources afford them the luxury of never having to experience healthy limits," remarked the evaluator one afternoon to the supervisor.

"Just so," he replied. "Fortunately for Hope and the church her core values are positive and will be somewhat controlled by the stringent expectations of a religious community. If she can avoid being so deceived by her own sense of uniqueness she may also avoid flaming out via drug abuse or a clandestine affair."

"That would certainly provide the same drama as the stars and starlets in those tabloids," observed the evaluator. "I guess the best any therapist could do would be to stand nearby, wait for such a train wreck to happen and then try to salve the survivors. Usually the people who create such calamities emerge unscathed while those around them are the ones who carry the stain of such tragedy."

The church is not the sole venue in which such fair-haired children rise to prominence only to collapse in a fiery ball of misfortune. The list of politicians, business heavyweights, artistic doyens, scientific and academic leaders whose lives move along this dazzling arc is legion. The list of those they stain is equally lengthy. Their underlying stain and the grime they leave on the citizens and systems they infect have the same heme as Hope's life. It is as ancient a theme as the ancient myths of Greece or Africa. It is as contemporary a story as the latest darling of the media's 24/7 news cycle.

This stain is what provides the poison at the heart of those 'deadly' sins and what signals the 'original' in our basic alienation from the Creator who gave that first eternal boundary we forever choose to ignore. (1) It is why an angel with a flaming sword prevents us from ever acquiring the fruit of the tree of life despite our broken perception of some that they are truly god-like. (2)

At this point in the diagnostic enterprise, Hope's diagnosis would look like this, utilizing both the formal DSM-IV system and my multi-axial system of diagnosis:

DSM-IV Diagnosis:

Axis I – Depressive Disorder NOS – 311.0

Axis II – Dependent Personality Disorder with

Narcissistic features – 301.60

Axis III – None Reported

Axis IV – Vocational Difficulties

Axis V – GAF Current: 55   GAF Last Year: 55

Spiritual / Theological Multi-axial Diagnosis:

Axis I- Guilt: Realistic failure of prior efforts at finding work; subjective belief that she is flawless.

Axis II – Idolatry: Mythic-literal level of faith with high need to see self as special agent of God. No tolerance for ambiguity of divine purpose.

Axis III – Dread: Fixation on particular vocation that reinforces primitive structure of self-identity.

Summary and Conclusion

Diagnosis remains an art and on-going process as much as it is an objective task that calls for making difficult decisions. Sometimes the initial decisions are made under the constraints of time and circumstance, as in a crisis care center or at the front end of an emergency admission to a hospital. Equally pressing in terms of time but not in terms of severity to the person is the initial diagnosis that must be made in order for the client to utilize their mental health insurance. In both settings the clinician must be accurate enough to provide effective care without saddling the individual with a diagnosis so severe that their future is compromised or so vague as to be unhelpful in their care.

These five vignettes do not comprise the entire landscape of diagnosis. They do comprise some specific examples of five major areas that mental health clinicians or providers of human care routinely face regardless of their setting: a mood disorder, a relational collapse, a child with serious developmental concerns, concerns regarding end-of-life care and vocational assessment. I have purposely avoided some areas so that I could cover them in more depth in the section that follows. But even there, the topics are limited more by my interest and expertise than by the range of problematic concerns of the heart or the severity of topics.

What I have hoped to show in these preceding vignettes is the way diagnosis remains reflective of the larger conversation that takes place between a suffering heart and a salving intention of two human beings. There are times when one must remain silent in the presence of profound suffering, much like the initial stance of Job's three friends. But there ultimately comes a time when words must somehow be spoken, the pain at the core of our existence must be named however tentatively and the trek toward health engaged. This is especially so if the ultimate goal is only to prepare the suffering heart for an encounter with the Divine Presence whose efficacy to bring healing is beyond all words. (3) *Selah!*

Part V – Special Considerations for Special Cases

Chapter 17: What About Children?

The prior installment of this volume had not been on the shelf one month before someone asked me the question that forms this chapter's title. Since approximately one-third of my clinical work is with children or adolescents, it was not an oversight. I believe the diagnosis and care of children, along with their overall spiritual formation, requires special consideration. While children are potential adults they are not little adults. Thus deciphering their sometime unusual efforts at expressing their concerns, along with their dependency on the very people who frequently are conflicted about how to proceed, makes this entire area quite a thorny thicket.

I want to recognize at the outset that the DSM-IV-T-R has an entire section devoted to this topic. Along with the more ordinary concerns of counseling children such as depression, anxiety, and interpersonal conflict that this section of the DSM-V identifies there are also the more complex developmental disorders and information processing disorders. It is an essential starting point for anyone who seeks to work with children or adolescents. Simply because all of us were once children, all of us are not cognitively or psychologically suited to work with children or adolescents in a therapeutic environment.

Therapeutic work with adolescents is even more difficult than children. Their growing physical strength and mobility, coupled with their access to mind-altering substances and the Internet compounds the effect of psychological and spiritual distress. Their role of being the foundation of the next generation insures a certain degree of inevitable conflict. This further complicates the task of discerning the distinction between these well-known millennial birth pangs and more serious disorders. Assisting parents and educators in striking the right balance between retaining the boundaries still necessary for their healthy development and joining with the adolescent's push for more independence requires wisdom as well as clinical perspicuity.

This is a way of saying that this chapter is nothing more than a beginning. Each of the following sub-sections to this chapter is worthy of an entire part in a much longer work. Yet there are three or four main considerations in working with youth that comprise at least the starting point of much of the therapeutic work with children and adolescents. I hope to address these overall concerns rather than delve more deeply into specific developmental or psychiatric disorders. The first area is that of recognizing genuine distress from the ordinary challenges of growing up. The second area is helping children negotiate through parental divorce or the death of a member of their immediate family. Thirdly the most troubling challenge appears to be working with oppositional or conduct-disordered adolescents. Finally, there are times when a clinician may be placed in the uncomfortable role of advising the courts on the termination or limitation of parental rights.

"How Did We Survive Childhood?"

"If you lived as a child in the 40's, 50's, 60's or 70's how did you survive? Looking back, it's hard to believe that we have lived as long as we have," begins one of the lists of wisdom posted on the Internet. The list reminds those of us now reaching retirement age just what we actually did during our childhood. The posting ends with this note, "Tests were not adjusted for any reason. Our actions were our own. Consequences were expected."

This is not the inevitable grousing of an older generation about the softness of the next generation. Roughly half of my clinical work with children amounts to relieving parents of their anxieties about what is essentially either normal childhood conduct or the normal push-and-pull between a parent and a developing child. This is especially true of boys, who have become the most over-medicated group of people in American society.

There are several pro forma 'pains' that bring these parents and their children into therapy. Academic performance in the form of average grades or an assessment by a teacher the child 'is not working up to his / her potential' will do it. So will repeated conflict over doing homework or the child hiding notes sent home by the teacher. The 'pain' here is the parental assumption that their child should be 'above average' just like everyone else's, that homework should be done flawlessly and without conflict or that the child should actively assist in what the child knows will be another harangue about their grades.

The 'pain' here is the parent's and not the child's, at least initially. This pain is driven by the parent's unrealistic expectation and conveniently flawed memory of his or her own childhood. The expectation of educators appears to be equally inconsistent. Obviously not everyone can be 'above average.' The educational assumption appears to be that if a student fails to achieve excellence it is a reflection on the teacher. The teachers, not wanting to admit a lack of excellence in themselves, pressure the students toward an unobtainable level of achievement.

A similar pro forma pain is acted out in the tableau around family chores and privileges. The variation here is not that parents expect flawless obedience but more that parents are unsure of how much discipline to enforce on their children. The parental fear of having someone, or even their child, complain to social services *and be taken seriously* about the consequences they impose for a child's resistance to standards makes them unsure about just how forceful to be with their child. In my experience the child quickly picks up on this parental uncertainty and exploits it as far as they can. There is genuine child abuse that is extraordinary and I will address such concerns below. But much of this pain could be corrected for if parents would follow this simple prescription: square your shoulders and be a paragon of virtue rather than caving in or coddling your son or daughter. In short, let the child experience early the exact behavioral consequences of their conduct. (1) Thus much of the care a clinician can provide in these circumstances has to do with normalizing the conduct of the child as well as reinforcing, in the presence of the child, the realistic expectations of their parents for respectful conduct.

A third area that is somewhat routine but much more serious for the child is when they encounter bullying. Typically this happens at school although bullying can occur within a neighborhood setting. Bullying has a corrosive impact on the very core of a child's personality. Unfortunately by the time a parent learns their child is the target of bullying much damage has been accomplished by the bully. The victim's sense of guilt and shame reinforces the secrecy on which the bully depends. Left undiscovered or unchecked, bullying usually results in long-term damage to the child.

Unfortunately the administrative leadership in specific schools often adds to rather than ameliorates the problem. Parents who finally learn of their son or daughter's victimization suddenly finds educators retreating behind administrative protocols that replicate the tactics of the bully: the victim's behavior becomes the first thing scrutinized and the bully's behavior the last to be contained. In my clinical practice I have seen more than one case where a teacher joins in the bullying by making degrading comments about the child's classroom performance or social appearance. This may be hard for a clinician to comprehend because the educational environment seems to be overwhelmingly focused on themes of acceptance, diversity and multi-culturalism. But these code words and the administrative protocols developed within public schools only serve to deepen the stain that bullying can produce within a child.

What can be therapeutically accomplished to relieve this pain? A clinician must take a dual approach of shoring up the self-image of the child and reinforcing the parents when they take a no-nonsense approach with the local school. The child needs an immersion into activities where they can rediscover their core competencies along with assertiveness training. Simply telling the child they are a good person or teaching them to be non-confrontational is insufficient. Physical competency through individual sports or emotional competency through engagement in the arts or their religious community will help. The parents likewise need encouragement to retain an aggressive and competent attorney who accompanies the parents to their very first meeting with school officials. Some therapists may view this as an unnecessary escalation; my clinical experience is that nothing else focuses the attention of the local school administrators to take the assertive action necessary to curb the conduct of the bully.

Most community-based or school-based anti-bullying programs also emphasize working with the bully and the bully's parents. Clearly the boy or girl who bullies others needs some type of assistance. But I have not seen these programs be very effective in stopping a bully. More to the point, in nearly thirty years of clinical experience I have yet to have a parent bring in their child for counseling because they were concerned their child was bullying others. Perhaps other clinicians have a different experience. But my guess is that these are the individuals who fill juvenile 'learning centers,' adult anger management classes, and whose marriages fail because of significant physical or emotional abuse.

"If You're Not Divorcing Me, How Come You're Not Around Much?"

The financial and emotional cost of divorce on children is immense and long-term. Minus egregious emotional or physical abuse, parents who remain married 'for the sake of the children' do, in fact, wind up having children who perform better in the major ways in which success is gauged. This is not to say there are not exceptional cases of children who seem to defy these odds along with heroic single parents who achieve sterling post-divorce success. But we name them as 'exceptional' and 'heroic' expressly because they defy these grim averages. (2)

Bringing healing to children of all ages affected by divorce is the number one task of any marriage and family clinician. This involves direct work with the child as well as with the parent(s). In the best situations both parents – and stepparents – can become involved in the healing of a child devastated by divorce. In the worst situations no parent is involved and the therapist becomes one of several instruments of the social welfare system and court's efforts to protect the child as an agent of healing focused on restoring joy to a youthful soul. I will address this latter development below; for the moment, let me turn to focusing on what seems to being healing the child's pain.

The core pain in a child's heart is the broken attachment with their parents. They grieve the loss of emotional warmth and spiritual security provided by an effective family. They have conflicted feelings toward both parents, especially the parent who has 'left,' regardless of the reason for the divorce. Research strongly suggests that even adults whose parents divorce in later life feel some of this loss even if their own marriage is stable. At the heart of this pain is the rupture of the marital covenant. The factual reason for the rupture appears to be much less significant. The spiritual reality is that the child believes the divorce is their fault, no matter what the parents say.

Thus the first therapeutic task is helping the child or young person give voice to this fundamental division of their family. With the very young child this will take the form of expressive drawings and play therapy. With older children this will grow into more verbal forms. In both cases it is likely that the child will act out their distress in some manner. Poor academic performances, social withdrawal, gravitation to different peers, sexual misconduct or outright flight are the most common melodies of distress. Only the most well adjusted child will readily express their heartache of loss in a direct manner.

A child's response to extreme parental conflict and divorce reverses the diagnostic pattern we have followed thus far. The child goes immediately to the experience of stain, primarily because they lack the ethical sophistication to express their pain in terms of guilt. Even when their fundamental assessment of parental divorce looks ethical, e.g. "It is my fault," or "I'm a bad person," the true consequence can be observed by their frequent existential follow-up to this self-image, "I want to kill myself" (in young children) or "I am living in Hell" (teenagers).

Divorce also shatters the idealism necessarily inherent in healthy childhood development. Parents are god-like to their children. When parents fall from the sky like Icarus a loss of eternal proportions that the child feels but cannot express erupts in their soul. To speak of this loss as somehow only introducing them to the reality that 'life is tough' or that 'people are cruel' is equally heartless. The empathy of a clinician toward this loss must frequently counter a wounded parent's own agonized expression of life's fundamental lack of fairness that the divorce exemplifies. The reversal of parent-child roles that frequently accompanies the coping of during must not be allowed to become the child's permanent role.

Guiding the care of a specific child requires paying attention to two things: the age of the child when the divorce occurred and their current age. While there is a gap between the ways a child initially reacts to the divorce and whatever problems develop later, the clinician must first address the child who was wounded at the time of the divorce. Using empathy, evocative stories, and the emerging insight of the adolescent a therapist can help the child befriend their earlier self who remains locked inside.

Therapists and pastoral professionals must also guide all adults to maximize healthy coping parenting strategies and relational postures toward one another. These strategies include, but are not limited to, an authoritative parenting style, repairing the broken attachment with the child and minimizing parental conflict. (3) Parenting classes that focus on healthy ways to resolve conflict are especially helpful for divorced parents, assuming the parents are mature enough to truly act out the easy pronouncement that forms the title of this sub-chapter. Of course if there were this type of maturity in both parents, the likelihood of divorce would be reduced in the first place.

"Get Outta My Life But First Can You Drive Me to the Mall?"

I stumbled across this book and its evocative title while browsing in a local bookstore. "This is spot-on," I thought. After reading it through I tried just the title out on several beleaguered parents. Their reaction was identical with mine.

Purchasing the book has done more than help them understand the contemporary struggle they face raising an American adolescent in today's entitlement-rich environment. The author's practical suggestions equip parents to regain their legitimate authority. When parents do so, adolescents regain an appropriate level of dependency that nurtures their emotional and spiritual development.

In clinical care, the pain of the parent(s) initiates this treatment. The initial challenge to any therapist is to establish control over the therapy session. I always begin the initial hour by allowing the parents to make their case, stopping the adolescent firmly but kindly if they interrupt. This takes roughly ten minutes.

During these ten minutes I am gauging the reaction of the teen. If they are able to contain themselves, I commend them as I turn toward them and say something like this, "Is Mom / Dad talking about someone we all know or did they make all this up?" The teen then gets roughly the same amount of time and I do not hesitate to quiet the parent who usually tries to respond to the adolescent's casting of events. This builds trust with both sides of the conflict, although it doesn't always proceed smoothly. More about what happens when it does not in a moment.

I then dismiss the parents to the waiting room and spend the next twenty minutes with the teen. I take a few notes, but basically I put the notepad away and try to use both my empathy and my smart-ass side to enter their world. I always end this time explaining to the teen just how much confidentiality they have with me and then I add a statement something like this: "toward the end of our time, I'm going to ask you 'is there anything else I should know?' If there is and you haven't told me, your parents are certainly going to tell me. You'll look foolish and they'll stay in the role of being your cop. If there is and you tell me about it, your parents will ask me if you told me. I want to be able to say 'Of course she did and here's what we decided to do about it.'"

Then I look the adolescent right in the eye and say, "Now, is there anything else you want to tell me?" Teens usually test this boundary at least once. When they do, I congratulate them for keeping their parents in the very role they alleged they hate – 'running my life and making me live like a prisoner.'

When this initial conversation goes well, all parties leave having had the experience of their particular pain being named and with a sense of hope that the underlying tension and conflict will abate. But the conversation doesn't always go well. Adolescent girls can be just as combative with their parents as adolescent boys in the first session. More seriously, their parents can be just as wimpy as Neville Chamberlain with the same devastating consequences for the life of the family and, sadly, ultimately for the teen.

"Grandpa scares me," said the fourteen-year old boy when I asked him why he was so respectful to his grandfather but so much 'in your face' with his mother (Grandpa's daughter). "He just looks at me and I tremble inside. So I do exactly what he says." The child's grades had improved steadily, his clothes had gotten increasingly more appropriate and his mouth had suddenly remembered vocabulary not used since turning twelve.

"My daughter has treated him more like a little man or pal than as her son," Grandpa had commented on the phone in setting up the counseling session. "When he turned twelve she began letting him run with his friends while she stayed out to party. He's a bright boy but if he doesn't turn around soon, there's going to be trouble. Her ex-husband had some problems, but Brett doesn't act that way with him; just with my daughter."

Mom was a competent professional woman who oversaw a department with a $2.3M budget. She knew how to set firm and fair boundaries with other adults, dress appropriately and speak well. The clinician has to make a choice in such settings: spend time analyzing Mom's unresolved 'childhood issues' or help her and her son regain their mutual self-respect. Taking the former only continues to feed the adult's narcissistic wound, once again abandoning the child to their own pain. The child in such circumstances is at risk for greater damage.

I always make the decision in favor of the adolescent. While a clear secondary gain of the parent becoming more authoritative is the resolution of their own childhood concerns, focusing on the young person models for both the appropriate level of interdependency that is such a challenge with today's teen whose parents frequently have more money than good sense. It also makes the point to the parent that their childhood is, indeed, over.

The key facet of guiding the care with this type of adolescent is reinforcing an appropriate level of discipline and respect. "By pushing back against your parents, you're doing the job of being a teenager," I tell them. "Your parents have to do their job as well, which involves pushing back. I can help you push away from your parents in a way that won't get you grounded for*ever* and I can help your parents set limits that won't get them thrown in jail."

What usually occurs is the adolescent calms down pretty quickly once the boundaries are reset and they've realized I'm going to be just as firm with them on keeping their promises as their parents. "You've done your job," I congratulate them. "You've not only gone back to being a teenager, you've also made it possible for me to focus on your parents underlying problems. They're the ones who really need the help in this situation. They either want to be too cool or try to be drill instructors." This paradoxical gambit appeals to the adolescent's natural belief that all parents are crazy, monstrous and completely irrelevant. Their improved behavior does, in fact, allow a therapist to turn the attention toward the parents and whatever unresolved issues from their own childhood or divorce or substance abuse have hampered their effectiveness as adults.

"The Court is the Meat Cleaver Once the Scalpel of Therapy Fails"

Just as there are some males who are simply sperm donors and some females who are merely brood mares, so there are some adolescents who are thugs and some adolescents who are tough girls. While these failed parents and tragic youth constitute a minority of the population they consume a major portion of the national treasure spent on mental health care judicial process and penal control. You might not believe this unless you walked through the halls of any juvenile and domestic courthouse or obtain your impression of the culture solely from the 'lead with what bleeds' media.

Perhaps few readers of this volume will come into contact with children or youth whose ignoble lives constitute these tragic tableaus. But there is some benefit in being exposed to the clinical histories of individuals: they illustrate the limits of empathic care and underscore the necessity for some individuals to live with firm and inviolable behavioral and legal boundaries. These realities go against the native optimism that is inherent in most clinicians and pastors who provide humane and compassionate care.

Yet some adolescents take a very dark path toward adulthood. The two teens who wreaked havoc upon their Colorado high school grabbed national headlines. There are many more whose violence and nihilism is less extreme but whose capacity to terrorize their peers is nevertheless significant. Within the clinical realm we focus on their conduct, naming their distress a Conduct Disorder. But the conduct we seek to control is fueled by despair from a misplaced sense of failed entitlement or a craving for structure that leads to gang membership. Such individuals have experienced a gross failure to thrive on all three axis of spiritual life. They have committed realistic acts of lawlessness for which the only hope is the strong social control of a restricted environment. They have placed the acquisition of material wealth, significant drug use, promiscuity or sadistic power as the center of their meaning. They have concluded they are stained beyond redemption.

A stance of soft optimism with such youth is neither helpful nor loving. Those who can be salvaged must endure the tough strictures of a controlled environment. Unfortunately the reality of such an environment is that it frequently places the adolescent among the very people who can hone her skills in crime rather than redeem her soul and redirect her steps. Thus for the average clinician and member of the clergy this step is distasteful because we recognize the inherent paradox that results from consigning a person to such a setting.

The same is true for adults. Indeed there yet remains cases of egregious miscarriages of justice where the desire to rehabilitate repetitive offenders overrides not only a lengthy criminal record but also solid clinical experience with the resistance of some behavioral patterns to any therapeutic intervention. Thus protecting children from adults who are sexual predators mandates the necessity to thoroughly restrict their access to children. If we would care for children, therapists must be ready to make such clear-eyed assessments based on an adult's – or an adolescent's – actual history of conduct rather than our hope that somehow 'one more chance at therapy' will suddenly help them to change. Recidivism of such children in late adolescence would not be such a problem if they had received direct, firm and effective behavioral care in early childhood rather than the vain hope that 'one more chance at caring' would somehow awaken a level of conscience that is sadly entirely absent for a few children.

Putting aside these extreme cases, the question remains of how to make the determination of the imperative necessity to terminate the parental rights of adults who otherwise appear to be socially successful and have adequate financial resources. "This is the realm of social workers and county departments of human services," private practice clinicians may say. Pastoral clinicians and general practice psychiatrists may likewise abhor having to render such a professional opinion with such permanent consequences.

I can tell the reader from personal experience that rendering such an opinion is not the hardest part of this task. Watching the child or adolescent continue to suffer while obtaining enough factual and clinical evidence to make such a determination while they are in your care is the most heart-wrenching part of this treatment. Providing the necessary nurture while documenting the child's level of pain reverses our traditional understanding of how healing should proceed. This is not a matter of withholding succor in order to play 'gotcha!' counseling. Rather, it is a matter of documenting what the child says about her treatment as she learns to trust you and stepping far enough from behind the fictive mask of neutrality so that she experiences a genuine therapeutic alliance.

The challenge for a clinician is to rightly distinguish between a truly abusive parent and a parent who is targeted by the virulent hostility of an aggrieved former spouse. The clinician must also discern the difference between a parent who is setting realistic standards of conduct and tough consequences on an oppositional adolescent and a parent who is overtly brutal or predatory. The clinician must assess the capacity of a young child to tell the truth independent of the influence of either parent as well as the ability of an adolescent to give up the fantasy of getting everything their heart desires if they can only be allowed to live with the *other* parent. This is not work for the faint of heart. Here are some of the guidelines within which I make an initial determination.

➤ Age – the child's age corresponds with the level of detail in their story and the child can explain the difference between truth and make believe.

➤ Consistency – the child's report of each event remains consistent over time.

➤ Spontaneity – the child volunteers statements about the parent's abuse without prompting by either therapist or custodial parent.

➤ Embarrassment – the child at first becomes uncomfortable when asked directly about abuse.

> ➤ Comorbid mood disorder – depression or anxiety in a heretofore healthy child, evidenced through drawings, conduct and affect.
> ➤ Reduced academic achievement – usually a clear signal of affective distress, especially if there was no prior indicator of a learning disorder.
> ➤ Social dyscontrol – striking other children or adult caregivers by a heretofore respectful child or regression in conduct; inappropriate sexual interest or speech.
> ➤ Bowel dyscontrol – enuresis or encopresis in a child who has achieved bladder and bowel control.

This is not an exhaustive list of criteria. There is also one other criterion: my appraisal of both parents, even if my only contact with the non-custodial parent is via telephone or e-mail. But a clinician who works in this area must be willing to trust their relational intuition outside of their office and the sacred clinical hour. A clinician who would truly be an advocate for children must also be willing to speak for them in the one venue that is truly the 'court of last resort' where the rules of evidence will work against them unless their therapist speaks with cogency and clarity. As I said above, this is not work for the faint of heart.

This leads directly into the notion of the Parental Alienation Syndrome advanced by Richard Gardner. While a thorough treatment of Gardner's positing of this syndrome is beyond the scope of this chapter, I would urge clinicians and caregivers to become familiar with the symptoms of this syndrome. (4) Gardner is a serious clinician of lengthy experience who worked effectively with numerous children and adolescents throughout his career. His insights should not be dismissed out-of-hand simply because the syndrome is not in the DSM-IV-TR or likely to make it into the DSM-V. (5)

Having said this, I would hasten to add the following. Gardner is clear that all factors of this syndrome must be present in order to make an accurate diagnosis of this syndrome. To supplant a child's natural affection for a parent in the absence of abusive conduct by that parent takes considerable effort on the part of the other parent. It is not a condition easily planted or quickly installed into the mind and heart of a child. (6) Thus this is the last conclusion a diagnostician should appeal to rather than the first syndrome on the diagnostic checklist when a child expresses fear of a parent. Even a law journal that is supportive of the concept of Parental Alienation Syndrome concludes with this caution:

All the criteria listed above can be found independent of each other in highly contested dissolutions, but remember that the appearance of some of them does not always constitute PAS. When all four are clearly present, however, add the possibility of real abuse has been reasonably ruled out, the parental alienation process is operative. (7)

The literature in this area is extensive but outside the purview of the average clinician. The best inoculation against this syndrome becoming the debating point in court is the involvement of a several independent clinicians known for their impartiality as well as character witnesses who can appear in court on behalf of the parent targeted with the charge of this syndrome. (8)

Finally the clinician must be certain enough of both the harm done to the child and the parent's inability to change that they will state it clearly in court. Typically this is not work one seeks but work which comes to a care provider. It is imperative that clinicians are thoroughly acquainted with their state's requirements for recognizing, documenting and reporting abuse so that they can reach the proper balance between a prudent caution that protects the well-being of children and a wise recognition that insures the ability of an effective parent to apply appropriate boundaries.

Conclusion

As noted at the outset of this chapter, we have barely touched the surface of the complex work of clinical interventions with children and adolescents. They certainly bring their own concerns, increasingly so as they mature, in addition to the events that occurs within their families. A child's spiritual life is either nurtured or neglected throughout their development. Just as with adults it is true that children who belong to an active religious community fare better as they face the hurdles of maturation. Children feel appropriate and inappropriate guilt. Children discover people and ends that are worthy of devotion as well as recognizing the inadequacy of some ends and the dishonorableness of some people. Children have their destinies shaped by significant trauma no less than adults. Indeed, while we rightly desire to protect children from catastrophic distress and dread disease, I am amazed continually at the resilience that children exhibit when faced with profound loss, even when their basic needs for shelter, food and warmth are met inadequately.

I am mindful of this resilience each time I look at a photograph taken by a fellow Marine in 1969 at Da Nang's Sacred Heart Orphanage. Amid the ravages of war, I am holding one little three-year old girl who weighed no more than thirty pounds and would likely not survive. Another Marine is holding a somewhat older boy whose blindness was caused by the rifle stroke to his skull of an NVA soldier after witnessing the death of his parents. He would need to live in a sheltered environment the rest of his life. A third Marine is lifting up a boy who wants to explore the roof of the hut that was sheltering us. A fourth child rests his arm on that Marine's knee and stares directly into the camera with an engaging curiosity. These latter two children will survive quite well, given their resurgent curiosity and physical health.

All four children had endured the uncertainties and cruelties of war yet had found some degree of comfort in an orphanage run by a religious community.

Given what eventually happened in South Vietnam, they endured more hardship and uncertainty on their way to adulthood. Nevertheless the literature of humanity is as filled with accounts of adults who trace their initiative and industriousness to triumph over childhood trauma as who trace their meager adult achievements to succumbing to similar trauma. Exposure to a vibrant religious community appears to be one of the determining variables. Thus in this week's clinical practice I am working with an adolescent girl who struggles to cope with a mother's chronic pain while she also tries to define herself within a strict religious school; a six year old boy who is grieving the loss of his grandmother who told him she was getting well and would not die; a pastor whose class of sixth grade boys have decided to challenge the leadership of their female teacher and a nineteen year old college student struggling to leave behind his dependence on marijuana. All of the individuals believe in God and express their faith readily albeit in very different terms given their diverse ages and distinct religious traditions. Helping them understand their pain and move toward health within their distinct religious traditions in ways that enhance their spiritual growth is as much a legitimate clinical goal as assisting them in their grief, their bulging testosterone, and their addiction. *Selah!*

Chapter 18: What About Substance Abuse and Addiction?

As I was completing my internship in 1985 one of the places I interviewed for work was a new residential substance abuse treatment center. In 1985 the twenty-eight day in-patient program was the gold standard for substance abuse treatment. Whether you were a substance abuse clinician in Indianapolis or Phoenix or Miami, you began treatment by recommending the client undergo such an in-patient program.

Within one year the insurance industry began instituting managed care guidelines. The twenty-eight day substance abuse treatment regime was one of the first casualties. Currently if someone wants to receive what is still the gold-standard and most effective way to begin breaking the back of substance abuse, you are likely to have to pay for it out of your own pocket. It remains my belief that such a program is ultimately more cost-effective than what is currently the industry standard, especially when followed up by an intensive outpatient program for structured aftercare and participation in one of the many Twelve Step groups.

Current substance abuse treatment now focuses on an intensive outpatient program plus involvement in a Twelve Step group. What is missing is the absolute break with the peer group and family that enables substance abuse to continue. Nevertheless when one wishes to redeem an adolescent who is trapped by their poor choices, parents readily turn back to an inpatient program that is frequently months long. These programs are intensive and expensive yet the power of addiction is so great that even these programs produce only modest results.

Naming the pain of substance abuse remains the hardest hurdles in diagnosis. The grip of addiction is so thorough on the mind that the individual's capacity to deny the obvious wreckage of their life is initially almost absolute. Guiding the care of recovery becomes a life-long enterprise. The spiritual, emotional and social skills necessary to maintain sobriety must be applied with disciplined integrity by the individual and by those who love them. In addition to these resources there are now powerful medical tools that assist clinicians in both tracking the consequences of addiction as well as portraying the hope inherent in abstinence.

A thorough review of the entire field of substance abuse treatment is beyond the scope of this chapter. The focus of this chapter will be much more narrow. The diagnostic indicators of substance abuse, dependence and the general resources necessary for effective treatment of addiction will be the foci of this chapter. For the pastoral counselor and religiously oriented clinician there are two significant tools that have become available both on-line for individual study as well as in print format for use in graduate-level education. These will be covered in some depth. But first we must turn our attention to the primary diagnostic task.

"Tryin' Out Tailor-Mades Like Cigarette Fiends"

When Professor Harold Hill sought to rouse the citizens of River City, Iowa to recognize the 'caliber of disaster indicated by the presence of a pool table in your community,' one of the consequences he warned parents of was their children would be trying out Bevo and begin smoking. Not only that (gasp!) but they would then brag 'all about how they're gonna cover up a tell-tale breath with Sen-Sen.' *The Music Man* is a wonderful story of how a scoundrel redeems a town and a town redeems a scoundrel.

But all too frequently the drug use, deception and disrespect begun in adolescence continue into adulthood with devastating consequences. Recovery and redemption from the corrosion of soul and ravages of the diseases that come from chronic substance abuse take more than joining the River City Boy's Band. The health costs alone to the individual, their immediate family and society are immense even if the person never 'graduates' from cigarettes and above-average beer drinking to harder drugs and certifiable alcohol dependence. (1) When the law-enforcement costs are added into this figure we are quickly talking about 'real money.'

Diagnostically two things are true. First, substance use that begins in adolescence is a rite of passage. Second, substance abuse that begins in adolescence is illegal. Because of the former being true, parents tend to adopt a 'what can I do?' stance, especially with teen smoking. 'Just don't smoke in the house,' usually becomes the resentful armistice worked out between teen and parents. But it is a deadly compromise even if using the 'nicotine delivery system' of cigarettes doesn't lead to the use of marijuana, cocaine, heroin, Ecstasy or methamphetamines. This compromise is deadly because it allows the brain to become attenuated to nicotine's siren song of life changing power. This is a deluded agreement for regaining control that spirals downward toward eventual addiction.

Diagnostically two more things are true. Substance use promises to change a person's life with little personal cost. This promise is true and it is the promise of every idol. Substance abuse does change each user's life but not in ways that the person foresees. This is the truthful reality of every deal we sign with who religious tradition calls The Adversary or The Father of Lies. Facing this idolatry requires the admission that one's life has 'become unmanageable,' if not from the total ruin of Skid Row then at least from the economic havoc literally gone up in smoke and down the drain. This requires a spiritual integrity that must accompany the physiological cleansing and the psychological reconditioning required in breaking the bondage of addiction.

Diagnostically two final things are true. Substance use stains the person and the environment in which they live. This results from the odors and the tainted fluids that come to be associated with the chronic substance abuser. Substance abuse also marks the individual for life if left unchecked. They are now banished from many public establishments and viewed as something of social if not moral lepers by others. The sacrifices associated with this alienation are profound if not always evident to the observing eye or listening ear.

Thus the pain that must be named in any case of substance misuse crosses all three diagnostic axes. There is both realistic guilt and subjective guilt. There is idolatry with all of the terror and rage that both defends the rites associated with addiction as well as results from the effort required to transcend the idol. There is defilement of physiology, psychology, spirituality and sociology in ever-widening circles around each addicted or abusing person. Whether named early in life or near the end of life, naming these various arenas of pain requires the courage to surrender as well as the humility to begin living each day with newly recognized gratitude.

"We Admitted We Were Powerless Over Alcohol"

Thus begins the first step of diagnosis in substance addiction. This is followed by the admission 'that our lives had become unmanageable.' This original confession of Alcoholics Anonymous has been changed by Narcotics Anonymous, but only by the substitution of other drugs of choice or destructive compulsion for the word 'alcohol.' The fundamental insight is two-fold: I have no power over my addiction and my addiction has made my life unmanageable.

This operational definition of addiction or compulsion gets us away from discussions over when, how, where, with whom, how long or what that takes up so much time during the initial arguments over substance abuse. I use a variation of this diagnostic clarity by making this statement: "If (insert your drug or habit here) is causing problems in my life, (insert your drug or compulsion here) is a problem." I usually follow this definition up with this diagnostic question, "How long do you want to continue living with these problems?"

Two other simple diagnostic screens can be used during the initial interview as soon as substance abuse has been identified as a feature in the person's reason for seeking help. One is the CAGE test. It involves leading the person through this serious of four questions:

> ➢ Have you ever tried to **Cut Down** on your drinking and failed?
> ➢ Have you ever gotten **Annoyed** or **Angry** with people who express concern about your drinking?
> ➢ Have you ever felt **Guilty** about your drinking?
> ➢ Have you ever needed an **Eye-Opener** drink to get going in the morning after a night of drinking?

Of course this assumes that the individual is willing to acknowledge the use of a substance. So much secrecy and deception are associated with substance abuse that the individual may never acknowledge their behavior, let alone the devastation their addiction imposes on others.

I see this basic denial regularly in the weekly psycho-educational classes provided under one of Virginia's Alcohol Safety Action Programs (ASAP). This is a court-mandated series of weekly group meetings for individuals convicted of driving under the influence of alcohol or being found driving with illegal drugs in their automobile. The Early Intervention program requires sixteen weeks of meetings, eight concurrent A. A. or N. A. meetings, at least two random urine screens in addition to weekly Breathalyzer tests. The person is allowed only two absences. Total abstinence from alcohol and drugs is required.

They may also be assigned to attend either an Intensive Outpatient Program or a Relapse Prevention Program. This depends upon the severity of the substance abuse revealed in their personal history. These are additional twelve week or twenty-four week psycho-educational programs that run sequentially or concomitantly with the Early Intervention Program. At the cost of $30 per group session, $25 per urine test and $75 per month for the ignition interlock they must have on their car for at least one year, the financial cost alone of this one program becomes extensive. Fines, court costs, lost income due to lost work or perhaps even losing a job if the DUI occurred while they were driving a company vehicle frequently makes that one arrest at least a $10,000 expense.

A person usually doesn't begin to claim their role in their arrest until the tenth week. The hard-core substance abuser usually becomes adept at saying what is expected by that point; the person who was 'simply in the wrong place at the wrong time' nevertheless has likely driven in an impaired condition at least four hundred times before they were finally caught. I will see the truly addicted person again after their second or third subsequent arrest and significant time in jail. Only then does the genuine addict begin to speak honestly about the difficulty they're having breaking free of bondage.

Programs such as this one are now nearly universal across the United States. Along with tough enforcement strategies and continued education of alcohol servers, deaths due to impaired driving are slowly falling. But these programs only touch the surface destructiveness that substance abuse exacts upon individuals, families and society. Hardly a week goes by without reading a news account of someone whose repeated failures to abstain from impaired driving produces consequences tragic enough for the court to finally impose a sentence lengthy enough to remove the individual from public for what amounts to the rest of their driving life.

My experience with both clinicians and with impaired individuals is that both communities have difficulty with such lengthy punishments. Our inability to place the deaths caused by impaired driving on the same plane as the deaths caused by a home invasion or a carefully constructed murder says much about our societal complicity in such deaths. It tells me that there is more than the addicted person who has trouble taking the first step of acknowledging 'powerlessness over alcohol.'

"Turned Our Lives Over to the Care of God as We Understood Him"

Five of the Twelve Steps of A. A. explicitly mention God. All other steps except the first one imply God or 'a Power greater than ourselves' as a necessary component in the task of recovery from substance abuse. The last three steps make the point that mending the damage from substance abuse and managing life as a now-clean addicted person is a life-long journey of care rather than merely a way station in one's life. This exhibits the essential distinction between care and cure as the second diagnostic task.

Thus it is not an accident that most Twelve Step groups meet inside a Christian church. Within the recovery community these groups are sometimes referred to as 'the church that meets in the basement of the church.' Few things in the spiritual life illustrate the journey of sanctification or self-transcendence so completely as the process of what A. A.'s second step calls being 'restored to sanity.' Other steps in recovery mirror this life of the Spirit that is acted out institutionally in many of the rites of the Christian faith. Self-examination is embodied in Step Four. Confession follows next in Step 5. Surrender takes two steps, 6 and 7.

The most thoroughgoing enactment of Steps 8 and 9 took place in nearby Charlottesville, Virginia recently. A man who had raped a fellow college student while both were at a drunken party eventually began facing the profound wreckage he had made of his life. In an effort to fully heal and conduct Step 9 he contacted his victim via e-mail, confessed his crime and requested her forgiveness. The woman went to the police with the e-mail. He was arrested, tried and eventually sentenced to two years in prison.

"I have just two questions for you to answer during the interview," said the television reporter who inquired with me about this case. "First, have you ever heard of anyone taking this step in recovery this far? Second, would you advise someone else taking such a serious step if they would likely wind up in jail?" Then his camera operator nodded, on went the red light and we began walking slowly toward the corner where the interview would occur.

"I cannot recall anyone taking their Eighth Step so seriously," I said. "If they were under my care in therapy I would insist they look first at how taking this public step of contacting the victim would affect the victim, followed closely by obtaining some legal advice about the consequences they would most likely endure." I followed up this comment by making an observation that I've had to embrace in my own life: "Sometimes the most powerful amend one can make is to rigorously allow the person you have wronged to live their own life free from the sound of your voice, the writing of your hand and the integrity of your word to consistently keep these promises with them." The essence of Step 9 is my ability to finally recognize that it is the peacefulness of the other person, and not my peace, which must eventually become my focus if I am to mature.

Within the various expressions of the Christian faith there is usually the rite of confession in any public liturgy. Private prayer likewise best begins with recognition of one's obvious failings. The most familiar form of this confession reads as follows:

> Almighty God, our heavenly Father, we have sinned against
> you, through our own fault, in thought and word and deed, and
> in what we have left undone. For the sake of your Son our Lord
> Jesus Christ, forgive us all our offenses and grant that we may
> Serve you in newness of life, to the glory of your name, Amen.

The priest or minister then pronounces a general absolution. The Tenth Step in recovery is much more specific, thorough and serious, although it has its roots in this rite's regularity.

Having made an initial 'searching and fearless moral inventory' in Step Four, this tenth step makes the point that whenever life is not going my way, it is incumbent for my growth that I acknowledge my role in the failure. Resentment is typically the key emotion that signals the necessity of 'taking an inventory.' An effective Tenth Step is not telling someone else 'I have some resentment toward you.' An effective Tenth Step is telling myself, "I am resentful because I feel threatened, or disappointed, or hurt because of my own selfishness, pride, envy or greed." A complete Tenth Step involves acknowledging this to God, myself, one other person.

Effective care of an addicted person involves guiding them to and through this type of maturity. This level of care takes time to appropriate and appreciate. It goes way beyond a politically correct *pro forma* admission that 'everybody is flawed' or 'it takes two to have conflict.' It is a surrender to the truth that my own self-will is the most destructive thing in my life, and that my self-will is the only thing I can submit to the loving care of God. It takes months if not years of therapy and regular involvement in a recovery group for this self-reflection to become a natural part of an individual's life. Thus this step directly challenges the idolatry of any addiction: that my life can become immediately better by taking a drink, swallowing a pill, or putting some mind-altering chemical into my body.

There are hundreds of books written on prayer and meditation. Step Eleven gets very basic, directing anyone who gets this far to focus on their essential status as a child of God: 'the knowledge of His will and the power to carry it out.' Whether working with addicted individuals or more generally with anyone who desires to develop a more satisfying life of prayer, I make one of two suggestions that elaborate on this basic stance. The first suggestion is that they adopt this prayer as a morning ritual for one month:

> Lord, take me where You want me to go;
> Let me meet who You want me to meet;
> Tell me what You want me to say, and
> Keep me out of Your way, Amen.

This was the prayer of Father Mychal F. Judge, OFM. He was the chaplain for the New York City Fire Department and the first official death of those who responded to the attack on the World Trade Center. Beginning the day with this brief prayer 'improves our conscious contact with God as we understand Him' while also placing us in the posture of humble surrender.

Another prayer that is simple, practical and powerful is called The Hand Prayer. In this prayer each finger reminds us of a distinct kind of prayer. You start with a closed hand, which is where we all start our walk with the Higher Power. Whether we elaborate on each of these statements or simply acknowledge Him quietly at the end of each statement, when the prayer reaches the final statement, our hand is open. Here is the prayer:

> I love you, God! (praise)
> I'm thankful, God! (thanksgiving)
> I'm sorry, God! (contrition)
> Help others, God! (intercession)
> Help me, God! (petition)
> I'm listening, God! (contemplation)
> Amen!

As I said there are countless other prayers and meditation regimes. But a person's emotional and spiritual development arrests at the age or stage where they began seriously abusing alcohol or using addictive drugs. So despite the individual's age, education and apparent social status, not only is the counselor working with a child but the damage of serious substance abuse takes anyone back to the basic status of a dependent child who must once again learn to crawl in all of their social, emotional and spiritual relationships. These prayers accomplish this goal.

"...We Tried to Carry This Message to Other Alcoholics..."

The clinician or clergy who works with substance-dependent individuals has a wealth of resources available to them. The Substance Abuse and Mental Health Services Administration (SAMSHA) has published a very helpful document that gives a brief but thorough overview of addiction as well as the attitudes and actions necessary for providing effective care. The *Spiritual Caregiving to Help Addicted Persons and Families: Handbook for Use by Pastoral Counselors in Clergy Education* is one volume that should be on every counselor's shelf, not just the clergy. It is available through their website, www.sahsha.gov.

Another document available by itself as well as being summarized in the above-mentioned volume is *Core Competencies for Clergy and Other Pastoral Ministers in Addressing Alcohol and Drug Dependence and the Impact on Family Members.* (1) This booklet identifies twelve core competencies ranging from basic awareness of the general definition of alcoholism and being aware of the benefits of early intervention to the competency of being aware of how to shape a congregation so that it welcomes and supports drug-addicted persons and their families. As a clinician I would not limit this document's usefulness to pastoral counselors or clergy. These are competencies that every mental health professional should be aware of if they interact at all with individuals affected by substance abuse. This document is available from the American Association of Pastoral Counselors website, www.aapc.org.

Counselors of all mental health disciplines who desire additional training in the Twelve Core Competencies have a very effective resource available to them. *Studies in the Twelve Core Competencies,* written and produced by Chris Bowers, is an interactive study that can be obtained directly from the author. This resource draws on the most current neurobiological research as well as providing clinicians with outcome based treatment options that, when the information is uploaded onto your desktop computer, become readily available to the client during the treatment process. Mr. Bowers is also the curriculum developer of the training manual *Spiritual Caregiving to Help Addicted Persons and Families.* Produced in cooperation with the National Association for Children of Alcoholics, this information is available through their website: www.nacoa.org. Mr. Bowers' resources are available directly from him through the website www.counselorandclergy.com.

These resources all point to the single most revolutionary tool now available for treating addicted individuals: spectral images of the brain. We now realize that while substance abuse affects all of an individual's organs and bodily systems, the brain is the primary organ damaged by substance abuse. The spectrographic images of the human brain document the ways in which specific regions of the brain are affected by substance abuse (something readily observable through seeing the behavioral consequences of substance abuse). More importantly, these images clearly portray the process of recovery, showing how lengthy and thoroughgoing the journey of healing takes. Simply put, when it takes months of abstinence from a drug before the region of the brain responsible for making effective decisions receives adequate blood flow, it is difficult if not impossible to make good decisions, resist cravings or otherwise maintain the quality of social relationships that enhance life. This does not remove the individual's responsibility for making good decisions. It provides the person, their family and clinicians with a tool that allows them to set realistic milestones for recovery and underscores the imperative for residential treatment if the individual is going to break the biochemical handcuffs that serious drug addiction places on the brain.

Dr. Daniel Amen is the seminal provider of the research. He has one of the most complete atlases of spectrographic brain images available on the World Wide Web. I have found that using these images directly in the counseling process helps the addicted individual face the ruin their habit produces as well as gives them a realistic measure of hope as they begin the task of rebuilding their life. This atlas portrays the alteration in blood flow patterns in numerous maladies and discrete injuries. This helps us comprehend the capacity of the brain of the afflicted individual to process the information and make the choices necessary for treatment to be effective. These photos also validate or disconfirm the efficacy of various medication in treating a host of mood disorders, whether those disorders are the result of substance abuse, brain lesions, or a basic organic fault within the brain's neurological structure.

As powerful as these spectrographic images are at convincing the ordinary individual that substance abuse carries long-term life altering consequences for them, these images are not in and of themselves curative. They are effective for the individual who is on the initial slope of Jellinek's famous chart of the addictive cycle. But for the individual who has reached the hellish proverbial bottom of addiction, these images underscore the simple fact that recovery will be a life-long battle fought out day by day if not hour by hour as the blood slowly returns to the brain's damaged regions and the neural pathways for making healthy decisions about peers and lifestyle slowly rebuild themselves. This reveals the inherent wisdom in many of the simple sayings of the various Twelve Step programs. They are the pitons necessary to hold one in place when the cravings would overwhelm us and the cairns necessary to guide us through the fog that inevitably clouds our best judgment. Only as we make this arduous ascent are we then able to complete the rest of the Twelfth Step's admonition, "…and to practice these principles in all our affairs."

Conclusion

The societal cost of substance abuse can be roughly calculated. But the individual expense of addiction is incalculable. Even the ten bullet points of these consequences just for children give one solemn pause:

> Children of addicted parents are the highest risk group of children to become alcohol and drug abusers due to both genetic and family environmental factors.

> Family interaction is defined by substance abuse or addiction in a family.

> A relationship between parental addiction and child abuse has been documented in a large proportion of child abuse and neglect cases.

> Children of drug addicted parents are at the highest risk for placement outside the home.

> They exhibit symptoms of depression and anxiety more than do children from non-addicted families.

> They experience more physical and mental health problems and higher health and welfare costs than do children from non-addicted families.

> They have a higher rate of behavioral problems.

> They score lower on tests measuring achievements and they exhibit other difficulties in school.

> Maternal consumption of alcohol or other drugs at any time of pregnancy can cause birth defects or neurological deficits.

The careful reader will notice there are only nine bullet points. The tenth major point bears directly on the topic of diagnosis and treatment: *Children of addicted parents may benefit from supportive adult efforts to help them.*[i] Thus the question 'what role does alcohol or some other drug play in your concern?' should be a routine part of any initial interview or psychological assessment. It is imperative that some form of this question be asked in the assessment of a child *after trust has been built and the parents are absent from the interview.* Most parents who are addicted start to recognize the impact their substance abuse is having on their children once the drugs leave their system. These adults also benefit from continued supportive and lifelong intervention once they leave a controlled rehabilitation or intensive outpatient environment. Their struggle to achieve sobriety and begin a lifestyle of recovery is still possible but much more difficult absent such an intensive intervention. One fifty-minute hour a week is seldom effective.

In a significant number of instances recovery from active substance dependence is only the first phase of a thorough healing. Frequently the substance addiction overlays a more primary mood disorder and has become interwoven into the individual's financial stability and vocational expression. Just 'naming those pains' require great courage from the individual and their family. The journey of restoring sanity to those other primary areas of soul, mind and body is an ascent out of Hell as arduous and as fraught with danger as was the descent. But the doorway to this portion of life has a different plaque on its face: Welcome Home! *Selah!*

Chapter 19: What About Stress Disorders?

The photographs now have the sepia tone that comes with age. Young men in boxing shorts are surrounded by their cheering supporters. Sometimes their arms are crossed in studied nonchalance. Other times their arms is raised in victory. Everyone in the photos is smiling. The men who dislodged the Japanese from those Pacific island hellholes relieved their pre-assault anxiety and their post-war nightmare trips toward home aboard ship with well-organized boxing matches.

We now live in kinder and gentler times, so we offer our returning warriors counseling and drugs to numb their horrors of battles. The lingering stress from trauma ranges from post-reprimand timidity to post-catastrophic nightmares. The operative word in the formal definition of post-traumatic stress disorder is 'Post.' It is the one psychiatric disorder where there is an identifiable event of sufficient severity to produce symptoms within an ordinary person.

This area of care has undergone nothing short of a revolution in the last thirty years. Prior to the post-Vietnam War period we viewed the distress of individuals who suffered from stress-related pain in a piecemeal fashion. Providers of humane care would do well to become acquainted with the diverse history of this disorder, ranging from a description of survivors of the Great London Fire as early as 1666 by Samuel Pepys to the current efforts within the DSM-V committee to refine the original formal definition from the 1980 DSM-III. (1) The thirty-three pages of the double-column eight-point bibliography available in this work would probably be double or even triple if compiled today.

In addition to the just-cited work of Donald Meichenbaum, interested readers could also review the extensive seminal writings of Charles Figley. (2) A returned Vietnam veteran, Figley's earliest writing in the area of what has become his life's work illustrates the way in which the search for individual meaning in trauma also provided the entire human community with a matrix of care for PTSD.

Because of the all-inclusive nature of post-traumatic stress disorder (PTSD) and its frequent citation in legal settings as the grounds for significant awards by sympathetic juries, this chapter will first review the diagnostic criteria associated with PTSD. This chapter will then review the impact of catastrophic trauma across the three axes developed in this volume: guilt, idolatry and dread.

"I'll Give You Something to Really Cry About!"

The men who landed at Anzio and Okinawa, the women who bore the hardships of the Dust Bowl, the kids from Hell's Kitchen who fought at Bastonge and the wives who sleep next to the POW's who returned from any war know genuine trauma. As a result their parenting strategies tend to be rather blunt if not harsh for no other reason than an innate desire to build into their children the resiliency necessary to endure a similar degree of adversity. I cannot count the number of clients, acquaintances and friends from all walks of life who, in revisiting the wounds of their childhood, remember hearing a parent utter this phrase in response to their tears. These are people who are both well adjusted and those with significant developmental or personality disorders.

In an American culture that cannot currently distinguish between the pain of being burned on the lips from hot coffee and the devastation caused by a Santa Ana wind-driven forest fire, sentiments such as this appear cruel. Thus in clinical practice and in the popular media there is initial pressure to baptize any disturbing symptom from life's unfortunate events as PTSD. At the outset it is therefore helpful to review the actual criteria for the event that must serve as the catalyst to begin assessment for PTSD. While there is a host of other stress responses to life's indignities, **both** of these criteria must be met before a clinician can legitimately begin assessing for full-blown PTSD:

> ➢ The person has experienced, witnessed or was confronted with an event or events that involved actual or threatened death or serious injury, or a threat to the physical integrity of self or others;
>
> ➢ The person's response involved intense fear, helplessness or horror (in children, disorganized or agitated behavior).

Meichenbaum observers two truths about trauma that are worth recalling: "most people will experience a traumatic event at some point during their lives, often while they are still quite young. The exposure to traumatic events is neither rare nor unusual." (3) This recognition is an important qualifier because the physiological and behavioral symptoms that result from such exposure help both the individual and a caregiver assess the individual's resiliency.

There are two general types of trauma. Type I trauma is short-term and unexpected. While events such as these can be rare, they can be intense. While an individual may experience them only once in a lifetime, they will exert a permanent influence on the meaning they assign to whatever life they pluck from the wreckage of home and family. Type II trauma are sustained ordeals or repeated exposure to a prolonged traumatic event. The former can be something as expected as a tornado in Kansas or as unexpected as a rape. The latter can be chronic abuse of child or living in a war zone. Because trauma can be expected and human resilience is an unpredictable factor with genetic and gender variables there is a diagnostic range of stress disorders including Acute Stress Disorder, Partial PTSD and Complex PTSD including formal Post-Traumatic Stress Disorder. Formal PTSD may be acute, delayed chronic, or intermittent. (4) Thus frequently in assisting the person to 'name the pain,' the triggering event is a clearly recognizable life-threatening stressor. Much care is provided in these instances by normalizing the individual's reaction, informing them of the normal course of recovery from such an event and reminding them of how they recovered from stressors of similar intensity. But occasionally the person must be helped to 'de-awfulize' their reaction to a reasonably expected event. The inappropriate level of reactivity to a mild stressor is still diagnostically useful but it will take the thoughtful clinician more in the direction of a personality disorder rather than a true stress disorder. As a result, it does serve to keep in mind the title of this sub-section when gathering the data of an individual's history: do the intensity of the 'tears' correspond to the intensity of the event, are the tears those of a crocodile benefiting from secondary sympathetic gains or are the tears the consequence of an individual's resiliency finally collapsing as a result of prior injuries?

"It's Not Your Fault!"

Dr. William B. Oglesby spoke this simple sentence to me in 1985. Offered near the completion of my internship in the art of counseling, it shut the door on the guilt shoved upon me by my nation and church's dishonorable 'welcome home' to Vietnam veterans. The issue of guilt looms large in the both the immediate and the long-term aftermath of any trauma. Individuals look immediately at the question of their own responsibility for their misfortune. If the trauma is serious enough this question gets hashed out in media, court and culture. It is likely to be a question to which the person returns with some regularity.

Adequate assessment of responsibility for serious personal misfortune may so thoroughly affect the course of an individual's life that it becomes the criterion to which a person refers all future moral, spiritual and vocational concerns. This appears to be the case whether the trauma is as public an event as a regional hurricane or as quiet a disaster as catastrophic childhood abuse and neglect. While the victim may initially feel singled out for special punishment by the trauma, the fact is that suffering is a regular occurrence in the course of a normal lifetime.

There is also the issue of survivor guilt. The individual wonders not only 'was this my fault?' they may also wonder 'why was I spared?' This latter question gradually transmutes into a more basic examination of life's purpose and the transformation of the ordeal's stain. Since this theme will be addressed below, for the present I want to stay focused on the question of helping the survivor examine and come to some degree of peace with whatever guilt is produced by the trauma, whether that guilt rises from the issue of responsibility or the issue of their own survival.

In recent decades we have gained enough moral awareness about trauma that we generally no longer blame the victim for their suffering. Cognitive interventions help the individual recognize their status as a survivor rather than that of a victim. Thus in providing emotional and spiritual first aid in the aftermath of a trauma it is helpful to tease out what the individual **did** that enabled them to survive rather than allowing them to only focus on what they **did not** do or **could not** do that contributed to their injuries or some degree of injury to another. Typically a counselor may hear a survivor lament, "I should have followed my instincts." It is more helpful to the individual if we guide them in teasing out that instinct rather than allowing them to spiral downward into a morass of self-recrimination.

Another common angle of survivor guilt focuses on the sentiment 'I should have done more.' A paradoxical cognitive intervention such as 'you should have lifted the car off of your child?' or 'you should have held the roof down against 150 mile-an-hour winds?' allows the individual to recognize for themselves the limits of their physical abilities and moral obligations. This are tied directly to the task of addressing their spiritual limitations.

Of course a clinician must balance our empathic desire to soothe all wounds with our moral obligation to assist the individual in naming whatever pain they must legitimately bear. This includes any moral obligation that rightly must rest upon their soul from failure to perform a *prima facia* duty in any one of the five moral categories: justice, fidelity, non-malfeasance, beneficence, and autonomy. This exploration must be a cognitive or rational enterprise if one hopes to bring about any measure of healing. The efficacious strength of these categories is their capacity to place realistic limits on personal responsibility.

This kind of moral and ethical evaluation becomes an especially important exercise for returned combat veterans. The relationship between personal valor, inevitably based upon how the individual performed under the duress of battle, is inextricably intertwined with the politically charged political constructs of victory, treatment of returned veterans and ceremonies that honor the dead. This type of ethical examination by the veteran goes far beyond the clinical efforts to assuage the symptoms of nightmares and hypervigilance, although the relief of these symptoms is not unimportant for they speak of the combatant's continued suffering and survival.

Indeed the foremost requirement for the clinician will be their capacity to put aside their own political views of the particular war and allow the soldier, sailor, airman or Marine to review these themes. In most instances this is a repetitive enterprise for the therapist and for the veteran in one's wider life. This is due to the fact that the outcome of any particular war remains a topic of examination and discussion within the culture long after the final battle and therefore re-immerses the particular combatant in both his personal decisions while in battle as well as the necessity to account for himself within the changing political constructs and cultural values through which the war is viewed by others.

While this level of individual inquiry appears to be a moral or ethical exploration in a therapeutic context, the true personal focus is a life-long spiritual quest to resolve questions of betrayal, terror and rage. For this portion of the diagnostic enterprise we much therefore turn to the matters of idolatry more rightfully reserved for Axis II.

"Does Anyone Know Where the Love of God Goes..."

This query from Gordon Lightfoot's ballad *The Wreck of the Edmund Fitzgerald* is completed by the phrase 'when the waves turn the minutes to hours?' Whether the event is a tornado seeking to tear the roof from your shelter, floodwaters sweeping your child from your clutch, or warplanes diving out of the rising sun with havoc, this theological conundrum haunts the soul of every trauma survivor. Resolving this mystery is daunting in a world increasingly driven by sound bytes and media shout-outs. When photos of something you lived through can be doctored, replicated, distributed world-wide for maximum propaganda purpose and then commented upon while your soul still reels from the wind or ducking from the sniper's bullet, such reflection can become a lonely task of individual heroism.

Pastoral care is only one of the multitudes of treatment strategies clinicians and caregivers have employed to relieve the symptoms and resolve the ambiguity trauma can imbed in the soul. Yet in reviewing the seven pages of treatment alternatives two insights remain constant. First, no treatment or combination of treatments will **cure** PTSD although some interventions will relieve more symptoms than others. This includes pharmacological interventions. (5) Second, the goal of any effective treatment is 'to help clients, not only improve their behavior, but to also change the 'story' they tell to themselves and to others.' (6)

Viewed from this wider perspective of care, alteration of the 'story' an individual tells to themselves and to others involves questions of life's ultimate worthiness and meaning. This naming of the pain and guiding the care is an inherently spiritual enterprise whether or not the individual is overly religions and whether or not the therapist is a recognized religious professional. At the 1990 Harvard Trauma Conference, Dr. Judith Lewis Herman began her remarks with this observation: "every instance of severe traumatic psychological injury is a standing challenge to the rightness of the social order." (7) Her observation was that one begins with 'the moral world of the soldier – what his culture understands to be right – and betrayal of that moral order by a commander' cites the work of Homer's *Iliad*.

This 'betrayal of the moral world' is a politically loaded phrase when applied solely to the world of the soldier. When affixed evermore narrowly to the world of the Vietnam veteran, it continues the stigmatization of those individuals. This viewpoint subtly pushes the political viewpoint that all commanders are somehow corrupt and that men enter the military and go to war lacking a full understanding that they will participate in both creating and witnessing death, destruction and suffering at close-order. Nevertheless, Ms. Hennan's observation makes a more general point about trauma generally: we do experience trauma as a betrayal of what we believe to be both 'right' in our world's order and a fundamental loss of our innocence.

We believe we have the 'right' to live without being raped, robbed, or assaulted when walking in our community or bullied in our public schools. We believe we have the 'right' to live without our home being destroyed by earthquake, fire, flood or tornado. We believe we have the 'right' to live without our community being afflicted by a toxic chemical spill, a radiological incident, an airline crash, or train wreck. But when somewhere between 40% and 70% of individuals in the US have been exposed to some type of crime along with the 69% of the women over the age of 18 in the US who are exposed to some type of traumatic event during the course of their life it behooves clinicians to have a more realistic view of the extent of trauma so that we can provide care that equips individuals to endure ordinary life rather than continuing to support a naïve expectation that life will be totally free from trauma. (8) Religiously oriented therapists in particular should be both willing and able to help clients explore both the existence and meaning of evil in the world and in their own lives.

In discussing the extent of trauma and its overall impact on the human mind, Donald Meichenbaum draws the following conclusions. "It is **not** just the objective features of the traumatic event but also **the meaning the trauma holds for the individual** that can put someone at increased risk for developing PTSD." (9) Moreover, it appears that the individual's membership in a supportive community and having obtained a realistic appraisal of the actual threats which come from living on planet Earth mitigate the impact of specific trauma through providing the individual with an interpretive framework through which to understand specific trauma. This is not a license to subject our children to beatings and stress-exercises or other inappropriate transgressions of their soul to somehow 'harden' them. There is, nonetheless, both a professional and ultimately parental obligation to provide those we care about and for with both a realistic matrix of meaning through which to understand life's stressors and explicit coping skills for reducing the after-effects of trauma one can reasonably anticipate.

Within the specific task of therapy this can include teaching behavioral skills such as deep breathing, meditation, encouraging aerobic exercise or yoga and developing greater situational awareness. Teaching cognitive skills such as reframing, reducing all-or-nothing thinking, challenging overgeneralizations, embracing rather than disqualifying the positive and avoiding emotional reasoning will also inoculate against stress. Parents can involve children in skill activities that develop physical strength and also teaches children to cope with physical discomfort and disappointment. Participating in a religious faith provides people with both the blessings and the challenges of living within a supportive community as well as a millennial spanning framework of belief that maintains resilience to ordinary stress and increases the likelihood of identifying positive benefits from stress.

Here is the some of the news from today. One hundred forty people died this morning in a plane crash in Jarkata, Indonesia including several Australian diplomats. Survivors were taken to a nearby hospital. Five Shiite pilgrims were killed in Karbula, Iraq in homicide bombings. People have a reasonable expectation that when they board an airliner they will arrive safely at their destination. It is questionable whether Shiite pilgrims can have a reasonable expectation of safety in Iraq. Yet those who survive the crash and who now cope with the death of their loved ones will apply a range of legal, moral and religious resources to understand the trauma of their survival and the life they must continue with their wounds and their losses. These resources will perhaps range from assigning the deaths to 'the will of Allah,' the ineptness of the pilot, the perversity of the killer and perhaps even the apostasy inherent in a competing expression of Islam, workaholism within Australia's diplomatic staff and the presence of U. S. troops in Iraq.

Our initial reaction to trauma such as these just recounted is likely to be a form of terror or disgust if we take more than a moment from our busy life to reflect upon the catastrophes of a single day. Yet it is ultimately the expression of rage over the betrayal our child-like expectation of innocence that leads toward the acquisition of healthy meaning. The transition point between what can rightly be termed indignant rage and the acquisition of healthy meaning is emotional and spiritual withdrawal. The work *Achilles in Vietnam: Combat Trauma and the Undoing of Character* offers an insightful analysis of this withdrawal as 'the first and possibly the primary trauma that converted subsequent terror, horror, grief and guilt into lifelong disability for Vietnam veterans.' (10) The author is on to something here but this indignant rage is not limited to combat veterans nor is it the inevitable terminus for all who suffer profound catastrophic trauma.

The author is correct in this regard. The rage required to destroy one's heretofore spiritual and moral expectation of good order is specifically the kind 'that ruptures social (and spiritual) attachments.' In my experience it is this rupture of attachments that creates what we recognize as the avoidance symptoms of trauma as well as the hyperarousal symptoms. (11) Thus for care providers it is imperative they encourage survivors of trauma to develop spiritual disciplines or maintain connection with their religious community. It is therefore not unusual for those who endure catastrophe go on to become care providers, emergency responders, physicians, social workers, educators, legislators or clergy.

These vocations allow the survivor to recover the inherent human dignity that is betrayed and therefore tarnished by catastrophic trauma. Despite the media image of the contemporary combat veteran, it is the rare veteran whose withdrawal and loss of attachment spirals downward into berserk rage. Research is clear: those most susceptible to such dysfunction are those who enter the catastrophic experience with some more basic mental disorder or whose primary emotional defenses have already been transgressed by childhood trauma. Meichenbaum and others make this startlingly clear: "the presence of a PTSD following a traumatic event is the exception rather than the rule." (12) As a consequence, we now turn our attention toward the third and most profound effect of catastrophe, beginning with a quote from someone who serves as an enduring beacon of this life-long transformation.

"They Called Him Moishe the Beadle."

The title of this section comes from the opening sentence of *Night,* Elie Wiesel's autobiographical statement of survival of Birkenau, Auschwitz and Buchenwald. This book is required reading for anyone seeking to accompany a fellow human as they peer up from the depths of catastrophe's Hell and wonder if their soul can survive the journey. The short lesson of this volume and the lives of those who survive catastrophic trauma is singular if not simple: trauma stains the soul but need not remain the soul's primary focus.

It is a singular task but not a simple task to assess and respond to the long-term devastation of the soul that result from severe trauma and catastrophe. In recent years the secondary gains that come from portraying one's self as a perennial victim has increased within Western cultures. The media rush in along with political opportunists who utilize the catastrophe as an occasion to promote their own particular cause, whether it be to advance the story line ("Bush Lied! People Died!") or to identify the newest poster child for some demagogic cause (less government aid, more government aid, global warming, gay rights, or stem cell research).

These are perhaps fine causes in and of themselves. But they fixate the individual at the point of their wound rather than advance the individual or community's healing. The clinically and culturally responsible thing to do is to assess the positive adjustment following trauma. This step of naming both the post-catastrophe pain and guiding the post-trauma care is crucial if there is to be genuine healing. Meichenbaum notes the following imperative, "after reading the plethora of bad or traumatic events that individuals experience, it is quite easy to become distressed or to vicariously become traumatized…the story of how people handle traumatic events is **a remarkable tale of resilience and courage,** and a testimonial to the indomitable human spirit." (13) As the individuals who survived one of the previously mentioned 'catastrophes of the day' will go on with their lives in some manner they become literal embodiments of this remarkable resilience.

Citing other research, Meichenbaum observes that even 'heavy combat veterans believe that their experience engendered valuable coping skills, self-discipline and an increased appreciation for life' even though 'combat anxieties and nightmares often extend into later years.' (14) This other source documents a finding that must be remembered by care providers, especially contemporary Western ones raised in a culture that views anything less than perfect recovery as inherently evil: 'these memories of combat experience are independent of adjustment patterns.' (15)

Active religious faith plays a central role in pre-event stress inoculation and post-trauma reappraisal of the catastrophe. The system of diagnosis developed by psychologist Paul Pruyser suggested for ministers is particularly appropriate for clinicians seeking to enhance a client's recovery from trauma and helping them enhance their quest for post-trauma meaning. Pruyser recognized nine discrete stages of faith or themes of hope through which one naturally matures as well as ones we must revisit after catastrophe:

1. Faith is Awareness of the Holy (what is Holy to the individual?)

2. Faith is perceived as Trust (is the Holy trustworthy?)

3. Faith is perceived as Courage (does the Holy permit independence?)

4. Faith is perceived as Obedience (what does the Holy expect;

    is the Holy merciful?)

5. Faith is perceived as Assent (what can I know about the Holy?)

6. Faith as Identity (what does the Holy say about my identity?)

7. Faith as Self-Surrender (how do I worship and serve the Holy?)

8. Faith as Unconditional Caring (what is my obligation to my neighbor, who expresses the Holy?)

9.   Faith as Unconditional Acceptance (what is the Holy's wider purpose for my life?) (16)

Religious belief inoculates individuals against full-blown PTSD by providing a template of meaning at the earliest stages of a person's development. While various theological traditions may emphasize different themes in accounting for the way the world works and what to do when the world comes crashing down in chaos, all of them move the individual believer and the corporate community toward a posture of life that recognizes evil occurs in both the natural order and through human conduct *and that such evil is not the last word on human existence.*

Put into therapeutic language, mature religious belief encourages positive reappraisal and reanalysis of trauma. Healthy religion promotes active coping with life and seeks to discourage self-pity, personal neglect, passivity, withdrawal from the community and avoidance. The seminal work of Vicktor Frankel, *Man's Search for Meaning,* illustrates how greater self-knowledge can come from profound horror; assumptions that are shattered by trauma can be rebuilt through a thorough re-examination of one's existence. Mature religious belief can assist an individual, a community or an entire nation in such an appraisal.

At the end of his work, Elie Wiesel's acceptance speech for the Nobel Peace Prize is reproduced. He is not the only one who has risen so high above the ashes of personal trauma that results from organized human perversity, but his words bear remembering as we seek to not only guide people up from whatever level of Hell they reached but also to help those around them recognize if not fully understand the incredible energy that may forever pulse through them and around them for whatever days a gracious God permits them to walk upon His earth. For those who feel such energy there is the humble recognition that it comes from beyond the self and is not entirely a choice. I believe it is pure Spirit. Here are Wiesel's final words:

> But I have faith. Faith in the God of Abraham, Isaac and Jacob and even in His creation. Without it no action would be possible. And action is the only remedy to indifference, the most insidious danger of all. One person of integrity can make a difference, a difference of life and death...Our lives no longer belong to us alone; they belong to all those who need us desperately. (17)

It is equally significant that one of the final promises the Almighty makes to one privileged to overhear that Voice is that at the end of all time there will be no more night. (18)

"Rise, Let Us Be On Our Way!"

I have chosen this statement of Jesus of Nazareth for this chapter's summary and conclusion not just because I am a Christian. The recent Pope, John Paul II, chose this statement as the title of his final book. Published in 2004 as a retrospective summation of his life, early formation and ultimate pontificate, he symbolizes the maturity of spirit and the integration toward which each of us may journey with confidence. I chose this statement because it represents the essence of what a person must recover in their soul as they address the inherent stain of trauma.

Sometimes this rising is exceptionally personal, occurring in the private confessional of individual therapy over a period of years. Trust is slowly built up to where the exact nature of the wound finally surfaces to the healing light of insight and the restorative breath of Spirit. Sometimes the going on our way is rather public, taking place in courtrooms and in the formation of public corporations or humanitarian foundations. Sometimes one is fortunate enough to have a gifted therapist, a compassionate partner or an insightful mentor who serves as our Virgil through both the descent and ascent from Hell. More frequently we cobble together a mixture of relationships, beliefs, habits and times of sheer white-knuckled determination to keep our stain as a part of our soul rather than as the whole of our soul.

There are excellent practical resources available to guide those who provide care to the walking wounded. There are also exceptional resources of Spirit that comes unbidden to those who find themselves in an unknown wilderness of suffering and who wish only for relief. May that Spirit not tarry as you walk with those whom it brings to the door of your own heart. *Selah!*

Chapter 20: What About Mass Bereavement?

The reader may be surprised to have a chapter on this topic immediately following a chapter on traumatic stress. "Why not include this topic in the prior chapter," you might rightly ask? "Especially when there are other themes you have not addressed."

I will respond to the second half of this question in my next chapter. For now, let me respond to the primary question: why an additional chapter focusing on a topic so closely associated with post-traumatic stress disorder and the catastrophes associated with stress reactions? Not only is there more technical information to cover in this field when the catastrophe is wider than a single individual, there is also a second role that clergy and therapists perform in catastrophes that goes well beyond the privacy of a counseling office and the confidentiality of a confessional.

Some circumstances of trauma fall between personal tragedy and national catastrophe. Someone's death in their workplace or a local business having a 'reduction in force' that involves sometimes hundreds of people sends ripples into a community. The local outlet of an international corporation decides to leave a community. A tornado obliterates a rural town or an industrial accident provides the necessity of multiple funerals in a single weekend. These events and their aftermath linger long after the news crews leave, the business resumes its normal operation and a new person sits in a briefly empty cubicle.

There are occasions when it is imperative for clergy and clinicians to adopt a public role as an event unfolds. This is not something most ministers, psychologists and counselors are trained to do. We're much more comfortable quietly cleaning up the aftermath than providing media-promulgated public guidance in the heat of the moment. Knowing what to say as well as what not to say can be crucial in limiting the amount of post-event spiritual and psychological damage anyone has to endure. Such emotional first aid and community service are important if overlooked parts of our clinical and spiritual formation.

Local rituals mirror national days of mourning. May 30, September 11, November 11, and December 7 are four American days of national memory. Other nations have similar days where past catastrophes and extensive sacrifices are memorialized in public rituals. Clergy of various faiths are inevitably called to offer words at these ceremonies. Counselors are sometimes surprised that historical events fading in the rear vision mirror of memory nevertheless reawaken long-buried memories from survivors during these ceremonies and holidays.

Clergy who are called to take part in such moments face a unique opportunity to place an individual's personal pain into the context of national destiny or community history.

I have had both the honor and the obligation of providing care in these circumstances. Thus this final chapter on special circumstances draws on my experience in such occasions of response to mass bereavement, providing direct care to individuals, a community and to some degree the soul of the nation itself.

"They Took Away Our School!"

The remnants of a building stood across the road from the first church I served. A stairway that went nowhere ascended out of a pile of bricks alongside a chimney. It was such an obvious landmark that I asked about it during my first conversation.

His reply forms the title for this subsection. It took ten minutes before he realized he was giving me more details than necessary. The most significant initial detail was the intensity of this twenty-year wound. Three factions among several rural townships had spent enough money on competing architectural plans, lawsuits and political campaigns during the ensuing twenty years to build a new school. Helping the community find a way to remove the bricks, sow the land with a crop of winter wheat and almost literally bury the hatchet with other small towns so that a consolidated school could be built was a facet of my six years there.

There were other community-wide losses that signaled ways forces outside the community had moved beyond the life and values the village held dear. A covered bridge was closed to traffic and a gristmill was permanently shuttered. Some in the community saw these as potential landmarks for tourists while others viewed them as wounds over which to perennial grieve. Encouraging the seeds of those hopes was again a facet of my work that others who followed me continued to nourish; a recent visit to the county's website revealed these landmarks were now part of the region's charm. The healing of such a mass loss doesn't always proceed according to our personal timeline for when a community should 'get over it and move on.'

In two other communities I served national corporations went through a major financial crisis. Threatened with the closure of over one thousand jobs at assembly plants and additional losses to sub-contractors, one region faced a loss as significant and permanent as any natural disaster. Another region saw the major employer go through a series of corporate buy-outs that reduced the workforce by hundreds. Yet other communities face the closure of military bases or the complete relocation of a significant employer overseas.

In such cases individual families and local governmental structures are subjected to economic and political forces over which they have no control. Sometimes they can see such events as they take shape on the horizon, such as the closing of a military base by the Base Reduction Committee of the Congress. At other times there is near-complete surprise, as when the combination of bad weather, tragedy, financial mismanagement and world market forces totally suppress a commodity such as grain or oil – or a corporation such as Enron totally collapses due to criminal intention and mismanagement.

It is easy for those removed from such mass suffering by either distance or accident of birth to resent the repetitive nature of survivors' story telling. Thus Baby-Boomers tired quickly of their parents' stories of the Great Depression. Thus Generation X'ers tired just as quickly of their parents' immature flower-child attitudes that lingered long into the 1980's. In our current post-modern hyperbolic reaction to each and every disruption of our life, it is helpful for those in the therapeutic community to have some baseline understanding of mass suffering that is realistic. It is imperative that current members of the mental health community truly comprehend the scope of potential bereavement we now face in our interconnected global economy where both grievances and infectious disease can travel around the world in days rather than months..

I grew up in a northern Illinois community that still remembered, in 1948, the wagons of influenza victims from the 1918 flu epidemic that devastated the world. In Illinois the death rate per 1,000 births was 16.0, a rate not even closely approached ever again, including throughout the 1940's during World War II. Over 100,396 people died in Illinois in 1918, an increase of roughly 25% over preceding and ensuing years. (1) Commenting on a map of the United States showing this epidemic's eruption in 1918, an author makes this point: "the disease disseminated across the country with the population, with a few focal areas of massive epidemic." (2) We should remember that this world-wide pandemic spread at the pace of ocean liners and people walking; today it would spread at the pace of jet planes and automobiles.

I offer this historical perspective as we make efforts in 2007 to educate the world's population about the rise and possible consequences of a worldwide flu pandemic. One recent estimate used in a simulation with world leaders responding to an intentional use of smallpox by a terrorist organization conducted a worldwide death toll between 600K and 1M. (3) This is not so that therapists can minimize the suffering of an individual or so pastors can revisit Revelation's apocalyptic Four Horsemen. I do so in the hope that the therapeutic and religious communities can work in concert with the medical community to develop protocols for care that go well beyond conducting single funerals should such a God-awful plague once again scour the earth. In the just-cited simulation, Madeline Albright portraying the President of the United States spoke the challenge facing all leaders, not just political leadership, in providing responsible advanced preparation and reasonable post-event protection: "How do you prepare and inform your citizens so that we don't frighten them into inaction?" (4)

Twenty-eight countries in Africa now suffer under the scourge of a drug-resistant form of tuberculosis. More than half of those in Africa afflicted with HIV also carry the tuberculosis virus, according to a report today on National Public Radio. (5) Thus in some areas of today's world we do not have to wait for some AK-47 toting terrorist loon to release another grainy audio tape claiming 'responsibility' in the name of a twisted deity for initiating such a horror. Mental health providers and religious leaders have a dual obligation when facing both the likelihood and the present reality of such scourges and pestilence. We have a responsibility to urge our people to take such dangers seriously rather than accepting their potential affliction as 'God's will' or 'God's punishment.' We also have a responsibility to name as unequivocally evil the clandestine manufacture and intentional release of viruses such as smallpox or anthrax or tularemia to further their cause.

Since the majority of this book's readers are Americans, it behooves us to remember that in some portions of the world mass bereavement is a standard facet of life. In addition to natural catastrophes for which they must rely upon an international infrastructure for relief and recovery, numerous nations and entire regions have a level of political or social violence that produces heaps of bodies with each new dawn. A level of such societal pain and suffering cannot be assuaged by individual effort alone. It must be redressed through the stories, songs, and art that speaks both of the horror of such anguish as well as illustrates the resiliency of the people.

The level of societal chaos created by an intentional bio-terrorist action will not be stemmed by reasoned discussion in the 'fair and balanced' media or academia's fine-point discussions over open borders and free speech. Governments will have to act swiftly, collaboratively one hopes, but promptly nonetheless if they desire to survive such an event. It behooves care providers and religious leaders of all theoretical persuasions to become realistically informed about the scope of such an event rather than maintaining some type of studied neutrality or lending their voice to the political gamesmanship that characterizes the abstract discussion of the worried well. If such a horror is unleashed, regardless of the cause, we will be the ones conducting and attending the funerals as well as comforting the survivors; assuming we ourselves are not among the second wave of deaths.

If the nation or culture matures spiritually over the centuries these losses fade somewhat into the near-genetic memory of the people. They eventually take their place in the pantheon of the nation's self-understanding and perhaps their self-transcendence as a nation. This is not always the case. But when it happens it signals a shift in the consciousness of a entire peoples. As the West seeks to understand the chronic resentments that fuel sectarian hatred in the Middle Eastit is well to take seriously how long an entire region can draw its self-understanding from a massive fall from prominence or when hatred is intentionally stoked by carefully re-told stories. The length of time, treasure and talent it took to unravel the political and spiritual complexities of Northern Ireland to bring some measure of stability to that geographically contained and racially singular region should give therapists and politicians patience, creativity and courage in resolving such bereavement. Guilt, horror and dread are not assuaged through enacting revenge on the grandchildren of monsters. But dread does not turn to joy without undergoing the painstaking work of brushing away the dust from the graves and putting in place force structures that will neither tolerate savagery from erstwhile saviors nor confuse obfuscation for negotiation.

Nevertheless, a letter as recent as yesterday's newspaper underscores the uniquely personal nature of each heart for answers to a loved one's fate no matter how massive the horror or how long the search. The letter details a woman's search for her brother, one name from among the identifiable 6 million Jews systematically exterminated by the Nazi regime in World War II. We should expect no less of an effort or no shorter a memory of those who suffered under Stalin's Gulag, Pol Pot's Killing Field, or the mass graves that are yet to fully emerge from Rwanda or Sudan or Kurdistan or Iraq or Darfur or _____(the sensitive and informed reader may fill in this unending litany of horror and bereavement).

"So Now I Go to Funerals of Men I Never Knew..."

The events of September 11, 2001 were ultimately resolved around the empty spaces at dinner tables. Every disaster, regardless of scope and regardless of origin begins and ends at the local level. What the world saw on that day was the bravery of initially anonymous first-responders heading into an inferno that they clearly knew would very likely become their tomb. The lyrics cited above come from 'The Bravest,' a song by Tom Paxton. The rest of the stanza, along with the entire composition expresses his mixture of shock, horror, grief and admiration that living through such an event inevitably instills.

Just as the experts in the field of response to catastrophe are 'not in Washington' so too are the experts in the task of guiding the care for survivors of catastrophe 'not in Washington.' (6) Harrald's observation that the National Response Plan needs to 'include the private sector in preparedness and planning in a meaningful way' must necessarily include the faith-based and mental health service professions. The presence within the Department of Homeland Security of a 'Center for Faith-based & Community Initiatives' at the level of Deputy Director signals the federal level's valuation of the voluntary and mental health community. (7)

Within the faith-based community we have to go well beyond crafting encouraging sermons that instill resiliency within individuals. It must become a part of our stewardship to build physical and organizational structures that are resilient *so that* we can provide adequate care to people who necessarily look to us for post-catastrophe relief, support and restoration. The various denominations and congregations outside of the Gulf Coast region that stepped forward to form partnerships with afflicted clergy and devastated parishes have provided incredible sustenance to the region's suffering people. Just as Trinity Episcopal Church became the ad hoc site of respite for the rescue workers at 9/11's Ground Zero, the religious community instinctively steps forward into the breach when governmental structures are overwhelmed or frozen due to the complications of federalism. This takes place whether the catastrophe is local, regional, national or international. Yet in the security and emergency environment of the post-9/11 world, our voluntary deployment and assumed access to survivors will be severely limited. While there is still a strong need for volunteers, the requirement for voluntary organizations, non-profits and religious institutions to be affiliated with a recognized structure will soon become nearly absolute due to security concerns from follow-on terrorist attacks and media known to impersonate rescue workers in order to gain an edge over competitors.

We must become as resilient and agile in our response to catastrophe as we rightly expect from our local and regional governmental responders. When the disaster occurs on our doorstep it is now both unrealistic and insufficient to assume that help will immediately arrive from somewhere else and that our work will survive simply because our parishioners and staff are resilient people. As therapists we are skilled at building or restoring the resilience of individuals and families. Given the failure rate of our mainline pastoral counseling agencies and our individual practices, it is not likely structures of governance will turn to clinicians as primary sources of insight on how to construct resilient societal structures and institutions. But as we saw clearly throughout the Gulf Coast in 2005 it takes years, not days, to rebuild a counseling practice and a counseling center in a region that has lost all essential institutions and whose citizens have been dispersed to all fifty states.

Initial crisis counseling services were deployed to throughout the afflicted Gulf Coast region by public relief agencies and private insurers. These counselors and therapists provided much needed post-disaster first aid. But the process of recovery and long-term guidance of the care cannot ultimately depend upon what Scarlet O'Hara called 'the kindness of strangers.' One of the long-term lessons for the therapeutic professional associations and national religious structures has been the recognition for some type of financial and vocational reserve that can be tapped for its members to assist them in rebuilding their careers *within the afflicted* region even as they rebuild their homes and professional offices.

Shortly after September 11th there was a massive outdoor memorial service for all of the deceased. Apart from the heretofore multiple funerals that periodically happen in small communities where there is a mining disaster, chemical spill or in the aftermath of a forest fire that obliterates neighborhoods, the majority of people in this nation had not witnessed such an event within our conscious memory. Only the fast-fading members of the Greatest Generation could recall a time when there were multiple funerals in the same community on the same day. But even that event exposed the political and theological divides within this nation: one sitting Senator was heckled for her opportunism and one minister lost his credentials for appearing on the same platform with other members of the American religious community.

The first anniversary of September 11th saw two events that signaled the actual beginning of the period of recovery: last firefighter to perish in the collapse of the Twin Towers was buried and The Pentagon's restoration was officially declared completed. Several religious bodies published volumes of poetry and offered suggested liturgies for that day. Newspapers ran anniversary retrospectives and did so again on the fifth anniversary of 9/11/01.

But other events have begun creeping into the anniversary memorials of that day and, given the increasingly partisan nature of our public ceremonial discourse and the continued role of media attention such vitriol attracts, we are likely to see this tone creep into public remembrances of other catastrophes. (8) Therapists and clergy tend to view these demonstrations as outpourings of corporate grief and thus legitimate them by our professional posture of civility if not genuine acceptance of what is disruptive or boorish conduct at a public memorial.

I do not believe the grief of a single individual or a sub-group should become the focus of a community's anniversary memorial. Once an individual or a sub-group of individuals within a community or nation use their personal loss to catapult themselves onto the public stage or insert themselves into the public debate, it is poor community care when their status as a public figure is allowed to become a primary focus of a community memorial. Cindy Sheehan is not the only parent to lose a son or daughter to war, or even the battles in Iraq. The Widows of 9/11 are not the only wives to lose husbands in the collapse of the Twin Towers.

Within my own community of loss, that of the Vietnam veteran, we had to face this concern around an issue that was deeply divisive for a period of time: the return of Prisoners of War from Vietnam and the subsequent recovery and return of remains. The public ceremonies conducted within the first fifteen years after that war's conclusion was rife with politicized speech, especially on the issue of whether or not there were still living POW's left behind in North Vietnam. Along with the continuing anguish over the Vietnam War, the public ceremonies became theater for the media. However, the large wheel of public history and the private wheels of individual grief gradually turned these ceremonies into more dignified if nonetheless still heart-felt events.

Several factors played roles in this gradual transformation. One factor was the simple fatigue of intense grief driven by the passage of time. Another factor was the perspective history provided on that particular war, one gradually provided by more genuine information about the events in that war if not yet a genuinely balanced presentation in the media and in academic venues. These latter discussions continue to this very day. Yet a third factor was the intentional imposition of decorum on public ceremonies by the sponsoring associations – the more garish displays of 'free speech' were gradually moved out of the National Mall, the *de rigueur* prominence supposedly combat-crazed veterans was replaced by veterans who are community leaders, and balanced public statements were crafted that recognized the need for mutual respect for competing viewpoints. Not surprisingly as these events became more dignified the video media disappeared, eventually followed by the radio and print media. Exposure of the status of many of the supposed 'war crazed veterans' as outright frauds and the complicity of the national media in promoting their fraud helped reduce these individuals' appeal and increase the decorum at public ceremonies.

In planning for a community's ceremony of memory, pastors and therapists who are asked to speak need to be mindful of our public responsibility. In this venue it is the community who is our 'client.' We need to observe the same level of restraint in our public remarks, with an eye toward promoting healing, that we would observe in a private counseling session with someone whose conduct we might find personally reprehensible but whose need for healing is nevertheless genuine. We have the same obligation to decline speaking at a public forum where we are at odds with the purpose of the ceremony as we have to refer a client with whom our own values conflict. A public ceremony of mass bereavement is an inappropriate venue in which to be 'prophetic.' Such prophecy usually meets our own need rather than speaks a true word from the Lord. The Lord typically urges genuine prophets to speak words of comfort to the bereaved widows and orphans.

These concerns for the overall decorum at a public ceremony, the truthfulness of other speakers, mindfulness about the role of the national or regional media and the need for decorum and restraint in public ceremonies are not typically the focus of mental health providers and ministers. But such events have the role of helping an entire community or even a nation to name its collective pain in a way that is distinct from the privacy of a counseling room. If we are to be instruments of care for the community, it is imperative we adopt a stance that is therapeutic for the community rather than assuming that the most dramatic emotiveness is necessarily the most helpful.

"Why are There Helicopters Over Your Office?"

Many readers outside of the well-traveled corridor from Baltimore to Richmond will not remember the fall of 2002. But those of us who live in this region remember it well. Two men with a rifle in a nondescript car whose trunk was modified into a shooting platform paralyzed the entire region. Schools were closed. Parents kept their children inside. Police presence was increased in local shopping malls and public parking lots. Drivers endured random roadblocks and vehicle searches. Set against the recent anniversary of September 11th and the snipers' public statements identifying themselves as agents of Allah's wrath, their actions exacerbated tensions between Muslim citizens and wider communities. They demonstrated how much panic two determined terrorists could inflict on a region.

The two men continue to await various trials five years later for the various deaths even though several jurisdictions have found them both guilty of capital murder. When arrested plans were discovered in their vehicle for travel to other cities to widen their circle of terror. The events of those days offer two other layers to our topic of mass bereavement: the public role of a therapist or minister in providing on-air guidance to a terrorized community and the lingering impact of such an event on children long after an event such as this comes to a conclusion.

First there is the matter of how to become a credible source of information during a community's crisis or in the aftermath of a disaster. The most obvious way is when the therapist or minister is in the wrong place at precisely the right time: the emergency happens in your location and the news crew shows up looking for someone to interview. You may not have time to prepare any statement or develop talking points at all. So if your public presentation is thoughtful and your bearing is professional, you have established some instant credibility with a single reporter. It is important to review how much of your interview is actually aired and for you to check it for accuracy. If you are presented accurately, drop the reporter a brief note acknowledging this and thank them for their professionalism. If not, it is important to also write the reporter expressing your concern and re-stating your viewpoint.

It will help your professional development to purchase a copy of the actual interview as aired to review your remarks. Share it with a colleague for critique in the same way you would review the audiotape of a counseling session with a supervisor. Think through how you could have stated the same remarks more concisely or more pointedly because the 'hot' media do look for the pithy comment.

In the case of an on-going community concern such as the snipers, you may also have the opportunity to put out a press release or speak with a reporter that you have established a prior relationship with. This is not something most therapists or clergy consider because we do not usually consider the community as a 'client' or view the community-as-a-whole as our 'parish.' Yet this step can provide a helpful level of care to our community by helping individuals effectively marshal their emotional and spiritual resources as well as their spare batteries and canned food. This is particularly important when the pain in a community is created by a human actor rather than by a natural disaster. With a human actor such as at Virginia Tech there is always the additional factor of helping individuals interpret the threat and place the evil conduct into some framework of understanding. The full portrait of the assassin at Virginia Tech as well as his motivation and the community's response is evolving at this writing.

In my view these are times for moral clarity and emotional calm rather than political correctness and emotive grandstanding. It is imperative in such situations that you make an effort to become a credible source of reliable information on both how to care for those you love and also rebut the fear-mongering opportunists who inevitably seem to show up to conduct some variation of race baiting or demagogue the tragedy in your community for their own selfish ends. Not only are the actions of people such as the snipers evil, the character of such individuals is evil. Saying so clearly helps people marshal their resolve; saying so in a way that protects the perpetrator only weakens the tenacity of the very people you are primarily called to serve: your neighbors. It is important, as feminist theorists insist, on naming the reality of evil not just identifying goodness.

The impact of these two individuals on our region lasted well beyond the immediate events and their eventual trials. Counselors in our city experienced a spike in children exhibiting anxiety. This pattern intensified as the next fall approached and was further exacerbated by Hurricane Isabel in the fall of 2003.Only in the fall of 2006 was there a bit of relief in demand for therapists. This systemic anxiety in children creates a public opportunity for a therapist or community-oriented minister to serve as a public educator. In addition to assisting an individual child and their parents develop the resiliency necessary to reduce such worry, you may wish to consider providing the community-at-large with information that places an interpretive framework around the consequences of such background apprehension.

I must give credit here to a six-year-old boy whose moods alternated between mild but uncharacteristic aggressiveness with siblings and what looked to everyone else like school phobia. When I asked him to draw a picture of anything he liked, he drew a characteristic six-year-old boy sketch. There were plenty of planes, guns, monsters, tanks and explosions. When I asked him, "Can you tell me about this drawing," he replied, "It looks like the whole world is crazy! Everybody is fighting, there are big storms and bad people that want to hurt me."

This was not a psychodynamic transmutation of family violence. This was how the world looked to him and to many of us in the summer of 2004. Thus his 'pain' was caused primarily by real events plus exposure to too much television news that amplified the impact of real events. Helping his family take realistic steps to redirect his attention, rather than reporting the family to a Department of Social Services' child protective unit, was the appropriate way to provide care for this child. I then took the additional step of putting out a press release on this general topic timed to become part of the community's normal 'get-ready-for-school' programming. Helping all of the community's families cope effectively with the social context of their children is a responsible facet of guiding care.

From a Day of Infamy to a Journey Home and Beyond to April

They gather every year at the Virginia War Memorial on December 7th. They are proud men and women whose shoulders may now stoop but whose resolve has not stopped. In a dignified ceremony they lay wreaths at the Statue of Memory to call out the names of Virginians who perished on that day in 1941 at Pearl Harbor. A bell is rung as each name is called. Prayers are offered. A military rifle salute is fired, followed by taps.

A few days later, a letter appears on the Letters to the Editor page of the local newspaper. If the event did not receive proper advance notice or coverage by the paper, the writer takes the editor to task. "How could you forget?" is usually the tone of the letter. If the event was mentioned in the paper, and especially if there is a photograph, the letter is appreciative. "Thank you for remembering us," is usually the tone of this letter.

Unlike Memorial Day or Veteran's Day or July 4, Pearl Harbor Day marks a specific event in the life of this nation and the individual lives of those who endured that attack, whether they survived or whether only their spouses and progeny survived. For these individuals even more than for the nation as a whole there is a deep part of their soul where it is always December 7th, 1941 – A Day of Infamy. I do not know when the last bell will be rung on this ceremony, perhaps in 2011, seventy years after that bloody dawn or in 2021.

Some of us have gathered every year the first weekend in February, the date of Tet – the Lunar New Year. The Tet Offensive and Counteroffensive remains the signature event of the Vietnam War. Although a complete military defeat for the forces of the North Vietnamese it marked a turning point in American consciousness, thanks primarily to Walter Cronkite's negative assessment of the attack on the American embassy in Saigon. For those who lived through those days of fire, who preceded them during the build-up or followed them in until April 1975, The Tet Offensive of 1968 symbolizes much that was right and much that went awry in that war.

Although the initial attack in 1968 began with some local Viet Cong units getting an early start on January 31, the original offensive began on February 1st because the Lunar New Year happened to fall on that date. A group of us who formed a Vietnam veterans reunion group in 1986 decided instinctively to hold the reunion during the weekend closest to the start of the Lunar New Year rather than to pin the event to a fixed date. This shifting anniversary provided a symbolic parallel to a ten-year war whose conduct shifted so much within the American consciousness and ultimately the way the nation has come to be viewed in the world.

This memorial weekend and reunion functioned a bit differently from Pearl Harbor Day in several other ways. Although it always began with a religious service that focused on remembering and honoring past losses, the major portion of the weekend was spent educating ourselves about aspect of the Vietnam War and spending time in fellowship with others who had served some portion of their military career in Vietnam. Thus while there was a facet of the reunion weekend that allowed for bereavement and the specific naming of this pain, the direction of the event was not to wallow in the past but to guide us as we matured over the lifespan.

Serving as the chaplain for the board and event, I saw our care of one another transform over the twenty years. In the earliest years the bereavement truly focused on two topics: the sense of betrayal felt by the nation's despicable treatment of returning veterans and the yet unanswered question of returned prisoner's of war. While these remain themes within the consciousness of the Vietnam veteran community to this day, they receded somewhat from the memorial service. Instead, the Friday night memorial service increasingly became an opportunity to express bereavement for all deceased comrades, whether they died in battle or died at some point later in their life. This shift was gradual but it was intentional on my part as I watched us mature. This larger focus became more pointed after the deaths of three board members over the twenty years of the organization's life.

The remainder of the weekend was focused on education. We would have speakers that presented some historical perspective on some aspect of the Vietnam War. We would also raise money for college scholarships that we awarded to the winners of an essay contest. In the twenty years we provided 120 scholarships to the children or step-children of Vietnam veterans to the tune of $86,000.00. This focus on education is not unique to the Vietnam veteran community; it is something common within the wider community of military veterans, especially providing financial support for the next generation's higher education.

Unlike the generation that still recalls Pearl Harbor, our reunion board decided to conclude our activities after twenty years. Thus the final reunion was held in during the 2007 weekend of the Lunar New Year. We were quite intentional about not becoming a 'last man' club nor putting on an event that deteriorated as we aged. It also became apparent that the children and step-children of the Vietnam generation was rapidly finishing their high school career. Thus bereavement for this generation will increasingly focus on our own aging and demise rather than on recalling the losses of the past.

This brings us to what may turn out to be the most bereaved five days in this generation of America: April 16 through April 20. The first event of the period occurred in 1995 with the destruction of the Murrh Federal Building in Oklahoma City, followed in 1999 by the shootings at Columbine High School near Denver, Colorado. Ironically the first event that will be remembered in this five day period is also the most recent, thus far: the Virginia Tech massacre of 32 students and faculty by a lone gunman in 2007, literally on the day when I thought I had concluded writing this chapter. 168 people died in Oklahoma City, 12 in Columbine High School in addition to the individuals in Blacksburg, Virginia.

The most recent mass carnage reawakened the wounds from the prior two events amongst those directly affected by the events in their cities as well as within the nation's consciousness. Unfortunately given the psychology of individuals who perpetrate such horror, we are likely to witness yet other similar types of events now growing up around this period in a macabre desire to enhance an impoverished psyche by association with other mass killings. This copy-cat element is one well-known to law-enforcement and mental health professionals who must cope with the events surrounding such mayhem. What mystifies the broader mental health community, those whom I call the 'professionally sensitive class,' appears to be a chronic unwillingness within their profession to recognize the core of ontologic evil that pulses in the heart of individuals who plot and execute such an event.

This is always a factor in the bereaved aftermath of such events: the effort that is made to discern the motivation behind an individual who visits such slaughter on their neighbors. In this sense society as a whole needs to understand and name the 'pain' of the perpetrators as a part of acknowledging its own losses. Thus whether the motivation appears to be the settling of a political grievance (Oklahoma City), a social grievance (Columbine) or an expression of mental illness (Blacksburg), the tableau remains fairly predictable. As media rush in while the bodies of victims are still being discovered, efforts are made to not just find out the facts but also explain the event according to one of these three templates: the 'angry male template,' the 'gun control template,' or the 'mental health template.' The effort to fix blame takes place even as mental health professionals arrive to assist victims and their immediate family members. Impromptu memorials quickly follow soon after the yellow crime-scene tapes are removed, followed shortly by several public memorials attended by a mix of religious and political officials.

While the conclusion of this public ceremony officially marks the conclusion of the event, the efforts to understand the perpetrator's motivation and help the survivors heal continue. These occasions of mass bereavement fade rather rapidly from the national focus even though they will not fade from the consciousness of those directly affected by such an event. One of the many challenges for both survivors and those who live with them is to help them cope with this shift in attention. Everyone else appears to 'move on' while their souls remain deeply afflicted by grief. They are forever bonded with those who shared the horror of such an event and with that particular date on the calendar. Markers, memorials and anniversary reminders help with their healing but we must recognize there will never be a time for these individuals that somewhere in their souls it is not December 7th, the first weekend in February, April 16th, April 19th, April 20, September 11th or some other anniversary of corporate bereavement. One thing that does not help survivors is to affix blame for such evil onto their souls. It is not just December 7th that remains forever a 'day of infamy.'

Conclusion

Naming the pain in a mass casualty situation requires more than affixing blame or determining responsibility. Guiding the care in the aftermath of mass bereavement additionally requires more than holding annual memorials. Nevertheless both of these activities are aspects of helping survivors and the nation as a whole build the resiliency necessary to overcome such tragedies. Try as much as we like, we cannot remove all risk from human life. As compassionate as we may like to be, no amount of monetary compensation will either replace those loved one we lose nor salve the ache in our collective heart. We may compute the metrics of risk assessment down to the third decimal point, yet lightning will still strike when and where we least expect it to strike.

   We have limited physical resources and these must be placed in venues most likely to receive a deadly blow. We have limited analytical resources and we must learn to accept some measure of uncertainty in our daily affairs. We have no guarantee of happiness, prosperity or longevity from either the Creator or from human governance. We have only the opportunity to pursue these goals with whatever courage, resiliency, and other virtues we can marshal. Those of us in the mental health and religious professions can help our neighbors develop these resources. But at the end of the day the responsibility for utilizing these resources effectively must remain with the individual. To believe otherwise is to claim for ourselves a power we do not have and will have the effect of keeping those we hope to help at a level of immaturity that in the end will do them more harm. *Selah!*

Part VI – Summary

Chapter 21: Wither DSM V and Axis VI?

The current *Diagnostic and Statistical Manual* (Fourth Edition) is the first manual to officially recognize religious or spiritual distress as a legitimate focus of humane psychological care. (1) The diagnostic criterion is quite simple: the focus of the counseling is some type of explicit religious or spiritual matter. As I have noted in many articles, classes and public lectures on this topic, the likelihood is greater of a particularly warm region of the netherworld sending a request for snow shovels than for an individual to walk into a counselor's office and say, "I am having trouble believing the universe was created in seven literal days" or "could you help me understand the difference between Calvin's and Luther's doctrine of Real Presence?' The diagnostic criterion for *Religious or Spiritual Problem* is so large as to be virtually worthless.

This is not to imply that these concerns are unimportant. This is not to suggest that these concerns are unaffected by depression, anxiety, trauma, addictions or physical illness. Indeed these resources can either create and enhance personal resiliency or contribute directly to our difficulties in responding to life's exigencies and emergencies. Thus professionals within the fields of pastoral counseling, hospital chaplaincy and theology join with professionals in the fields of psychiatry, psychology, social work and nursing to produce diagnostic models that take seriously the significance of religious belief or agnosticism in all cultures and in all people.

The purpose of this chapter is not to revisit this concern from the standpoint of our shared professional history. Rather, I hope in this chapter to look forward toward the diagnostic horizon of DSM-V and the status of religious or spiritual diagnosis in the years beyond 2010. Professionally the issue remains the same as for the past quarter century: will there be any intentional integration of spiritual or religious diagnosis within the official lexicon of diagnosis? Answering this question is the focus of this chapter.

Personally the issue remains more complex: how will we maintain a vibrant spiritual core in our culture as we become more pluralistic in our religious identity? I begin to provide my answer to this second question in the next chapter. If this nation is to survive as a religiously vibrant culture with a spiritual core that transcends petty partisan concerns and sectarian Balkanization, then we must find a way to acknowledge such matters when they enhance health as well as when they degrade well-being. We will not thrive if we continue to enact a politically correct attitude that either banishes spiritual discussion from the public square or views all religious language as equally healthy and inevitably helpful.

DSM-V: The Current Status

In the research that will lead up to the formation of the *Diagnostic and Statistical Manual (Fifth Edition),* religion and spirituality are covered in Chapter Six. Entitled "Beyond the Funhouse Mirrors: Research Agenda on Cultural and Psychiatric Diagnosis," the power of religious belief 'and its spiritual component' is recognized to 'influence mental status, the experiencing of illness and disease, coping styles and even clinical outcomes.' (2) Religion is viewed as one of the cultural variables that any clinician or health care provider must consider with conducting diagnosis. Along with ethnicity, language, education, gender and sexual orientation, the authors make this point about religion:

> Religion is one of the cultural values that 'influence age group and family dynamics, beliefs about health and health care, social networks; and perspectives on migration, acculturation patterns, socioeconomic status, and occupational hierarchies that also have a definite impact on psychiatric diagnosis. (3)

This document provides a well-written theoretical precursor to the eventual DSM-V. It also marks a further step away from a purely Western oriented psychodynamic or medically oriented neurological understanding of diagnosis. This chapter makes a pointed reference to the paucity of cultural insight in manuals prior to the DSM-IV. It also observes that even in the DSM-IV 'the dynamic role of culture, intricately tied to the social world of the patient, (nevertheless) it tended to exoticize the cultural approach by ascribing it only to ethnic minorities.' (4) I would add the vast majority of clinicians still exoticize people who are religiously faithful rather than seeking to discern whether the person's spiritual approach to life improves or hampers their overall adjustment. Citing several sources, the writers of this chapter are unblinkingly blunt in their assessment of the need for further research:

> Comorbidity may be determined by as-yet unidentified cultural factors that contribute, for instance, to the internalization of personality features or the externalization of clinical syndromes. The clarification of terminological distinctions has not been exhausted from the perspective of culture and must be considered a worthy research topic. (5)

Significantly for the purpose of this volume, the very first research question raises the concern addressed by this writing and that of other religious theoreticians: 'has the right nosologic system been conceptualized?' (6) The writers continue this strong endorsement of research by noting the arrival of an accurate nosology is more than 'editorial convenience.' An inaccurate nosology 'may obscure important cultural dimensions.' I would add that an accurate nosology might also enhance cultural, and particularly religious dimensions of human distress and human equanimity. (7)

The other research questions posed in the volume's chapter are worthy of consideration by the readers of this work. Academicians, clinicians within the disciplines of pastoral theology, chaplaincy, pastoral care and pastoral counseling would do well to conduct their own research on these questions. They would also do well to directly engage the psychiatric community with the results of their research and thus continue the diagnostic conversation well into the publication of DSM-VI. As a way of furthering this effort, I am listing the research questions here for the interested reader:

- Are the right diagnostic criteria and categories being used?
- Has the diagnostic threshold been set at the right level?
- Has the course and characteristics of the disorder been correctly typified?
- Are existing diagnostic criteria being employed in an unbiased and culturally appropriate way? (8)

Graduate students in the aforementioned fields have here ready-made foci for their masters and doctoral projects. The chapter outlines appropriate research methodology, suggests assessment instruments that may be helpful in conducting research, and identifies initial epidemiological concerns related to cultural and anthropological research. The authors are pointed in their assessment of the need for further research stating, "Obviously clinical, health services and outcomes research can be better only if the diagnostic bases of such endeavors are sound, valid and reliable." (9)

Nevertheless, while the interested reader should take my words as nothing less than a strong endorsement of the direction the research for DSM-V appears to be heading, the interested reader should not be disillusioned. This chapter and the entire volume overall continues to demonstrate the very institutional and clinical bifurcation noted throughout the past twenty years. In the two paragraphs that explicitly address religious and spiritual concerns, this chapter cites only two sources, the most recent one from 1995 that makes this point: "Religion is to be examined in the history-taking and cultural formation processes, and spirituality becomes a paramount component of self-identity, self-care, insight, self-reliance and resiliency in the treatment arena." (10)

One searches in vain within the bibliography of suggested research for DSM-V for any of the theoreticians or sources cited who have written about religious or spiritual diagnosis, developed assessment instruments for use in hospitals or outpatient counseling centers or published topical articles in professional journals that are specific to these disciplines. The appendix to this chapter, noted as a preliminary research agenda for areas of cultural and psychiatric diagnosis, suggests only two research areas:

- Religions and spirituality as pathologenic / pathoplastic and interpretive / explanatory factors in psychiatric diagnosis
- Transgenerational similarities and differences of religious and spiritual issues across ethnic and cultural groups (11)

While this is a helpful start, it is a meager start. It does not take seriously the research already available in these areas and readily available to any individual willing to go beyond the current DSM's biopsychosocial model of diagnosis that the authors of this solitary DSM-V research chapter rightly identify as 'disease centered, essentializing, individual-based and driven by biomedical technologies.' (12)

Axis VI: The Suggested Addition

In 2003 a packet arrived from the managing editor of The Journal of Pastoral Care & Counseling. Inside was an article for editorial review entitled *A Proposed Diagnostic Schema for Religious / Spiritual Concerns*. My assessment was that this article was worthy of producing a supplemental issue of the journal, replete with respondents, rather than burying the article among many other concerns that necessarily compete within any professional journal. I initiated a back-channel contact with the article's author, Wesley L. Brun, in the hope that collaboration about his schema would eventually break the logjam within our own discipline about this topic and eventually produce consensus between psychiatric and pastoral clinicians. Indeed this is Brun's primary hope:

> I am pressing my colleagues in pastoral counseling and psychotherapy to settle on categories by proposing a set for consideration. We have been considering Pruyser's and others' categories for some time, but without ever codifying or settling on anything. (13)

I was particularly impressed by Brun's holistic approach that defines healthy religious expression in addition to codifying dysfunctional religious practice. Like him, I believe the debate needs to be moved forward rather than to continue one more round of discussion. I am less hopeful than Dr. Brun. It still appears the religious providers of humane care would rather continue to debate one another about the fine points of diagnosis rather than act to build a bridge to the psychiatric community and the wider community of emotional and spiritual care.

Nonetheless, I want to provide the interested reader with a brief overview of Brun's system. It does represent a step forward in both the enterprise of religious or spiritual diagnosis as well as a step forward in creating a common resource for diagnosis that can be used in a clinical setting by both religious and secular providers of care. The proposal that a sixth axis will produce a 'metaspirituality' whose 'underlying assumption that all religious expressions and spiritualities have some dimensions and / or issues in common' will not please the orthodox of either the religious or secular communities. But both Wesley Brun and I believe it is a conversation that must continue to go forward. (14) So do the other respondents to his proposal, albeit in varying degrees of strength. (15)

One respondent provides a succinct summary of Brun's proposal. I am reproducing it here in an effort to acquaint interested readers with some of the other major pastoral theorists in on-going conversation. Dr. George M. Fitchett offers this abstract:

> Brun's model has ten categories or types of religious / spiritual concern. He acknowledges that any set of categories are imposed on experience, but notes they also permit a more focused understanding of the clients religious / spiritual issues. The seven dimensions in Pruyser's important model for pastoral diagnosis are evident in these categories and Brun acknowledges this influence. Like Pruyser, these categories have a functional focus on how spirituality or religious shapes our life. (16)

To give the reader of this volume a brief feel for how these ten categories appear, let's look quickly at one of those categories. Brun describes one concern as *An Awareness of Providence / Grace and a Capacity for Dependence.* He describes the concern both in its healthy and unhealthy dimensions. A healthy sense of providence 'has a feeling of receiving good things, of being blest with what one needs to flourish. In its unhealthy form, 'this concern might take one of two basic expressions' a feeling of entitlement or a feeling of being deprived. Thus far, Brun's schema is very similar to other developmental models. (17)

What is new are Brun's *Proposed Diagnostic Criteria* for this concern. He notes, "People with an unhealthy or faulty awareness of providence, grace and / or dependence will exhibit at least four of the following:

1) They tend to feel deprived / needy regardless of their level of wealth; enough is never enough.
2) They feel diminished by their dependence.
3) They feel a certain 'entitlement' about what is due / owed them.
4) They have a sense of desperation about needing to be taken care of.
5) They lack any sense of gratitude or thankfulness; they do not feel 'blest' by their level of comfort.
6) They tend to depreciate that which they do have
7) They have not had, or cannot recall any experience of 'grace' (being given to without one's deserving). (18)

The other diagnostic entities are:

- A Sense of the Holy / Numinous and a Capacity for Reverence
- An Appreciation of the Earth and a Capacity for Stewardship
- A Sense of 'Self' and a Capacity for Solitude
- A Desire for Community / Belonging and a Respect for Authority
- A sense of Values / Morality / Ethics and a Capacity for Guilt / Repentance/ Forgiveness
- A Sense of Vocation and the Capacity for Meaning
- A Need for Leisure / Self-Care and the Capacity to Play
- A Desire for Companionship and a Capacity for Intimacy
- An Appreciation of 'Time' / Finitude and a Capacity to Face Death
- Religious / Spiritual Concerns Not Otherwise Specified

In each category the person must meet at least four of the seven criteria. Each category has a positive description of health, a decided boon to those who feel unqualified to gauge an individual's spiritual health. Failure to meet four of the criteria obviously signal a baseline of health if not saintliness in each area.

One respondent to Brun's schema worried the proposal is 'premature.' He 'would have preferred that he formed a working group to develop this model before he set it before us.' (19) That both Brun and this particular respondent were unfamiliar with the twenty-year efforts of The Working Group on Pastoral Diagnosis within the American Association of Pastoral Counselors underscores the tendency of pastoral clinicians to produce theories in isolation from their colleagues. It also underscores the Group's inability to come to any consensus or sustain any research in this area.

As Brun notes in his Response to the Responders, the chair of The Working Group on Pastoral Diagnosis has been quite supportive of his effort. Indeed the group invited Brun to present his schema at their meeting during the 2006 Louisville conference where it was received with strong support. However, no research task force has yet coalesced around his categories. Most individuals in that small Working Group are practicing clinicians who have precious little time to write professionally let alone conduct research on this model sufficient enough to propose it to the American Psychiatric Association.

The Two Percent Solution

Most professions appear to proceed based on the research conducted by roughly two percent of their colleagues. With the aid of doctoral assistants and research grants researchers in all fields have the opportunity to test and refine the insights developed by practicing clinicians as well as other researchers. Having chaired the *Working Group on Pastoral Diagnosis* for twenty years, I have struggle with the need for primary research in this field while also maintaining a demanding clinical practice. So have my other colleagues. Nonetheless, without such research, the wider mental health community is likely to be roughly where I anticipated it being at the conclusion of my first volume on this topic. The religious community will have produced more models that are unique to either theological viewpoint or specific clinical venue. The psychiatric community will have eventually produced some type of diagnostic model without the benefit of input from the religious community.

The four research questions noted above in Chapter Six of *A Research Agenda for DSM-V* set the proper place to begin. The fact that these questions are being raised within the psychiatric and psychological communities rather than the religious communities underscores the observation made by Dr. Bruce Hartung, "The time in our culture is right; interest in spirituality is on the rapid rise; attention is increasingly moving toward an assessment of both the healthy and pathological components of spiritual and religious experience." (20) This is precisely the point made at the conclusion of chapter six in the research agenda. (21)

Thus my proposal is singular if not simple: that research projects be undertaken to test the categories and criteria proposed by Dr. Brun against the questions offered by the authors of Chapter Six in *A Research Agenda for DSM-V*. Neither the seminaries nor the professional pastoral organizations have the financial resources, the political clout or the abiding academic interest to conduct this research. This will of necessity involve the development of new psychometric instruments, a refinement of the definitions surrounding religious health and integration of spiritual concerns within the other dimensions of cultural psychiatry that Chapter Six lays out. Such research will also ultimately produce clinicians within the broader field of humane care who are able to assess spiritual or religious concerns with some degree of confidence rather than continuing yet another generation that falls victim to either uneasy silence about these matters or baptizing all vague statements of transcendence as health.

The resolution of this challenge will not occur in time for DSM-V. Given the way that research proceeds, I would anticipate some reworking of the initial scales along the lines proposed by Dr. Brun to be ready for trial when DSM-VI is published. So by the half-century mark when DSM-VII is published, 2050, we may finally have a diagnostic and statistical manual that adequately contains the rubrics for a bio-psycho-social-spiritual diagnostic model.

In the meantime, I would urge my clinical pastoral colleagues to take the multi-axial model I offer in this volume, along with the schema outlined by Dr. Brun, and conduct front-line research within your own caseloads. Become able to articulate the concerns of your clients in the language of ethics, idolatry and dread. Include this language in your case notes, in your submissions to insurance companies and in your professional case consultations. Do the same with Dr. Brun's schema. Build on his definitions and refine his criteria. Conduct small research studies within your own caseloads and present his schema within the educational offerings of your centers and regional gatherings.

Conclusion

I developed a grudging respect for Richard J. Daley, "The Boss," of Chicago. After every election won by the Democrat Machine, some reporter would inevitably come forward and gush this question, "Mr. Mayor, why do you think your party won?"

Without skipping a beat, Mayor Daley would say, "We got more votes." No mention was ever made of how those votes arrived in the ballot boxes, whether through attractive policies or jiggered voter lists! His party had simply out-hustled their opposition.

I share this example by way of making this point. The inclusion of an effective and thorough going category for religious or spiritual assessment in some future diagnostic manual will be achieved only when professionals within the various clinical disciplines doing a lot of hard work and hustle. As I have said numerous times, for secular clinicians this means finally becoming acquainted with the diagnostic literature within the community of pastoral care and counseling. It is insufficient to acknowledge that religion plays a crucial role in how disease is understood and addressed but then to avoid engaging the very resources that religious care providers utilize to address human pain.

For the pastoral clinicians this means doing the political work of making themselves known to the medical-psychiatric community. This means conducting academic research of sufficient strength and interest for inclusion in medical journals. This means forming professional relationships across associational boundaries. This will entail having speakers at our conferences from within the medical-psychiatric community rather than constantly listening to 'one of our own.' We will have to demonstrate in our daily contact with the medical-psychiatric community that we work just as hard as they do to provide effective care. All of these avenues are primarily political and social in nature rather than clinical. They are nonetheless the avenues that must be taken if the end result is a system that adequately recognizes the spiritual underpinnings of our secular society. *Selah!*

Chapter 22: Secular Counseling in a Spiritual Society

We are children of the planet's soil empowered with the breath of heaven, according to one of our most ancient stories. Placed in a benign environment and given the capacity to name reality, we quickly demonstrated our capacity to exceed those divinely imposed limits of existence. According to the story, the Divine sought us out, described the consequences of our failure, and then joined in helping us cover our shame. We continue to this very day writing the follow-on chapters to this basic dynamic: we are spiritual beings having a physical experience, neither able to transcend the limitations of our bodies nor betray our creaturely consciousness without profound consequences.

This basic dilemma expresses itself through a variety of fault lines or dyadic tensions in our effort to name reality, relieve human suffering and live responsibly within the limits of our existence. Formal religion and informal spiritual practices have sought throughout the ages to provide some measure of assistance and control in this enterprise. So has science and social policy struggled to find both specific answers to life's most disabling diseases and challenges as well as afford the masses of people with access to those solutions. While none of these solutions have been flawless, and not a few of them have been abject failures, there have been enough successes overall to advance human survival and lift human eyes toward the heavens than leaving us mired in primal muck.

This journey has frequently been violent and mean spirited. Religion, science, and social policy has each done singly and collectively as much to damage as to promote human progress. Our ancient stories remind us that no arena of human existence will be pristine. There is no sterile ethical field. None. Yet at our very best nature we feel the obligation to choose right over wrong, promote health over disease and affirm the right of our neighbor to live as unmolested as we desire to live. So while we can readily find contemporary examples of our failures at achieving utopia for ourselves or delivering it to our neighbors, there are also significant moments of individual compassion and corporate humane care that are true examples of saintliness.

These United States continues to be one of the premier arenas in which these diverse tensions lead to both great achievement and great acrimony. Organized religion and private spiritual practice is as much a part of these tensions are the cultures who come to these shores and the other institutions that shape our efforts in this evolution of human consciousness. Thus in spite of efforts to banish overt discussion of religion from the public square, explicit religious faith and private spiritual practice remain key factors in how people live their daily lives, make important decisions, raise their children and bid farewell to one another at death's doorway.

The notion that the United States is a secular society is over-sold. Just as our greatest lights strongly suggest we are spiritual beings having a physical experience, so the data more accurately reveals we are a Christian society that is benign toward those who have no explicit religious practice. Here is the challenge for the future: how will we maintain a vibrant spiritual core in our culture as we become more pluralistic in our religious identity? More pointedly, how will providers of humane care utilize this nation's spiritual resources effectively as people cope with significant cultural change and personal identity?

We may not have a religious litmus test for our friendships and hair-stylists, but with the exception of a group such as the ACLU neither do we seek to sterilize religion out of public life and spirituality out of our most closely held moments. The tensions inherent in this cultural and religious pluralism remain significant. They thus affect how and why people come to counselors of all theoretical persuasions and throughout caring venues. There are several fault lines along which these cultural, religious and emotional forces collide. Providers of humane care must do more than simply succor the casualties. Assisting our culture to name these pains and guide the care of our society is part of our obligation as healers. The following tensions press us particularly hard as providers of humane care.

Assimilation and Globalization

While I was still in college I helped a local church conduct some primary outreach to Hispanic immigrants moving into the nearby apartments. The year was 1973. When one of my sons moved into a apartment in the same region while attending the School of the Art Institute twenty-five years later, this well-defined Hispanic enclave was starting to feel pressure from the students and young professionals moving in to change the face of this community once more. The Roman Catholic Church across the street from his apartment not only had services in Spanish; it also touted a 'Saturday night contemporary service' on a banner hung outside the building. A drive down the length of Chicago's Western Avenue will still take you through the rich diversity of cultures that make the city work.

Religion is one place where the ultimate questions of 'who am I, why am I here and what is my future?' meet with the practical concerns of how to live out the answers of these eternal questions within a particular culture and nation through a distinctive piety. Thus the church I grew up in still featured had a Christmas Eve service spoken entirely in Swedish because the initial founders of that congregation were Swedish. This service was ended sometime in the early 1970's as that founding generation faded away. When I served a church in rural Indiana, the Old Order Baptists who lived among us kept their traditional dress, drove buggies and had no telephones. Both the evangelicalism of my youth and my Indiana neighbors who still farmed with horses believed that living out those eternal questions through divergent pieties expressed their understanding of traditional Christian identity: they were to be 'in the world but not of the world.'

If you asked anyone in either of these sub-groups 'are you Christian or American?' the vast majority would have probably answered one of two ways. "If am a Christian who is an American" or "I am an American who is a Christian," would be the likely reply. The tension between Christian identity and American citizenship is a perennial topic of some discussion that usually revolves around the display of the American flag in the sanctuary.

This rather heart-felt but benign discussion has exploded with America's newest immigrants. A recent survey released by Pew Research Center, *Muslim Americans: Middle Class and Mostly Mainstream,* provides some disturbing statistics. The executive summary of the research paints an accurate but somewhat muted portrait of the Muslims who live in America:

> Muslim Americans have a generally positive view of the larger society. Most say their communities are excellent or good places to live. As many Muslim Americans as members of the general public express satisfaction with the state of the nation. Moreover, 71% of Muslim Americans agree that most people who want to get ahead in the U.S. can make it if they are willing to work hard. (1)

In a follow-on chapter that addresses religious identity, the report draws parallels between the religious practices of this newest population of immigrants and certain sub-groups of American Christians:

> Muslim Americans have distinctive beliefs and practices; their religiosity is similar to American Christians in many respects. For example, U.S. Muslims are a little more likely than American Christians to say religion is "very important" in their life (72% and 60%, respectively) but a little less likely to say that they pray every day (61% vs. 70%). The two religious communities are about equally likely to attend religious services at least weekly (40% for Muslims vs. 45% for Christians). Thus in terms of the broad patterns of religiosity, American Islam resembles the mainstream of American religious life. (2)

While the report continues in this overall vein when discussing assimilation, the cultural expression of some of these statistics is quite disturbing. For starters, a twelve percent difference is hardly 'a little more.' Moreover, a full thirteen percent of Muslims living in America who consider themselves Muslims first 'believe that suicide bombing to defend Islam from its enemies can often or sometimes be justified.' Forty percent of this population who consider themselves Muslims first believes the attacks of September 11th were not carried out by groups of Arabs. Most interestingly, 'nearly half of African-American Muslims are more likely to argue against new arrivals fully assimilating into American life.' Only thirty-one percent of African-American Muslims believes new arrivals 'should try to assimilate.' (3)

These are sobering statistics. While they are sobering for reasons of public policy, because these statistics illustrate the practical piety of a significant segment of American Muslims, these statistics also point directly at those of us who provide humane care and are viewed as resources for addressing the religious, spiritual, emotional and social aspects of the complex process of assimilation. Remember, it is through religious piety that theological principles are made real.

The dominant religious perspective within the over 2,000 mosques in America is Wahhabi Islam. In the first task of diagnosis, naming the pain of assimilation experienced by a Muslim in a non-Muslim nation is generally viewed as an illustration of the *host culture's* lack of religious faithfulness. Thus piety's care plan for such pain is not one of adaptation to the new culture. The pietistic care plan for a practitioner of Wahhabi Islam in non-Muslim nation appears to one of converting the host nation to Wahhabi Islam.

From a standpoint of religious diagnosis, practical piety and overall faith development, the level of sophistication of the majority of imams from Saudi Arabia who promote Wahhabi Islam appears at best to be the mythic-literal level of faith. James Fowler describes individuals at this level of faith development as

> Both "carried and 'trapped' in" their own narrative. Stage two can be dangerous because the relentless belief in reciprocity forces the individual into a strict, over-controlling perfectionism; their religious system will without doubt be either legalistic or else, in the case of abuse, the child may be convinced of his or her own irredeemability. (4)

This religious rejection of assimilation is generally viewed through the lens of fundamentalism. As a spiritual viewpoint, fundamentalism is a rejection of the dominant culture coupled with an piety driven with an authoritarian zeal to force the fundamentals of *their* faith upon others either 'to save your soul' or 'for your own good.' So thorough is the fundamentalist's theological belief in the eternal value of their worldview that others hope in vain for the main body of such a worldview to vanish as a movement through maturation. This transformation will take centuries, not decades.

Even Fowler's next stage, *synthetic-conventional faith*, appears to be somewhat meager in its ability to reflect upon life critically and adopt the 'live and let live' perspective that is necessary for assimilation in today's pluralistic

Western culture. (5) Thus in the best of possibilities the majority of American Muslims are very likely to undergo a profound religious crisis within the next twenty to forty years. What makes this a matter of concern for mental health professionals is not just the necessity to help specific individual's make this transition. This particular expression of Islam encourages, and a percentage of adherents clearly *believe*, that one expression of religious faithfulness includes a piety that permits the forced conversion of those viewed as infidels or 'other' rather than taking the path of assimilation through personal change. Where Islam is the dominant religion, non-Muslims face growing levels of persecution based on principles 'that have been part of Islam for more than 1000 years.' (6)

This is only one-half of the challenge presented by the tensions of assimilation and globalization for mental health providers. There is another type of fundamentalism that is as every bit as virulent as Wahhabi Islam in its intensity and use of force to impose its worldview. This is liberal fundamentalism and it is the dominant paradigm within the mental health community. It also shares much of the basic alienation from the values of Western culture as the Wahhabi Muslim albeit from what appears to be a mostly secularizing point of view. My concern is this: because the dominant paradigm of the care providers shares the same alienation from Western values as the people who will be attempting to cope with assimilation into those Western values, the caregivers are likely to confuse their shared cultural alienation as empathy and thus reinforce the very rejection and alienation in the Muslim community they are partly responsible to assuage.

Liberal fundamentalism is self-identified as 'progressive' by its adherents. Its detractors call this paradigm 'secular progressivism'. I prefer the name of 'liberal fundamentalism' since this label clearly signals the alienation and evangelistic zeal that is otherwise masked by the softer features of its external appearance and its apparent acceptance of diversity. This label also helps express the confiscatory authoritarianism liberal fundamentalism shares with its more primitive cousins. The only genuine difference between these two worldviews is the means through which they seek to limit individual freedom, self-determination, respect for the rule of law and other basic human rights. While the primitive fundamentalism may use swords and burkas to oppress infidels liberal fundamentalism utilizes tax policies and unending group process to suppress dissent. Birkenstocks are optional for this latter group of fundamentalists.

Both types of fundamentalism abhor individual freedom, believing they have a god-given right to rule others. Both types of fundamentalism corrupt common language and public education, using shame and guilt to manipulate how a nation's history understood. Both types of fundamentalism focus on the primacy of emotion over reason. Thus the much-vaunted 'Muslim street' shares a basic similarity of worldview with anti-global Green anarchists and the pro-choice activists whose screed is abortion on demand. The assumption here is this: either a mass of people shouting in the street or continuing to talk until everyone 'feels good' inevitably must trump genuine democratic process. Emotionally and spiritually there is very little difference between the fundamentalist Muslim offended by a scantily clad Western woman and a fundamentalist Green offended by that same woman driving solo in her Chevrolet Suburban. Both would forcibly change her conduct if they had the means to do so.

My diagnostic and care concern here is not primarily for the people of either type of fundamentalism who take to the streets in demonstrations. Demagogues will always exploit the pain of such individuals by offering them care disguised as confiscating the property or otherwise punishing the 'others' whom fundamentalists of all stripes view with self-righteousness and envy. My concern is for those within the care-providing community who remain home from the demonstration but whose worldview and access to the direction of public policy makes them capable of translating this shared fundamentalism into laws. These types of policies will be named as 'progress' but actually embody a new Dark Age in which junk science, political correctness and unending class warfare will likely inhibit the spiritual transformation necessary for the human race to truly become a world in which we can all live. In short, both types of fundamentalism believe their worldview is capable of building a tower to reach their own view of heaven. One of our most ancient stories tell us that such an effort is an expression of human pride and thus ultimately doomed to fail, a story we neglect at our corporate peril. (7)

Lifestyle and Responsibility

Our oldest story of bearing the consequences of our choices speaks the language of curse. Because of the First Couple's transgression, humanity now has the responsibility for discerning the difference between good and evil, according to the story. The consequences of their lifestyle choice include the pain and suffering the normal processes that begin and nourish life: childbirth and work. As the follow-on stories amply illustrate, raising children, getting along with in-laws, cooperating in public work projects and finding hospitable communities are likewise now arenas for figuring out the dividing line between good and evil. In all venues we humans bear the responsibility for our lifestyle choices. (8)

Medically speaking much of our care is devoted to repairing the damage we do to ourselves and to others through our lifestyle choices. As our diagnostic enterprise grows in sophistication, thanks to advances in the sciences of genetics and neurobiology, we have a greater ability to relieve human suffering as well as to gain clarity about the exact etiology of such suffering. Thus while we no longer blame the whims of the gods for our genetic time bombs, we also increasingly struggle to discern how much our own conduct contributes to our physical and psychological pain. Even more important, we increasingly face the opportunity to amend our lifestyle in ways that reduce if not thoroughly preclude the likelihood of our contracting a dread disease or bearing with a profound mental disorder.

Yet this increasing sophistication nonetheless carries with it increasing levels of personal and corporate responsibility for our lifestyle choices. In the realm of physical disease the linkage between cigarette smoking and either lung cancer or chronic obstructive pulmonary disease is nearly a one hundred percent certainty. So what role does personal responsibility play when a smoker of forty years contracts lung cancer? Psychologically, how does one truly understand such a person's depression and anxiety as they face the demanding treatment regime required to extend their life? Spiritually, what are the dynamics of forgiveness and mercy one may offer to someone whose nicotine addiction conquered them so thoroughly? Communally, how do we balance public health and personal freedom for those who not only chose 'to not smoke' but whose own health status renders them vulnerable to other illnesses when they are exposed to second-hand smoke?

This is just one small area where lifestyle choices intersect with mental health, spiritual vitality and public policy. Unplanned pregnancies, work that requires lengthy and regular familial separation, e.g. an off-short oil-rig worker, PTSD as a consequence of serving as a first responder, parents who serve their children alcohol at graduation parties, media celebrities whose virulent language reduces respect for public decorum, corporation decisions that leave entire communities bereft of a major employer and public officials whose pride or greed leaves communities vulnerable to foreseeable disasters is but a very short list of such arenas. The diagnostic challenge to the provider of humane care is complicated by these lifestyle factors, sometimes profoundly so. For each of these life circumstances and lifestyle choices there is an increased likelihood of a diagnosable psychological disorder: depression, anxiety, or substance abuse on Axis I of DSM-IV perhaps followed by a more severe personality disorder such as narcissism, sociopathy or paranoia on Axis II of DSM-IV.

Thus on the one hand of this dyadic tension between lifestyle and responsibility we have the Hippocratic Oath in all of its various permutations. Care is to be given to suffering individuals without regard to their own role in producing their maladies. Care is to be provided in moments of extreme need even without consideration for the person's ability to pay for the care, so great is the moral and spiritual imperative of this dictum. Another aspect to this tension is that of a growing cultural insistence in the West to *not* bear the cost or consequences for someone else's poor choices or poor circumstances through the growth of both means-based and needs-based assessments. Whether through a criminal justice system that says 'three strikes and you're out,' a medical system that says 'no second liver transplant if you continue to drink,' or a social relief system that says 'no help rebuilding if you return a second time to live on a flood plain,' the mood now clearly is one of recognizing some resources for care are finite.

The other extreme in this dyad's tension is the lifestyle of selfishness that asserts one can say 'whatever I want to' without having to endure the consequences of such unbridled speech or 'its my body, I can sell it if I want to' without the community having any role in saying 'but not on our public street or through out public airways.' Again, diagnosable psychological distress can be recognized at each point along this lifestyle and responsibility continuum. There is in this absence of individual responsibility a desire to carry the social privilege of childhood well into adulthood. An increased percentage of humanity appears to desire the irresponsible lifestyle of social boors such as Paris Hilton and Mel Gibson.

When reality imposes its own limitations, as reality eventually does, there usually is a dysfunctional emotional or social response within the individual and sometimes throughout their family system. But do we want to label someone as with an Adjustment Disorder with Depressed Mood because their employer has fired them for chronic tardiness? Remember, the criteria for an adjustment disorder is the normal mood or conduct response of a normal person to an abnormal situation. Timely appearance for an employer is not an abnormal situations.

The driver arrested for the offense of driving while intoxicated has done so at least fifty times prior to their first arrest. Yet some helping professionals in addition to many in the public worry about hurting the individual's feelings when a clinician identifies them as being alcohol dependent. Or do we as clinicians take the easy way out and help the person examine how their current dilemma is *really* the result of poor parenting rather than something for which they are ultimately responsible and should be held accountable?

The tension inherent in this dyad has been in existence for millennia. So I do not believe there is a final definitive solution to this tension. But as we continue to address the consequences of peoples' lifestyle choices in our societies, families, and cultures as well as in our consulting rooms, places of worship and hospitals, we have to find a better way to identify the individual's responsibility in their painful circumstance and guide them toward an effective regime of behavioral change and moral responsibility.

Security and Privacy

Recently a man infected with a strain of multi-drug resistant tuberculosis coupled with an indication of pulmonary tuberculosis created an international frenzy. After being advised by the Centers for Disease Control to report to a hospital for treatment rather than fly, he boarded an international flight to France. In the ensuing days he was again instructed to report to a hospital in Europe; an order he again dismissed. He boarded another flight in the Czech Republic and arrived in Canada. What was his explanation for his defiance? "I didn't think I was that contagious," he said. "I'm sorry for the inconvenience I caused everyone," he said from his quarantined hospital room in Denver, Colorado.

Few things highlight the diagnostic and lifestyle challenges of our global culture than reading the transcripts of the daily news conferences from the Centers for Disease Control while watching the instantaneously available surveillance camera photo of the man crossing into the United States. There is a surreal quality to the CDC following the HIPAA guidelines to protect his 'privacy' while the patient himself is giving interviews and releasing partial transcripts of his conversations with CDC officials from his isolation room in Denver while avoiding accepting responsibility for his travel placing at risk the health status of upwards of 80 people in a profound violation of their 'privacy.'

In a similar vein, those of us who sought to gain access to the mental health records of the individual who slaughtered 32 people at Virginia Polytechnic University ran into a similar Kafkaesque conundrum. Suddenly this now-deceased person's mental health history trumped the need to understand his motivation as well as revisit guidelines that might prevent future horrors. Confusion over privacy guidelines emerged as the single most critical area needing redress in the national investigation aftermath of the shootings at Virginia Polytechnic University. (9) Just as there appears to be no way to prevent a determined individual from amassing 400 rounds of ammunition to wreak havoc on an unsuspecting community, there does not appear to be a way to prevent a determined patient from eluding international no-fly or no-leave orders issued by the either the World Health Organization or national health departments.

Whether we speak of putting in place a security apparatus to prevent mass violence or health guidelines to preclude the spread of virulent disease, we quickly run into spiritual, ethical and psychological concerns as evidenced by these remarks from the CDC's Media Relations Tele-briefing. Dr. Martin Cetron, Director of Global Migration and Quarantine, is speaking. He cites Dr. Gerberding, the Director of the CDC:

> In many ways we balance individual freedoms and public good. And we depend on a covenant of trust, … in the vast, vast minority of situations of infectious tuberculosis drug resistant or otherwise, require legal restraining orders to keep people from moving, in order to encourage them to do the right thing. The preferred approach is to work with that covenant. And as she indicated in this case, the individual had a compelling interest from his own perspective to initiate that travel out of the country. (10)

So when facing a potentially devastating public health concern the governmental agencies charged to protect international health at present relies on a spiritual constraint (covenant) and ethical persuasion 'to do the right thing.' As is now evident, a personal 'compelling interest' easily trumps these restraints. Not only did the perpetrator of the massacre at Virginia Polytechnic have a 'compelling interest from his own perspective' to lie about his mental health status on the Federal form required of everyone who intends to purchase a handgun, so did Adam and Eve have a 'compelling interest' when they decided to violate an earlier covenant of trust. (11)

As the inevitable Congressional hearings and media editorials either illuminate or obfuscate these specific concerns, providers of humane care may wish to reflect on this more basic concern regarding security and privacy. These concerns are made especially complex by the realities of international travel and inter agency jurisdictions as well as the aforementioned tensions around assimilation and lifestyle. What if the challenge we face here is not a psychological diagnosis but a theological diagnosis? What if we face in all these concerns not narcissism, a basic lack of common sense or naiveté but an idolatry of the self? (12) What if we face in both these individuals and structures that have caused so much suffering not an identifiable mental illness or a lack of some 'controlling legal authority' but a manifestation of evil?

The majority of our mental health and religious professionals have a basic paradigm that fails to account for the dynamic of active evil. They thus do not take evil seriously in their efforts to name human pain accurately and relieve human suffering adequately. They assume that everyone shares their own urbane brand of reasonableness. This also makes it difficult for mental health professionals and others within the social disciplines to accurately assess the presence of an active threat to security. This too was underscored in the aftermath investigation of the Virginia Polytechnic University shootings:

> Of course, a predicate to sharing information is recognizing when individuals pose a threat to themselves or others, and when intervention to pre-empt the threat is appropriate. In this regard, participants flagged the need for effective, evidence-based, inter-disciplinary tools to conduct a reliable assessment of the degree, type, and immediacy of safety risk the individual poses. (13)

A primary contributor to this lack of ability to recognize such individuals is a worldview that prefers to see guilt and responsibility within the collective rather than recognizing an individual's capacity for doing great unilateral harm. This worldview responds enthusiastically to discussion and accepts the excuse 'but I didn't intend to hurt anyone' as being more significant than the actual consequences of an individual's conduct.

Absent such a tepid apology when a perpetrator is presented with the cost and consequences of their breaking such a 'covenant of understanding,' it is unlikely the majority of people providing humane care will be able to hold the individual fully and solely accountable for their conduct. It remains to be seen whether or not the mental health community and mainline religious community can ever regain the philosophic integrity to recognize the primary value of subsuming personal privacy to the more pressing needs of community security, especially when it comes to concerns of controlling the spread of virulent disease or preventing the community from someone who has the willpower necessary to slaughter the innocent neighbor. When facing the tension of security and privacy, the mental health community prefers to blame the communal victim for somehow inviting the trespass rather than look at the responsibility of the perpetrator for incurring the moral debt. It is significant that the report to the President *On Issues Raised by the Virginia Tech Tragedy* highlighted both the necessity for mental health providers and teachers to be instructed in the warning signs of someone on the cusp of committing a violent act so that appropriate pre-emptive action can be taken as well as noting, *"it is critical that states have adequate systems for monitoring and following up, particularly where a legal ruling mandates a course of treatment"* (emphasis added). (14)

Conclusion

The work of providing counsel and care that relieves human suffering while also protecting human dignity continues. We are more than a complex collection of neurons yet our neurons hold many keys to relieving our anguish. We are less than divine yet our great religions, at their best, speak of our collective promise and individual responsibilities within a matrix that takes seriously our chaotic origins. One source describes our situation in these words:

> Life is a gift to be received with gratitude and a task to be pursued with courage. Man is free to seek his life within the purpose of God: to develop and protect the resources of nature for the common welfare, to work for justice and peace in society, and in other ways to use his creative powers for the fulfillment of human life. (15)

The introductory letter of the Report to the President *On Issues Raised by the Virginia Tech Tragedy* echoes these sentiments in the language of public policy, stating, "the report serves to focus our attention on the issues that must be a part of the ongoing national dialogue as we continue to protect the freedoms we enjoy in our society while appropriately minimizing risks to public safety." (16) Another great writer puts the challenge thusly, reminding us of what our religions and our desire to care for one another must embrace, "Beginning with Abraham, the faith of each of his sons represents a constant leaving behind of what is cherished, familiar and personal, in order to open up to the unknown, trusting in the truth we share and the common future we all have in God." (17)

There is significant pain in the human condition that we seek to leave behind. Some of this pain rises from the limits of existence and lurks as a malevolent force within our genetic structure or as a blind consequence of our planet's tectonic structure. The vast majority of our pain comes from our fellow travelers upon this sparkling globe of water-drenched rock. Or it is self-inflicted. There is also considerable care and cure that rises from our human endeavor. We continue to learn ways of reducing the acrimony between people and one of our signature qualities, as the planet's premier toolmaker, remains successful in the quest alleviate suffering and disease.

The resource of the Spirit remains an indispensable ingredient in this healing endeavor. Whether expressed through the great religions or enacted quietly through the heroism of a single soul, our best efforts to name disease and to reduce if not turn back its devastating consequences ultimately draws upon the history of our most ancient ancestors. Those ones who stood at the doorway to some long-forgotten cave to defeat a pair of glowing eyes outside in the darkness or who bent over a fevered companion with only their cool hand were the forerunners of those today who guard our liberties and inspire our best efforts to lengthen life. What was said by President George W. Bush in the aftermath of the Virginia Polytechnic tragedy can be said of the wider human family in these efforts, "We reflect on what has been lost and comfort those enduring a profound grief. And somehow we know that a brighter morning will come. And we know this because Americans have overcome many evils and found strength through many storms."

The two tasks of diagnosis, naming the pain and guiding the care, not only help us reflect on these losses, they help us identify the cause of our losses. These two tasks also guide us in our efforts to defeat various evils and rebuild after many storms. *Selah*!

Epilogue

The matters of spiritual maturity and emotional health contribute directly to individual well-being, family stability and the destinies of nations. Having a unified method for describing the challenges humans face and the suffering we endure is an essential factor in helping all three arenas contribute to human wholeness. A spirituality or theology that fails to take account of ordinary human development is cruel just as a psychology or sociology that omits humanity's religious practices is barren. It is my hope that this volume will enrich the collaboration between these two efforts at naming and reliving human pain.

I recognize this volume is incomplete. Specialists and advocates in various sub-fiends of humane care will inevitably say that I did not include a chapter on their area of interest. I would encourage each reader to analyze their own clinical care through the matrix of guilt, idolatry and dread whether or not I addressed your specialty. There is plenty of anguish readily available for analysis.

I also recognize this volume assumes a clinical setting. While this is the primary place of my own work, it is not the only place or even the primary locus where the effort to relieve the heart's distress and the mind's confusion occurs. Local religious communities, volunteer relief organizations, spontaneous support groups, the various Twelve Step programs and ordinary people provide significant respite to others caught in the grip of anxiety, depression, addiction and outrageous fortune. These inevitably anonymous angels face the ravages of defilement, betrayal and punishment. I hope this volume will make their flights of mercy a bit more effective. *Selah!*

Abbreviations

BTM	-	*Behind the Mask: Personality Disorders in Religious Behavior*
JPCC	-	*The Journal of Pastoral Care and Counseling*
MAD	-	*The Minister as Diagnostician*
PNFCMH	-	*President's New Freedom Commission on Mental Health*
RADSM-V	-	*A Research Agenda for DSM-V: Summary of the DSM-V Pre-planning White Papers Published in May 2002*
RDSS	-	*Religious Diagnosis in a Secular Society*
TSISP	-	*Treating Spiritual Issues in Secular Psychotherapy*

Notes

Foreword

1. Kendler, KS. Reflections on the relationship between psychiatric genetics and psychiatric nosology. Am J Psychiatry 2006;163:1138-1146.
2. McHugh PR, Slavney PR. The Perspectives of Psychiatry, 2nd Edition, Baltimore, Johns Hopkins University Press, 1998.
3. Morrison J. Diagnosis made easier: Principles and techniques for mental health clinicians. New York, Guilford Press, 2007.
4. Compton WM, Guze SB. The neo-Kraepelinian revolution in psychiatric diagnosis. Eur Arch Psychiatry Clin Neurosciences 1995;245:196-201.
5. First MB, Pincus HA. The DSM-IV text revision: Rationale and potential impact on clinical practice. Psychiatry Serv 2002; 53:288-292.
6. Kirmayer LJ, Rousseau C, Jarvis GE, Guzder J. The cultural context of clinical assessment. In: Psychiatry, 2nd Edition (Tasman A, Kay J, Lieberman JA, Eds.), Chapter 2, pp.19-29. Chichester, Wiley & Sons, 2003.
7. American Psychiatric Association. Diagnostic and Statistical Manual of Mental Disorders, 4th Edition, Text Revised. DSM-IV TR. 886 pages. Washington DC, 2004.
8. Kupfer DJ, First MB, Regier DA (Eds). A research agenda for DSM-V. 307 pages. Washington DC, American Psychiatric Association, 2002.
9. DSM-V research planning activities: DSM-V Prelude. Available in: http://www.dsmiv.org/planning.csm
10. Kendler KS. Toward a philosophical structure for Psychiatry. Am J Psychiatry 2005;162:433-440
11. Eisenberg L. Does social medicine still matter in an era of molecular medicine? J Urban Health 1999;76:164-175.
12. Denton WH. Issues for DSM-V: Relational diagnoses: An essential component of biopsychosocial assessment (Editorial). Am J Psychiatry 2007;164:1146-1147.
13. Charney DS, Barlow DH, Botteron K, et al. Neuroscience research agenda to guide development of a pathophysiologically-based classification in DSM. In: A research agenda for DSM-IV (Kupfer DJ, First MD, Regier DA, Eds.) Chapter 2, pp. 31-75. Washington DC, American Psychiatric Association, 2002.
14. Ustum PB, Sartorius N (Eds). Mental illness in general health care: an international study. Chichester, John Wiley and Sons, 1995.
15. Alarcón RD, Westermeyer J, Foulks ES, et al. Clinical relevance of contemporary cultural psychiatry. J Nerv Ment Dis, 1999;187:465-471.
16. Engel GL. The need for a new medical modal: a challenge for biomedicine. Science 1977;196:129-136.
17. Bickle J. Philosophy and neuroscience: a ruthlessly reductive account. Boston, Klauwer Academics, 2003.
18. Alarcón RD, Bell CC, Kirmayer LJ, et al. Beyond the fun house mirrors: Research agenda on culture and psychiatric diagnosis. In: A research agenda for DSM-V, (Kupfer DJ, First MV, Regier DA, Eds). Chapter 6, pp. 219-281. Washington DC, American Psychiatric Association, 2002.

19. Bartocci G, Dein S. Detachment: Gate to the world of spirituality. Transcult Psychiatry 2005;42:545-569.

20. Henig RM. God has always been a puzzle. The New York Times Magazine, pp. 39-43, March 4, 2007.

21. Bathgate D. Psychiatry, religion, and cognitive science. Australian NZ J Psychiatry 2003;37:277-285.

22. Boehnlein JK. Introduction. In: Psychiatry and Religion: the convergence of mind and spirit (Boehnlein JK, Ed), pp. XV-XX. Washington DC, American Psychiatric Press, 2000.

23. Baca E, Lázaro J (Eds.) Hechos y Valores en Psiquiatría. 581 pages.   Madrid, Triacastela, 2003.

24. Boehnlein JK. Religion and spirituality in psychiatric care: Looking back, Looking ahead. Transcult Psychiatry 2006;43:634-651

25. Mohr S, Brandt PY, Borras L, et al. Toward an integration of spirituality and religiousness in the psychosocial dimension of schizophrenia. Am J Psychiatry 2006;163:1952-1959.

26. Koss-Chioino JD. Spiritual confirmation, relation, and radical empathy: Core components of the ritual healing process. Transcult Psychiatry 2006;43:652-670.

27. Frank JD, Frank JB. Persuasion and Healing: A comparative study of psychotherapy, 3rd edition. 343 pages. Baltimore, Johns Hopkins University Press, 1991.

28. Hackney CH, Sanders GS. Religiosity and mental health: a meta-analysis of recent studies. J Scient Study Religion 2003;42:43-55.

29. Koenig HG. Religion and future psychiatric nosology and treatment. In: Psychiatry and Religion: A convergence of mind and spirit. (Boehnlein JK, Ed), pp. 169-185 Washington DC, American Psychiatric Press, 2000.

30. Rieff P. Charisma. The gift of grace and how it has been taken away from us. 271 pp. New York, Pantheon Books, 2007.

31. Caldwell C. Falling from grace. The New York Times Book Review, page 25. March 4, 2007

32. Okasha A. Globalization and mental health: a WPA perspective (Editorial) World Psychiatry 2005; 4: 1-2.

33. Kirmayer LJ. Beyond the 'New Cross-cultural Psychiatry': Cultural Biology, Discursive Psychology and the ironies of Globalization. Transcult Psychiatry 2006; 43: 126-144

34. Kleinman AM. Experience and its moral modes: Culture, human   conditions and disorder. In: The Tanner Lectures (pp. 357-420). Stanford University, 199

Introduction

1. Donald Denton, *Religious Diagnosis in a Secular Society* (Lanham, MD: University Press of America, 1998), Xv (hereafter cited as *RDSS*)

2. Wesley Brun, "Response to the Responders,"
The Journal of Pastoral Care & Counseling,
Vol. 59, No. 5 (Supplement 2005): 452.

3. RDSS, Xviii.

4· Michael B. First, *A Research Agenda for*
DSM-V: Summary of the DSM-V Preplanning
White Papers Published in May 2002.
(http:aadsm5.org/whitepapers.cfm) (hereafter cited as *RADSM-V*).

5. RADSM-V.

6. *RDSS* , Xviii.
7. *RADSM-V*

Part I

Chapter One

1. DSM-IV, pg. Xxi.
2.   P. W. Pruyser, *Dictionary of Pastoral Care and Counseling.* 1990 ed., s.v. "Evaluation and Diagnosis, Religious," 371-373.
3.   President's New Freedom Commission on Mental Health (www.mentalhealthcommission.gov/reports/Finalreport/FullReport) (hereafter cited as *PNFCMH*).
4. Genesis 3:1-24.
5. Shomer S. Zwellin, *Quest for a Cure: The Public Hospital in Williamsburg, Virginia, 1773-1885.* (The Colonial Williamsburg Foundation: Williamsburg, Virginia, 1985).
6. *PNFCMH*
7. Zwellin, *Quest,* 2.
8. *Ibid.* 10f.
9. *PNFCMH*
10. Zwellin, *Quest,* 11-13.
11. *PNFCMH*
12. Zwellin, *Quest,* 11f.
13. *PNFCMH,* Goal 4.3.
14. *Ibid.*
15. *Ibid.*
16. *Ibid.*
17. *Ibid.*
18. *RDSS* , pg. 104.
19. Zwellin, *Quest,* 48.

Chapter Two

1. John 4:1-30
2. *NeuroPsychiatry Reviews* (January 2006: Vol. 7, No. 1).
3. I Timothy 3:1-13.
4. Robert M. Kaplan and Dennis P. Saccuzzo, ed. *Psychological Testing: Principles, Applications and Issues.* (Belmont, California: Thomson Wadsworth, 2005).
5. *Ibid,* 393.
6. United Health Foundation. *Clinical Evidence Mental Health, Vol. 11.* (BMJ Publishing Group: Minnetonka, Minnesota, 2004).
7. *Ibid,* 114.
8. *Ibid ,* 115-116.

9. *Ibid*, 118, 152.
10. John J. Gleason, "Pastoral Research: Past, Present and Future," *TJPC*: Vol. 58, no. 4 (Winter 2004): 295.
11. *Ibid*, 296.
12. *Ibid*, 300.
13. *Ibid*, 301.
14. *RDSS*, 103.
15. *RDSS*, 98.
16. Lucy Bregman, "Spirituality: Multiple Uses and Murky Meanings of an Incredibly Popular Term, *TJPC* Vol. 58, no. 3: 157.
17. *Ibid*, 166.
18. Martin Rovers and Lucie Kocum. *Faith, Hope and Love: Towards a Holistic Definition of Spirituality and the Development of a Holistic Spirituality Scale.* (Ottawa, Ontario: St. Paul University, 2005).
19. *Ibid*.
20. George Fitchett, "A Response to 'A Proposed Diagnostic Schema for Religious / Spiritual Concerns," *TJPCC* 59, no. 5 (Supplement 2005), 444. "Most pastoral caregivers will probably be uncomfortable with the diagnostic labeling, not to mention the evaluative features of this model."
24. Wesley L. Brun, "Response to the Respondents." *TJPCC* 59, no. 5 (Supplement 2005), 454. "I fear that Dr. Denton may be correct when he observes that 'the religious community appears to still be debating the efficacy of diagnosis, let alone being at the point of agreement on anything approaching unanimity about a single diagnostic system.'

Chapter Three

1. Genesis 3:22-24.
2. Edward S. Neukrug and Charles R. Fawcett, *Essentials of Testing and Assessment: A Practical Guide for Counselors, Social Workers and Psychologists.* (Belmont, California: Thomson Brooks/Cole, 2006), 4.
3. Kaplan and Saccuzzo, *Psychological Testing: Principles, Applications and Issues, Sixth Edition*, 617.
4. Neukrug and Fawcett, 199.
5. *Ibid.*, 233.
6. David H. Olson and Amy K. Olson, *Empowering Couples: Building on Your Strengths* (Minneapolis: Life Innovations, Inc., 2000), 108.
7. *Ibid.*, 9.
8. Walter L. Larimore, "Providing Basic Spiritual Care for Patients: Should It Be the Exclusive Domain of Pastoral Professionals?" *American Family Physician* 63, no. 1 (January 2001): 5.
9. *Ibid.*, 2.
10. *Ibid.*, 1.
11. *Ibid.*, 4.

Chapter Four

1. Stephen G. Post, Christina Puchalski and David B. Larson, David B. *Annals of Internal Medicine* 132, no. 7 (April 2000): 580.
2. John 9:2.
3. Mark 2:10-11.
4. Exodus 20:1-17.
5. Exodus 20:6.
6. Don S. Browning, *Religious Ethics and Pastoral Care* (Philadelphia: Fortress Press, 1983), 55.
7. *Ibid.,* 16-17.
8. *Ibid.,* 16.
9. *Ibid.,* 53.
10. *Ibid.,* 99.
11. Kenneth Elzinga, "Interview with Kenneth Elzinga," interview with editor, *Region Focus,* 8: no. 3, (summer 2004), 36.
12. Wendell E. Miller, "Providing An Alternative that is Not an Alternative," (www.biblical-counsel.org/bes-04).
13. *Ibid.,* (www.biblical-counsel.org/bes-04).
14. *Ibid.,* (www.biblical-counsel.org/bes-04).
15. Richard A. Gardner, *Therapeutic Communication With Children: The Mutual Storytelling Technique,* (New York: Science House, Inc, 1971) .
16. Janice Goldman, "A Mutual Storytelling Technique as an Aid to Integration after Abreaction in the Treatment of MPD." *Dissociation* VIII, no. 1, (March 1995).
17. Janice E. DeSocio, "Accessing Self-development through Narrative Approaches in Child and Adolescent Psychotherapy." *Journal of Child and Adolescent Psychiatric Nursing.* (April-June:2005).
18. *Ibid.*
19. Gardner, 29.
20. Goldman, VIII: no 1, (March 1995).
21. Mark 4:1-9, Matthew 13:24-30, Matthew 18:23-35.
22. Paul Pruyser, *The Minister as Diagnostician* (Philadelphia: Westminster Press, 1976), 11.
23. *Ibid.,* 11.
24. Andrew J. Weaver, Kevin J. Flannelly, Harold G. Koenig, and Fred Douglas Smith, "A Review of Research on Chaplains and Community-Based Clergy in *The Journal of the American Medical Association, ,Lancet and The New England Journal of Medicine: 1998-2000. The Journal of Pastoral Care and Counseling* 58: no. 4, (Winter 2004), 348-350.
25. *Ibid* 349.
26. Thomas C. Ogden, *Care of Souls in the Classic Tradition* (Philadelphia: Fortress Press, 1978), 54.
27. Wayne Oates, *Behind the Masks: Personality Disorders in Religious Behavior.* (Philadelphia: The Westminster Press, 1987), 11.
28. *Ibid.,* 12.
29. *Ibid* , 119.

30. TJPCC, 58: No. 4, (Winter 2004), 349.
31. David R. Hodge, "Spiritual Assessment in Marital and Family Therapy: A Methodological Framework for Selecting from Among Six Qualitative Assessment Tools." *The Journal of Marital and Family Therapy* (October 2005), Retrieved from www.findarticles.com/p/articles/mi_qu3658/is_200510/ai_n15715462/ pg. 1
32. *Ibid* 3.
33. *Ibid* 7.
34. *Ibid* 9.
35. Robert T. Lawrence, "Principles to Make a Spiritual Assessment Work in Your Practice." *Journal of Family Practice* (August 2004). Retrieved from www.findarticles.com/p/articles/mi_m689/is_8_53/ai_n617884/

Part II

Chapter Five

1. Paul Ricoeur, *The Symbolism of Evil* (Boston: Beacon Press, 1967), 100.
2. Nicolai Hartmann, *Ethics; Selections from Classical and Contemporary Writers*, Oliver A. Johnson (Chicago: Holt, Rinehart and Winston, 1965), 383.
3. *Ibid.*, 394.
4. *Ibid.*, 392.
5. Immanuel Kant, *Groundwork of the Metaphysic of Morals* (New York: Harper & Row, 1948), 13.
6. James Gustafson, *Ethics from a Theocentric Perspective*, vol. 2 (Chicago: University of Chicago Press, 1984), 8-10
7. Matthew 22:37-39
8. Kant, 88.
9. Robert Lovinger, *Religion and Counseling: The Psychological Impact of Religious Belief* (New York: The Continuum Publishing Co., 1990), 91-139.
10, Ricoeur, 74.
11. Genesis 2:16-17.
12. Bernard Spilka, Ralph W. Hood, and Richard L. Gorsuch, *The Psychology of Religion An Empirical Approach* (Englewood Cliffs: Prentice-Hall, Inc., 1985), 66.
13. Genesis 3:10.
14. Don S. Browning, *Religious Ethics and Pastoral Care* (Philadelphia: Fortress Press, 1983), 18-30.
15. *Ibid.*, 54.
16. Edwin Herr and Spencer Niles, "The Values of Counseling: Three Domains," *Counseling and Values* 33 (1988): 4-16.
17. W. D. Ross, *Ethics: Selections from Classical and Contemporary Writers*, Oliver A. Johnson (Chicago: Holt, Rinehart and Winston, 1965), 401.
18. *Ibid.*, 402.
19. Edith Hamilton, *Mythology* (New York: Little, Brown & Company, 1940), 88.

20. Romans 12:19.
21. Romans 1:18.
22. James W. Fowler, *Becoming Adult, Becoming Christian* (San Francisco: Harper & Row, 1984), 50.

Chapter Six

1. Dorothee Solle, *Suffering* (Philadelphia: Fortress Press, 1975), 73.
2. I Corinthians 6:1-6.
3. Solle, 73.
4. Sheldon Zimberg, *The Clinical Management of Alcoholism* (New York: Brunner/Mazel, 1983), 120.
5. James W. Fowler, *Stages of Faith: The Psychology of Human Development and the Quest for Meaning* (New York: Harper&Row, 1981), 274.
6. 2 Corinthians 5:17.

Chapter Seven

[1] □□□□□□
2. Deuteronomy 4:41-43.
3. Julia C. Keller, "Busting a grudge clears way for health," *Science & Theology News* (www.stnews.org/php?article_id=763).
4. Thomas C. Fenter, et. al. "The Cost of Treating the 10 Most Prevalent Diseases in Men 50 Years of Age or Older, *The American Journal of Managed Care.* Vol. 12, no. 4, Sup. (March 2006) : 90-98.
5. www.spiritualityhealth.com/newsh/items/selftest/item_232.html
6. David Augsburger, www.journeytowardforgiveness.com/mapping/article4.asp
7. *Ibid.*
8. The Confession of 1967, *The Constitution of the Presbyterian Church (USA): Part I, Book of Confessions.* (Louisville: The Office of the General Assembly, 1967), 9.09.
9. Job 42:10-17.
10. Tsunami in Sri Lanka, democracy in Iraq and Afghanistan, recovery from hurricanes Katrina, Rita and Wilma.
11. Lucy Holmes, "Marking the Anniversary: Adolescents and the September 11 Healing Process," *International Journal of Groups Psychotherapy.* Vol. 55, no. 3, (July 2005): 441.

Chapter Eight

No footnotes.

Part III

Chapter Nine

1. Merle R. Jordan, *Taking on the Gods: The Task of the Pastoral Counselor* (Nashville: Abingdon Press, 1986), 18.
2. Howard Clinebell, *Basic Types of Pastoral Counseling* (Nashville: Abingdon Press, 1966), 118-19.
3. Acts 17:23.
4. DSM-IV, pg. 630.
5. Wayne E. Oates, *Behind the Masks: Personality Disorders in Religious Behavior.* (The Westminster Press: Philadelphia, 1987), 12.
6. Oates, pg. 14.
7. DSM-IV, pg. 176.
8. Edith Hamilton, *Mythology* (New York: Little, Brown & Company, 1940), 54f.
9. Peter Trachtenberg, *The Casanova Complex: Compulsive Lovers & Their Women* (New York: Poseidon Press, 1988), 28.
10. Substance Abuse and Mental Health Services Administration, *Core Competencies for Clergy and Other Pastoral Ministers In Addressing Alcohol and Drug Dependence and the Impact on Family Members* (HHS: 2003), Pg. 13.
11. Christina Hoff Sommers, *The War Against Boys.* The Atlantic Monthly, May 2000.
12. Frank Schaeffer and John Schaeffer, *Keeping Faith: A Father-Son Story About Love and the United States Marine Corps.* (Carroll & Graf Publishers: New York, 2002), pg. 172-173.
13. John McDargh, *"Concluding Clinical Postscript"* in *Exploring Sacred Landscapes: Religious and Spiritual Experiences in Psychotherapy*, Mary Lou Randour (New York: Columbia University Press, 1993), 178

Chapter Ten

1. Job 23:2.
2. Wayne E. Oates, *Behind the Masks: Personality Disorders in Religious Behavior,* pg. 120.
3. Oates, pg. 71.
4. Howard Cooper, *Psychiatry and Religion: Context, Consensus and Controversies*, Dinesh Bhugra (New York: Routledge, 1996), 76.
5. Howard Cooper, *Psychiatry and Religion: Context, Consensus and Controversies*, Dinesh Bhugra (New York: Routledge, 1996), 76f.
6. Paul W. Pruyser, "Religion in the Psychiatric Hospital: A Reassessment," *The Journal of Pastoral Care* 38(1) (March, 1984): 5-16.
7. Ellyn Spragins, "Shortchanging the Psyche," *Newsweek,* August 25, 1997, 78.
8. Nancy C. Andreasen, "Body and Soul," *The American Journal of Psychiatry* 153(5) (May, 1996): 589.
9. *Ibid,* pg. A22.
10. Job 2:10, 23:3.

11. Albert Ellis, "Rational-Emotive Therapy (RET) and Pastoral Counseling: A Reply to Richard Wessler," *The Personnel and Guidance Journal* 62 (1984): 266-267.
12. Job 7:11.
13. Job 13:25-28.

Chapter Eleven

1. Jeremiah 20:7
2. Psalm 51:10
3. Exodus 16:3.
4. James Fowler's Stages of Faith in Profile.htm
5. Luke 11:24-26.
6. Mark 9:29.
7. James Fowler's Stages of Faith in Profile.htm

Chapter Twelve

1. Mark 4:3-9.
2. Arthur C. Brooks, "Compassion, Religion and Politics." *Public Interest.* Vol. 157, No. Fall: pg. 57-66.
3. Hamlet (V, i.).

Part IV

Chapter Thirteen

1. Dan C. Pinck, "Prisoners and/of War," *Intelligencer: Journal of U. S. Intelligence Studies,* 15, no. 1 (Fall/Winter 2005): 59.
2. Genesis 3:22.
3. Anton T. Boisen, *The Exploration of the Inner World: A Study of Mental Disorder and Religious Experience* (Philadelphia: University of Pennsylvania Press, 1936), 53.
4. St. Anselm, *The Ontological Argument from St. Anselm to Contemporary Philosophers,* Alvin Plantinga (New York: Anchor Books, 1965), 4.
5. Paul Ricoeur, *The Symbolism of Evil* (Boston: Beacon Press, 1967), 33.
6. Genesis 4:10-15.
7. B. B. McKinney, Music Editor, *The Broadman Hymnal,* 1940 ed., s.v. "Love Lifted Me," 352.
8. Paul Ricoeur, *The Symbolism of Evil* (Boston: Beacon Press, 1967), 35.
9. Paul Ricoeur, *The Symbolism of Evil* (Boston: Beacon Press, 1967), 55.

10. *Diagnostic and Statistical Manual,* IV ed., s.v. "Personality Disorders," 629-30.
11. John 4:1- 26. The entire pericope illustrates pastoral conversation where healing symbol is embodied in presence of the counselor.

Chapter Fourteen

1. Ruth Hennesy, *Personal Bereavement and Its Effects on the Choice of Religious Vocation,* diss., Northwestern University, 1987 (Evanston: Northwestern University Press, 1987), 247.
2. Donald D. Denton, "The Warrior's Prayer: Combat Experience, Vocational Choice and Depth Relationships Among Vietnam Veterans Who Become Clergy," *The Journal of Pastoral Care* 45 (1991): 107-116.
3. Vance P. Davis, "Spiritual Assessment and Care for Veterans with Post-Traumatic Stress Disorder, *Plain Views*: Vol. 1, No. 12 (2004).
4. Dale A. Matthews, David B. Larson, Constance P. Barry, "The Faith Factor: An Annotated Bibliography of Clinical Research on Spiritual Subjects," (National Institute of Healthcare Research: Vol. 1 and Vol. 2), July, 1993.
4. Daniel A. Helminiak, "Treating Spiritual Issues in Secular Psychotherapy." Unpublished manuscript, State University of West Georgia. 1999 ((check date)) Hereafter cited as *TSISP*
5. H. Stifoss-Hansen, "Religion and Spirituality: What a European ear hears." *International Journal for the Psychology of Religion* 9 (1999): 25-33.
6. *TSISP,*quoting J. M. Holden, "Summit on Spirituality in Counseling," *Association for Transpersonal Psychology Newsletter* 14 (1996, Winter).
7. *RDSS,* 106.
8. *TSISP*, quoting J. M. Holden, "Summit on Spirituality in Counseling," *Association for Transpersonal Psychology Newsletter* 14 (1996, Winter).
9. *TSISP*
10. *TSISP*
11. *TSISP*
12. William Shakespeare, *Hamlet* (3.1.66).
13. Job 31:35.
14. R. C. Kessler, A. Sonnega, E. Bronmet et. al., "Posttraumatic Stress Disorder in the National Comorbidity Survey." *Archives of General Psychiatry*: 1995, 52 (1995):1048-1060.
15. Genesis 4:10.

Chapter Fifteen

1. Sam Shoemaker, *I Stand By the Door,* Faith@Work, 1926.
2. Philippians 2:12-13.
3. James 2:14-26.

4. Bonnie Heneson, "How a Life-Changing Event Led to the Spiritual Center." *Focus* (Fall, 2006).
5. Mark Twain (obtain full source).
6. Nicholas Warr, *Christmas, 1967: Anything But Merry*, The Old Breed News (November-December 2006), pg. 23.

Chapter Sixteen

1. Genesis 2:15-17
2. Genesis 3:22-24
3. Job 2:13, 38:1.

Part V

Chapter Seventeen

1. John Rosemond. Parenting Stories, www.rosemond.com. (accessed 12/24/04)
2. Susan Orr, Single Parenthood: Life Without Father, Family Research Council: www.familyresearchcouncil.org, 2000. (accessed 11/11/2003).
3. Richard Niolan, Children of Divorce and Adjustment, www.psychepage.com (accessed 5/27/00).
4. Rand, Deidre Conway. "The Spectrum of Parental Alienation Syndrome." *American Journal of Forensic Psychology.* (Vol. 15, No. 3, 1997).
5. Criteria for Parental Alienation Syndrome are: Access and Contact Blocking, Unfounded Abuse Allegations, Deterioration in Relationship Since Separation, and Intense Fear Reaction by the Child.
6. Leadership Council on Child Abuse and Interpersonal Violence. "Child Abuse Experts Applaud Legal Community for Rejecting Parental Alienation Syndrome." US Newswire (July 12, 2006)
7. Bone, Michael J. and Walsh, Michael R. "Parental Alienation Syndrome: How Conway, pg. 9. to Detect It and What to Do About It." The Florida Bar Journal (Vol. 73: No. 3, 1999), pg. 8.
8. Amy Johnson Conner. "Parental Alienation: The Latest Weapon in Nasty Divorces." Minnesota Lawyer: (Jan. 8, 2007), 1098-4410.

Chapter Eighteen

1. http://www.cdc.gov/tobacco/data_statistics/Factsheets/economic_facts.htm (accessed 8/5/07)
2. Woodruff, C. Roy.. *Spiritual Caregiving to Help Addicted Persons and Families.* (SAMHSA: 2006), Pp. 55-59.

Chapter Nineteen

1. Donald Meichenbaum, *A Clinical Handbook / Practical Therapist Manual for Assessing and Treating Adults with Post-Traumatic Stress Disorder.* (Waterloo, Ontario: Institute Press, 1994), 41 (hereafter cited as *CH/PTM*)
2. Charles Figley, *The American Legion Study of Psychological Adjustment among Vietnam veterans.* (Lafayette, Indiana: Purdue University, 1977).
3. CH/PTM, pg. 46.
4. CH/PTM, pg. 43f.
5. CH/PTM, pg. 284-297
6. CH/PTM, pg. 339.
7. Shay, "Achilles in Vietnam: Combat Trauma and the Undoing of Character," (www.buffgrunt.com/Achilles.html). Accessed 3/4/2007.
8. CH/PTM, pg. 29-30.
9. CH/PTM, pg. 31 (emphasis in original text).
10. Shay, (www.buffgrunt.com/Achilles.html). Accessed 3/4/2007.
11. CH/PTM, pg. 37.
12. CH/PTM, pg. 23.
13. CH/PTM, pg. 244 (emphasis in original text)
14. CH/PTM, pg. 244.
15. G. Elder and E. C. Clipp, "Combat experience and emotional health: Impairment and resilience in later life." *Journal of Personality* Vol. 57:336.
16. MAD.
17. Elie Wiesel, *Night.* (New York: Hill and Wang), 1972, 120.
18. Revelation 22:5.

Chapter Twenty

1. United States Bureau of Census Series P-25, Nos. 139.
2. Areas of the US where the flu first erupted (www.stanford.edu/group/virus/uda/flustat.html). Accessed 3/17/2007
3. http://www.npr.org/templates/story/story.php?storyId=9096726 (accessed 3/23/07)
4. Center for Biosecurity of UPMC. *Atlantic Storm Interactive.* (222.upmc-biosecurity.org).
5. Center for Biosecurity of UPMC. *Atlantic Storm Interactive.* (222.upmc-biosecurity.org).
6. John R. Harrald, "Hurricane Katrina: Recommendations for Reform." (March 7, 2006). Senate Homeland Security Subcommittee testimony.
7. DiNapoli, Greg. "Second National Comment Period on Revised NIM Document" (NIMS Working Group). U. S. Department of Homeland Security, Center for Faith-based & Community Initiatives. Broadcast e-mail.
8. Matthew Cooper, "Fallout From A Memorial." *Time.* Saturday, November 9, 2002.

Part VI

Chapter Twenty-One

1. DSM-IV, pg. 685.
2. A Research Agenda for DSM-V, Chapter 6, "Beyond the Funhouse Mirrors," pg. 221. (Hereafter designated as BFM-6).
3. BFM-6, pg. 221.
4. BFM-6, pg. 222
5. BFM-6, pg. 223.
6. BFM-6, pg. 223
7. BFM-6, pg. 224.
8. BFM-6, pg. 224-25.
9. BFM-6, pg. 237.
10. BFM-6, pg. 262.
11. BFM-6, pg. 289.
12. BFM-6, pg. 263.
14. PDS, pg. 426.
15. PDS, pg. 430.
16. PDS, George Fitchett, Bruce M. Hartung, H. Newton Malony and this author.
17. PDS, pg. 443.
18. PDS, pg. 431.
19. PDS, pg. 432.
20. PDS, pg. 445.
21. PDS, pg. 447.
22. BFM, pg. 262.

Chapter Twenty-Two

1. Pew Research Center, *Muslim Americans: Middle Class and Mostly Mainstream.* (May 22, 2007), pg. 1.
2. Pew Research Center, *Muslim Americans: Middle Class and Mostly Mainstream,* pg. 22.
3. Pew Research Center, *Muslim Americans: Middle Class and Mostly Mainstream,* pg. 24.
4. James Fowler, *Stages of Faith* (Harper & Row, 1981).
5. James Fowler, *Stages of Faith* (Harper & Row, 1981).
6. Hanna Allam and Leila Fadel, "Insurgents Threaten Baghdad Christians," *Richmond Times-Dispatch,* Sunday, June 10, 2007, sec. A.
7. Genesis 11:1-9.
8. Genesis, chapters 3 – 50.
9. Report to the President, *On Issues Raised by the Virginia Tech Tragedy* (Washington, D. C.: GPO, June 13, 2007), 11.

10. Centers for Disease Control. *Update on CDC Investigation Into People Potentially Exposed to Patient With Extensively Drug-Resistant TB.* (Wednesday, May 30, 2007). Accessed June 5, 2007.

11. Genesis 3:6-7.

12. Centers for Disease Control. *Update on CDC Investigation Into People Potentially Exposed to Patient With Extensively Drug-Resistant TB.* (Wednesday, May 30, 2007). Accessed June 5, 2007.

13. Report to the President, *On Issues Raised by the Virginia Tech Tragedy* (Washington, D. C.: GPO, June 13, 2007), 6

14. Report to the President, *On Issues Raised by the Virginia Tech Tragedy* (Washington, D. C.: GPO, June 13, 2007), 14

15. The Constitution of the Presbyterian Church (U.S.A.) Part I – The Book of Confessions, *The Confessions of 1967,* 9.17

16. Report to the President, *On Issues Raised by the Virginia Tech Tragedy* (Washington, D. C.: GPO, June 13, 2007).

17. John Paul II. *Rise, Let Us Be On Our Way.* (Libreria Editrice Vaticana, Citta del Vaticano), 2004, pg. 213.

Bibliography

Alarcón RD, Bell CC, Kirmayer LJ, et al. Beyond the fun house mirrors: Research agenda on culture and psychiatric diagnosis. In: A research agenda for DSM-V, (Kupfer DJ, First MV, Regier DA, Eds). Chapter 6, pp. 219-281. Washington DC, American Psychiatric Association, 2002.

Alarcón RD, Westermeyer J, Foulks ES, et al. Clinical relevance of contemporary cultural psychiatry. J Nerv Ment Dis, 1999;187:465-471.

Allam, Hanna and Fadel, Leila Fadel. "Insurgents Threaten Baghdad Christians," Richmond Times-Dispatch, Sunday, June 10, 2007, sec. A.

American Psychiatric Association. Diagnostic and Statistical Manual of Mental Disorders, 4th Edition, Text Revised. DSM-IV TR. 886 pages. Washington DC, 2004.

Andreasen, Nancy C. "Body and Soul," The American Journal of Psychiatry 153(5) (May, 1996): 589.

Augsburger, David. www.journeytowardforgiveness.com/mapping/article4.asp

Baca E, Lázaro J (Eds.) Hechos y Valores en Psiquiatría. 581 pages. Madrid, Triacastela, 2003.

Bartocci G, Dein S. Detachment: Gate to the world of spirituality. Transcult Psychiatry 2005;42:545-569.

Bathgate D. Psychiatry, religion, and cognitive science. Australian NZ J Psychiatry 2003;37:277-285.

Bickle J. Philosophy and neuroscience: a ruthlessly reductive account. Boston, Klauwer Academics, 2003

Boehnlein JK. Introduction. In: Psychiatry and Religion: the convergence of mind and spirit (Boehnlein JK, Ed), pp. XV-XX. Washington DC, American Psychiatric Press, 2000.

Boehnlein JK. Religion and spirituality in psychiatric care: Looking back, Looking ahead. Transcult Psychiatry 2006;43:634-651

Bregman, Lucy. "Spirituality: Multiple Uses and Murky Meanings of an Incredibly Popular Term. , The Journal of Pastoral Care & Counseling 58, no. 3: 157.

Brooks, Arthur C. "Compassion, Religion and Politics." Public Interest. Vol. 157, No. Fall: pg. 57-66.

Browning, Don S. Browning, Religious Ethics and Pastoral Care . Philadelphia: Fortress Press, 1983.

Brun, Wesley. "A Proposed Diagnostic Schema for Religious/Spiritual Concerns. The Journal of Pastoral Care and Counseling. 59 (2005): 425-440

_____ "Response to the Respondents." The Journal of Pastoral Care & Counseling. 59 (2005): 452-455.

Caldwell C. Falling from grace. The New York Times Book Review, page 25. March 4, 2007

Center for Biosecurity of UPMC. Atlantic Storm Interactive. (222.upmc-biosecurity.org).

Centers for Disease Control. Update on CDC Investigation Into People Potentially Exposed to Patient With Extensively Drug-Resistant TB. (Wednesday, May 30, 2007).

Charney DS, Barlow DH, Botteron K, et al. Neuroscience research agenda to guide development of a pathophysiologically-based classification in DSM. In: A research agenda for DSM-IV (Kupfer DJ, First MD, Regier DA, Eds.) Chapter 2, pp. 31-75. Washington DC, American Psychiatric Association, 2002

Clinebell, Howard. Basic Types of Pastoral Counseling (Nashville: Abingdon Press, 1966).

Compton WM, Guze SB. The neo-Kraepelinian revolution in psychiatric diagnosis. Eur Arch Psychiatry Clin Neurosciences 1995;245:196-201.

Conner, Amy Johnson. "Parental Alienation: The Latest Weapon in Nasty Divorces." Minnesota Lawyer: (Jan. 8, 2007), 1098-4410.

Cooper, Howard. Psychiatry and Religion: Context, Consensus and Controversies, Dinesh Bhugra (New York: Routledge, 1996).

Cooper, Matthew. "Fallout From A Memorial." Time. Saturday, November 9,

Davis, Vance P. "Spiritual Assessment and Care for Veterans with Post-Traumatic Stress Disorder, Plain Views: Vol. 1, No. 12 (2004).

Denton, Donald D. Religious Diagnosis in a Secular Society. Lanham, MD: University Press of America, 1998.

Denton, Donald D. "The Warrior's Prayer: Combat Experience, Vocational Choice and Depth Relationships Among Vietnam Veterans Who Become Clergy," The Journal of Pastoral Care 45 (1991).

Denton WH. Issues for DSM-V: Relational diagnoses: An essential component of biopsychosocial assessment (Editorial). Am J Psychiatry 2007;164:1146-1147.

DeSocio, Janice E. "Accessing Self-development through Narrative Approaches in Child and Adolescent Psychotherapy." Journal of Psychiatric Child and Adolescent Nursing. (April-2005).

DSM-V research planning activities: DSM-V Prelude. Available in: http://www.dsmiv.org/planning.csm

Elder, G. and Clipp, E. C. "Combat Experience and Emotional Health: Impairment and Resilience in Later Life." Journal of Personality 57: 311-341.

Ellis, Albert. "Rational-Emotive Therapy (RET) and Pastoral Counseling: A Reply to Richard Wessler," The Personnel and Guidance Journal 62 (1984).

Engel GL. The need for a new medical modal: a challenge for biomedicine. Science 1977;196:129-136.

Eisenberg L. Does social medicine still matter in an era of molecular medicine? J Urban Health 1999;76:164-175.

Fenter, Thomas C. et. al. "The Cost of Treating the 10 Most Prevalent Diseases in Men 50 Years of Age or Older, The American Journal of Managed Care. Vol. 12, no. 4, Sup. (March 2006) .

First MB, Pincus HA. The DSM-IV text revision: Rationale and potential impact on clinical practice. Psychiatry Serv 2002; 53:288-292

Fitchett, George Fitchett. "A Response to 'A Proposed Diagnostic Schema for Religious / Spiritual Concerns.'" The Journal of Pastoral Care & Counseling 59, no. 5 (Supplement 2005),

Fowler, James W. Fowler, Becoming Adult, Becoming Christian (San Francisco: Harper & Row, 1984).

Fowler, James W. Stages of Faith: The Psychology of Human Development and the Quest for Meaning (New York: Harper&Row, 1981)

Frank JD, Frank JB. Persuasion and Healing: A comparative study of psychotherapy, 3rd edition. 343 pages. Baltimore, Johns Hopkins University Press, 1991.

Frist, Michael B. A Research Agenda for DSM-V: Summary of the DSM-V Preplanning White Papers. (2002).

Gardner, Richard A. Gardner, Therapeutic Communication With Children: The Mutual Storytelling Technique. , New York: Science House, Inc, 1971.

Goldman, Janice Goldman, "A Mutual Storytelling Technique as an Aid to Integration after Abreaction in the Treatment of MPD." Dissociation VIII, no. 1, (March 1995).

Gleason, John J. Gleason. "Pastoral Research: Past, Present and Future," The Journal of Pastoral Care & Counseling. 58, no. 4 (Winter 2004): 295.

Hackney CH, Sanders GS. Religiosity and mental health: a meta-analysis of recent studies. J Scient Study Religion 2003;42:43-55

Hamilton, Edith. Mythology (New York: Little, Brown & Company, 1940).

Harrald, John R. "Hurricane Katrina: Recommendations for Reform." (March 7, 2006). Senate Homeland Security Subcommittee testimony.

Henson, Bonnie. "How a Life-Changing Event Led to the Spiritual Center." Focus (Fall, 2006).

Helminiak, Daniel A. "Treating Spiritual Issues in Secular Psychotherapy." Unpublished manuscript, State University of West Georgia. 1999

Henig RM. God has always been a puzzle. The New York Times Magazine, pp. 39-43, March 4, 2007.

Hennesy, Ruth. Personal Bereavement and Its Effects on the Choice of Religious Vocation, diss., Northwestern University, 1987 (Evanston: Northwestern University Press, 1987).

Herr, Edwin and Niles, Spencer. "The Values of Counseling: Three Domains," Counseling and Values 33 (1988).

Hodge, David R. "Spiritual Assessment in Marital and Family Therapy: A Methodological Framework for Selecting from Among Six Qualitative Assessment Tools." The Journal of Marital and Family Therapy (October 2005), (Retrieved from www.findarticles.com/p/articles/mi_qu3658/is_200510/ai_n15715462/)

.Holmes, Lucy. "Marking the Anniversary: Adolescents and the September 11 Healing Process," International Journal of Groups Psychotherapy. Vol. 55, no. 3, (July 2005):

John Paul II. Rise, Let Us Be On Our Way. (New York: Warner Books, 2004).

Jordan, Merle R. Taking on the Gods: The Task of the Pastoral Counselor (Nashville: Abingdon Press, 1986).

Kaplan, Robert M. and Saccuzzo, Dennis P. ed. Psychological Testing: Principles, Applications and Issues. Belmont, California: Thomson Wadsworth, 2005.

Keller, Julia C. Keller, "Busting a grudge clears way for health," Science & Theology News (www.stnews.org/php?article_id=763).

Kendler, KS. Reflections on the relationship between psychiatric genetics and psychiatric nosology. Am J Psychiatry 2006;163:1138-1146.

Kendler KS. Toward a philosophical structure for Psychiatry. Am J Psychiatry 2005;162:433-440

Kessler, R. C., Sonnega, A., Bronmet, E., et. al., "Posttraumatic Stress Disorder in the National Comorbidity Survey." Archives of General Psychiatry: 1995, 52 (1995).

Kirmayer LJ. Beyond the 'New Cross-cultural Psychiatry': Cultural Biology, Discursive Psychology and the ironies of Globalization. Transcult Psychiatry 2006; 43: 126-144

Kirmayer LJ, Rousseau C, Jarvis GE, Guzder J. The cultural context of clinical assessment. In: Psychiatry, 2nd Edition (Tasman A, Kay J, Lieberman JA, Eds.), Chapter 2, pp.19-29. Chichester, Wiley & Sons, 2003

Kleinman AM. Experience and its moral modes: Culture, human conditions and disorder. In: The Tanner Lectures (pp. 357-420). Stanford University, 1999.

Koenig HG. Religion and future psychiatric nosology and treatment. In: Psychiatry and Religion: A convergence of mind and spirit. (Boehnlein JK, Ed), pp. 169-185 Washington DC, American Psychiatric Press, 2000.

Koss-Chioino JD. Spiritual confirmation, relation, and radical empathy: Core components of the ritual healing process. Transcult Psychiatry 2006;43:652-670

Kupfer DJ, First MB, Regier DA (Eds). A research agenda for DSM-V. 307 pages. Washington DC, American Psychiatric Association, 2002.

Larimore, Walter L. Larimore. "Providing Basic Spiritual Care for Patients: Should It Be the Exclusive Domain of Pastoral Professionals?" American Family Physician 63, no. 1 (January 2001): 5.

Lawrence, Robert T. "Principles to Make a Spiritual Assessment Work in Your Practice." Journal of Family Practice (August 2004). (Retrieved from www.findarticles.com/p/articles/mi_m689/is_8_53/ai_n617884/)

Leadership Council on Child Abuse and Interpersonal Violence. "Child Abuse Experts Applaud Legal Community for Rejecting Parental Alienation Syndrome." US Newswire (July 12, 2006)

McDargh, John. "Concluding Clinical Postscript" in Exploring Sacred Landscapes: Religious and Spiritual Experiences in Psychotherapy, Mary Lou Randour (New York: Columbia University Press, 1993).

McHugh PR, Slavney PR. The Perspectives of Psychiatry, 2nd Edition, Baltimore, Johns Hopkins University Press, 1998.

McKinney, B.B. Music Editor, The Broadman Hymnal, 1940 ed., s.v. "Love Lifted Me," 352.

Matthews, Dale A., Larson, David B., and Barry, Constance P. "The Faith Factor: An Annotated Bibliography of Clinical Research on Spiritual Subjects," (National Institute of Healthcare Research: Vol. 1 and Vol. 2), July, 1993.

Morrison J. Diagnosis made easier: Principles and techniques for mental health clinicians. New York, Guilford Press, 2007.

Miller, Wendell E. "Providing An Alternative that is Not an Alternative," (www.biblical-counsel.org/bes-04).

Mohr S, Brandt PY, Borras L, et al. Toward an integration of spirituality and religiousness in the psychosocial dimension of schizophrenia. Am J Psychiatry 2006;163:1952-1959.

Neukrug, Edward S. and Fawcett, Charles R . Essentials of Testing and Assessment: A Practical Guide for Counselors, Social Workers and Psychologists. (Belmont, California: Thomson Brooks/Cole, 2006).

NeuroPsychiatry Reviews. 7, no. 1 (January 2006).

New Revised Standard Version, The Holy Bible. (Nashville, Tennessee: Thomas Nelson, Inc., 1990).

Oates, Wayne. Behind the Masks: Personality Disorders in Religious Behavior. Philadelphia: The Westminster Press, 1987.

Oden, Thomas C. Care of Souls in the Classic Tradition. Philadelphia: Fortress Press, 1978.

Okasha A. Globalization and mental health: a WPA perspective (Editorial) World Psychiatry 2005; 4: 1-2.

Olson, David H. and Olson, Amy K. Empowering Couples: Building on Your Strengths. Minneapolis: Life Innovations, Inc., 2000.

Pew Research Center, Muslim Americans: Middle Class and Mostly Mainstream. (May 22, 2007),

Pinck, Dan C. "Prisoners and/of War," Intelligencer: Journal of U. S. Intelligence Studies, 15, no. 1 (Fall/Winter 2005): 59.

Post, Stephen G. , Puchalski, Christina and Larson, David B. Annals of Internal Medicine 132, no. 7 (April 2000).

President's New Freedom Commission on Mental Health. www.mentalhealthcommission.gov/reports/Finalreport/FullReport)

Pruyser, Paul W. The Minister as Diagnostician. Philadelphia: Westminster Press, 1976.
_____. "Evaluation and Diagnosis, Religious." Dictionary of Pastoral Care and Counseling. (1990) : 371-373.

Rieff P. Charisma. The gift of grace and how it has been taken away from us. 271 pp. New York, Pantheon Books, 2007.

Report to the President. On Issues Raised by the Virginia Tech Tragedy (Washington, D. C.: GPO, June 13, 2007).

Ricoeur, Paul. The Symbolism of Evil (Boston: Beacon Press, 1967).

Ross, W. D. Ethics: Selections from Classical and Contemporary Writers, Oliver A. Johnson (Chicago: Holt, Rinehart and Winston, 1965).

Rovers, Martin and Kocum, Lucie. "Faith, Hope and Love: Toward a Holistic Definition of Spirituality and the Development of a Holistic Spirituality Scale." (Ottawa, Ontario: St. Paul University, 2005).

St. Anselm, The Ontological Argument from St. Anselm to Contemporary Philosophers, Alvin Plantinga (New York: Anchor Books, 1965), 4.

Schaeffer, Frank and John Schaeffer. Keeping Faith: A Father-Son Story About Love and the United States Marine Corps. (Carroll & Graf Publishers: New York, 2002)

Shoemaker, Sam. I Stand By the Door, Faith@Work, 1926.

Solle, Dorothee Suffering (Philadelphia: Fortress Press, 1975).

Sommers, Christina Hoff. The War Against Boys. The Atlantic Monthly, May 2000.

Spilka, Bernard, Hood, Ralph W. Gorsuch, Richard L. The Psychology of Religion An Empirical Approach (Englewood Cliffs: Prentice-Hall, Inc., 1985),

Substance Abuse and Mental Health Services Administration, Core Competencies for Clergy and Other Pastoral Ministers In Addressing Alcohol and Drug Dependence and the Impact on Family Members (HHS: 2003).

Spragins, Ellyn. "Shortchanging the Psyche," Newsweek, August 25, 1997, 78.

Stifoss-Hansen, H. "Religion and Spirituality: What a European ear hears." International Journal for the Psychology of Religion 9 (1999).

The Confession of 1967, The Constitution of the Presbyterian Church (USA): Part I, Book of Confessions. (Louisville: The Office of the General Assembly, 1967).

Trachtenberg, Peter. The Casanova Complex: Compulsive Lovers & Their Women (New York: Poseidon Press, 1988), 28.

Twain, Mark.

United Health Foundation. Clinical Evidence Mental Health. 11. Minnetonka, Minnesota: BMJ Publishing Group, 2004.

United States Bureau of Census Series P-25, Nos. 139.

Ustum PB, Sartorius N (Eds). Mental illness in general health care: an international study. Chichester, John Wiley and Sons, 1995.

Warr, Nicholas. Christmas, 1967: Anything But Merry, The Old Breed News (November-December 2006).

Weaver, Andrew J., Flannelly, Kevin J. , Koenig, Harold G. and Smith, Fred Douglas. "A Review of Research on Chaplains and Community-Based Clergy in **The Journal of the American Medical Association, ,Lancet and The New England Journal of Medicine: 1998-2000.**" The Journal of Pastoral Care and Counseling 58: no. 4, (Winter 2004).

Wiesel, Elie. Night. (New York: Hill and Wang), 1972.

Woodruff, C. Roy, Spiritual Caregiving to Help Addicted Persons and Families. (SAMHSA: 2006).

Zimberg, Sheldon The Clinical Management of Alcoholism (New York: Brunner/Mazel, 1983). .

Zwellin, Shomer S. Quest for a Cure: The Public Hospital in Williamsburg, Virginia, 1773-1885. Williamsburg, Virginia: The Colonial Williamsburg Foundation: Williamsburg, 1985.

Index

Index

Index

Index